A Chancellor's Tale

A Chancellor's Tale

TRANSFORMING ACADEMIC MEDICINE

RALPH SNYDERMAN, MD

Foreword by Darrell G. Kirch, MD

DUKE UNIVERSITY PRESS

Durham and London 2016

Printed in the United States of America on acid-free paper ∞
Typeset in Whitman by Westchester Publishing Services

Library of Congress Cataloging-in-Publication Data
Names: Snyderman, Ralph, author.
Title: A chancellor's tale : transforming academic medicine /
Ralph Snyderman, MD ; foreword by Darrell G. Kirch, MD.
Description: Durham : Duke University Press, 2016. | Includes
bibliographical references and index. | Description based on
print version record and CIP data provided by publisher;
resource not viewed.
Identifiers: LCCN 2016019476 (print) | LCCN 2016018393 (ebook)
ISBN 9780822361855 (hardcover : alk. paper)
ISBN 9780822373933 (e-book)
Subjects: LCSH: Snyderman, Ralph. | Health services
administrators—North Carolina—Biography. | College
administrators—North Carolina—Biography. | Duke
University. Medical Center. | Duke University Health System.
Classification: LCC RA982.D842 (print) | LCC RA982.D842 D857
2016 (ebook) | DDC 610.71/1756—dc23
LC record available at https://lccn.loc.gov/2016019476

Cover art: Ralph Snyderman in front of Davison Building, 1995.
Photo by Will and Deni McIntyre.

CONTENTS

Galleries appear after pages 120 and 186

FOREWORD

When Ralph Snyderman, MD, was elected chair of the Association of American Medical Colleges (AAMC) in 2001, he was at the forefront of leaders in academic medicine who were thinking about the changes looming in health care. In his chair's address at the AAMC annual meeting the next year, Dr. Snyderman discussed the great strides that medicine had made since World War II as a result of our country's investment in biomedical research and development. He described the sequential emergence of the fields of genomics, proteomics, and metabolomics—areas of study that would allow us to better understand, diagnose, and treat complex diseases. He also outlined a practice of medicine based in these discoveries—one that was proactive, predictive, team based, and customized for the individual.

At that time, these concepts had not yet attained the broad acceptance we see today. Perhaps most important, Dr. Snyderman then called on all those in academic medicine to "lead the transformation of American health care in the twenty-first century, as our predecessors did in the twentieth century." This call to action has resonated with the community in the ensuing years. As changes accelerate in health care, academic medical centers have been clearly positioned on the cutting edge of change.

Leading in a time of transformation is not a minor task. Successful leadership in our rapidly evolving health care environment requires individuals with both vision and flexibility, ones who can mobilize high-performing teams to find customized solutions to the unique challenges our institutions face. We need leaders who recognize and extend the talents of those around them rather than dictate a prescribed set of "one-size-fits-all" answers. As Dr. Snyderman writes, "high energy, drive, a willingness to listen and to learn, and a very high standard for success" produce the most successful and innovative leaders. You will see these qualities illustrated throughout the journey described in this book.

More than ever, American health care writ large and the academic medical centers that drive its innovations need forward-looking leaders to achieve the culture of personalized and patient-centered care that Dr. Snyderman called for in his address. In the years since he outlined his vision, we have made significant progress. The pace of scientific discovery has accelerated, bringing new tools that allow highly targeted diagnostics and therapeutics. Health care delivery systems have sharpened their focus on quality and safety programs to improve outcomes for both individuals and populations. And because of the leadership of institutions like Duke University in advancing personalized medicine, patients across the country are more actively engaged in their own care.

In addition, we have a greater ability than ever to determine the likelihood of a patient developing a certain disease, offer guidance on managing risks, and minimize the damage of disease through early diagnosis and intervention. We have enhanced and extended our partnerships with colleagues across the health care professions so that interdisciplinary teams of professionals ensure continuity of care for patients. Technological advances have improved patients' access to medical information, as well as to their own biological data, helping them make better-informed health care decisions to achieve their desired outcomes.

Hospitals across the country also are piloting new payment models to ensure that patients pay for value-based care rather than for individual services on a fragmented, fee-for-service basis. All these changes are being embedded in new delivery models such as the patient-centered medical home and are supported by tools such as telehealth to enhance patient autonomy and transform care. The result is unprecedented flexibility in how, when, and where patients can access and communicate with their physicians.

These delivery models not only are having a positive impact on individual patients but also are providing better health care access to entire communities, even those that historically have been underserved. Advancing personalized and holistic care requires enhanced, bidirectional community engagement to achieve greater health equity, a more diverse workforce, and care that truly meets the needs of each patient in our diverse and growing population. Patient-centered care requires cultural competence to engage in effective communication with patients and families, data to document and understand patients' backgrounds and preferences, and partnerships to connect patients with community resources, social services, and health care specialists so that care is holistic, linked to local assets, and responsive to patient needs.

Despite all these advances, the health needs of too many patients go unmet. As Dr. Snyderman noted in his AAMC chair's address in 2002, the growth of proactive and predictive care was the result of a half century of federal investment in cutting-edge research that vastly increased our body of medical knowledge. But more than a decade of divisive politics has put our government in a state of gridlock, with serious implications for academic medical centers. The Great Recession of 2008 resulted in declining state support for higher education, increasing the debt burden of those pursuing careers in the health professions. Stagnant federal funding for medical research has put hope on hold for millions of patients and their families suffering from chronic or life-threatening diseases.

Stable federal funding for medical research is vital—not only to find new cures and treatments for illnesses today but also to generate groundbreaking discoveries that will continue to transform how we practice medicine in the future. Ultimately, the only way to achieve better care for individuals, create healthier communities, and reduce health care costs is to invest in the education and research that will make these goals possible and will provide a platform for the next great transformation of medicine.

Physicians take an oath to respect a patient's autonomy and right to self-determination. This fundamental need to respect the outcomes that matter most to a patient is at the heart of many of the changes we see across health care. When the AAMC presented Dr. Snyderman with the David E. Rogers

Award in 2012, it was in honor of his role as the "father of personalized medicine," a concept he put into practice at Duke and one that has infused the way we think about proactive, patient-centered care. Dr. Snyderman's message of personalized care and academic medicine leadership is as relevant today as it was at the beginning of the century. I hope academic medicine will heed his call and continue to lead the transformation of American health care into a more equitable and patient-centered system.

DARRELL G. KIRCH, MD
President and chief executive officer
Association of American Medical Colleges
Washington, DC

ACKNOWLEDGMENTS

At the time of this writing, I have been a physician for fifty years and have been publishing scientific literature for forty-five of them. This is my first attempt at writing a book about something other than science. Moving beyond disciplined academic writing to a highly personal story without preconditioned boundaries has been a difficult challenge and one for which my professional career did not prepare me. Among the many things I've gained during the preparation of this book is a greater appreciation of how much I owe to others for the many opportunities I've had.

First, I'd like to mention my parents—Ida and Morris Snyderman—immigrants who fled the pogroms in the Ukraine in 1918 and ultimately made their way to Bensonhurst, Brooklyn, to what I realize in retrospect was a lower-middle-class neighborhood. In a one bedroom apartment, they raised my older brother Ted and me as best they could. My parents knew very little about scholastics or ways beyond the hardships they experienced, yet they raised me to understand that my future lay outside of Brooklyn. They taught me the importance of learning, integrity, persistence, high aspirations, and striving to do important things. The traits I learned from them and the rugged nature of my years growing up provided me with a toughness and determination that, for better or worse, have continued to shape me. I am grateful to my brother Ted, who tragically died when I was eighteen; my cousins Rachel, Jessie and her husband Dave, and Edith and her husband Sy, who helped guide me out of Brooklyn toward academic achievements; and my former wife Judith, who stood by me with great strength and supported me from residency training through most of my years as chancellor. I am fortunate that our son Ted, named after my brother, was able to navigate the difficult upbringing of a driven father to earn a BA from Duke University and MSW from Smith College. I am also grateful that I have connected with my first son Matt, who grew up without me but is now an important part of my life. Matt graduated from Brandeis University and has a successful marketing firm in New York. Matt, his children Davida, Josie, and Isaac, and Ted, his wife Amanda, their children Ariella and Mikayla create great pleasure and delight.

My wife of the last eleven years, Renée, has been a source of love, joy, advice, support and has provided valuable editing of this book. She has given me the stability, optimism, and comfort I needed for completing this endeavor. Renée and my family are my greatest sources of joy.

I was privileged to develop a deep lasting friendship with Robert J. Lefkowitz that has continued for more than forty years. Bob and I have been closer than most brothers, yet we have had no sibling rivalry. Bob's companionship helped sustain and guide me through many of my most difficult moments as chancellor. The Durham Beth El congregation has provided me with guidance and comfort as has my friendship with Joel Fleishman. I am grateful for the advice and friendship of David W. Martin, Jr., a resident when I was an intern at Duke. Dave influenced my decision to return to Duke for my first faculty appointment and enabled my decision to leave Duke for Genentech as vice president for medical research and development. Absent Dave's influence, I would likely not have been Duke's chancellor for health affairs.

I have been fortunate, actually blessed, to have had the support of Cindy Mitchell, my executive assistant for more than fifteen years. She deserves tremendous credit for her continued support, advice, and friendship during many hectic and difficult times. From the beginning of writing this book through its conclusion, her input has been critical for all the good parts; I take responsibility for the rest. She has helped organize, research, and edit extensively and has kept me focused on the task and coordinated the efforts of others involved. It is true and fair to say that I couldn't have written this book without her.

I had excellent assistance in preparing this book. Adam Garfinkle edited the manuscripts and provided guidance on their organization. Bobby Clark interviewed me in detail and compiled the stories in a useful way. Vicki Saito had been a colleague, adviser, and friend since 1992. During my time as chancellor, she oversaw the collection of information needed to create the history and she graciously helped edit the book. Vicki passed away in the summer of 2015, and I will deeply miss her. Gale McCarty, a former rheumatology fellow became a colleague and family friend, and she provided valuable feedback on the content of the book.

The members of the Duke University and Medical Center Library and Archives, especially Dawne Lucas, Amy McDonald, and Jolie Braun, as well as Chris Hildreth and Leslie Todd with Duke Photography spent many hours organizing and retrieving the material needed to reconstruct the events and to document the accuracy of stories created from my memory. I am also thankful for Duke University Press for its guidance and support in this endeavor.

I would like to acknowledge the many friends and relatives who have meant so much to me and have helped to shape my life. I cannot mention each by name but, perhaps, will do so in my next book where I hope to explore the trail that begins with my parents in Pechera, Ukraine, who traveled through the ghettos of Philadelphia, the Bronx, and Brooklyn and created a child whose life journey allowed him to see things they never could have imagined.

Finally, I will forever be grateful to Duke University for allowing me to have such a rich career and providing me the opportunity to be its chancellor for health affairs for fifteen and a half years. I cannot imagine having a more meaningful professional experience. Over the course of a fifty-year relationship with Duke, the institution has been inexorably imbedded in all of what I became and was able to achieve.

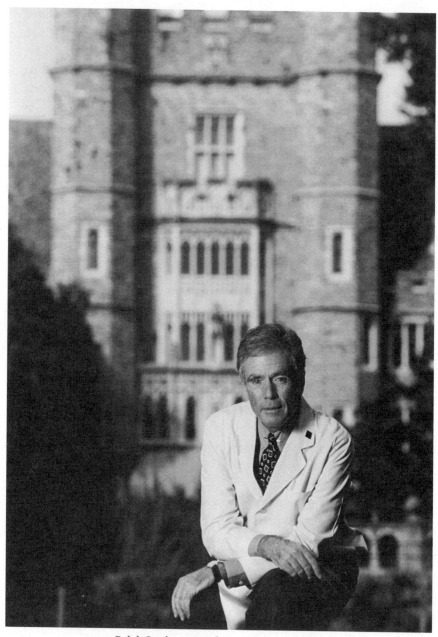

FIG. I.1 Ralph Snyderman in front of Davison Building, 1995.
Photo by Will and Deni McIntyre.

Introduction

I served as the chancellor for health affairs of Duke University from January 1989 until the end of my third five-year term on June 30, 2004. When I started, I had hoped to enhance the stature of an excellent medical school and university hospital. By the time I stepped down, we had accomplished this and much more. By 2004, the Duke University Medical Center and Duke University Health System represented a paradigm shift, having replaced one concept of an academic medical center envisioned a century earlier with something dramatically different. Duke created a vast, integrated health care delivery system, stood among the nation's largest academic biomedical research enterprises, and could claim a leading school of medicine, an innovative and growing graduate school of nursing, a satellite international school of medicine in Singapore, and a novel organizational structure to oversee the whole, multifaceted enterprise.

More important than institutional markers of progress, however, is that engagement in these diverse health-related activities enabled the creation of new models of health care delivery itself. Moving beyond the disease-oriented approach, Duke led the conceptualization and implementation of integrative medicine by focusing on the holistic needs of patients and engaging them actively in their own care. Then, from the merger of new science, advanced clinical methodology, and cutting-edge management design, the concept of personalized health care evolved. Fundamentally, personalized health care—a personalized, proactive, patient-driven approach to care as opposed to a disease-repair focus—is becoming recognized as a more rational approach to improve health and minimize the clinical, financial, and moral burden of disease.

While this book is a narrative of my experience as Duke's chancellor for health affairs and is relevant to all those interested in Duke University, it should also be of interest to those in academic medicine and health care delivery, as well as to developers of rational models of health care. It imparts leadership principles I've learned and, I hope, will serve as a guide for individuals bearing leadership responsibilities in academic medicine and health care delivery and for those aspiring to do so. Although this is not written as a how-to book, I hope that the reader will discern guidance on how to be a better leader and innovator by understanding what did and did not work well for me.

What follows is more personal than coldly observational or reportorial, but the personal and professional mix in all we do. Indeed, that inevitable mixing is one of the general lessons that come through the details herein. I take pride in the accomplishments achieved by the institution during my tenure, as is natural, but I am also mindful of what was achieved the "hard way," what could have been done better, and what remains to be done by my successors and all who work with them. As the admonition in the Mishnah states, "It is not your responsibility to finish the work, but neither are you free to desist from it." I'll add that, while you're not desisting, you should strive to do your best to make a positive impact.

I am a doctor, not a philosopher, but it is the philosopher's dilemma of parsing contingency and necessity that comes to mind as I struggle to analyze my tenure at Duke. At the outset of that period, no initial plan, whether my own or anyone else's, could have envisioned that by 2004, Duke's medical enterprise would be the twenty-first-century model of a comprehensive academic health system and that fundamental concepts developed there would be incorporated into practical applications that now form a basis of health care delivery. For more than fifteen years, the contingency inherent in decision making was my constant companion, yet these decisions unfolded into what now seems to be a grand vision for health care reform. Historical analysis, by its very nature, tends to render seemingly unrelated events into an orderly and purposeful narrative, often leading to explanations that present themselves as though what happened was planned or could not have happened in any other way. What seems contingent in the midst of living life ends up in retrospect appearing to have been part of a coherent plan pointing to an inevitable outcome. As it is for the history of nations and epochs, so it is for the history of individuals and the far more modest traces they make on earth in a lifetime. Trying to understand how a lifelong series of contingent decisions led to what was ultimately achieved is, I believe, worthy of explanation and the subject of this book.

— — —

The chapters that follow have a certain order to them, but not of the simplest sort, for they all are a mix of the chronological and the thematic. In chronological chapters there are thematic elements, and in thematic chapters there is relevant chronological narrative. It has to be that way as many different things were happening at the same time. Time may (or may not) be linear, but the substance of our professional and personal lives seems to dash about in circles, arcs, and comet streaks from one week or month or year to the next. Projects based on contingency start, swerve, stall, and stampede toward completion, weaving in and out of our lives without strict concern for parsimonious order.

The book is constructed in three related parts. Part I (chapters 1 through 8) is the chronology of my tenure as chancellor, with an emphasis on the first two terms. Part II (chapters 9 through 13) presents an account of five major initiatives that more broadly transformed Duke and affected academic medicine and health care. The final part (chapters 14 through 16) describes relationships, critical events, leadership, and reflections on learning.

Chapter 1 begins with my reflections on my path from being raised in Brooklyn to being offered the position of chancellor for health affairs at Duke. Chapter 2 provides a short history of medicine and the development of the academic medical center. The evolution of the Duke University Medical Center and what it was like when I became chancellor is the subject of chapter 3.

During my first five-year term, I initially delved into understanding the business of the medical center, namely, how the operations of this complex institution actually worked. My analysis presented opportunities for initial and obvious improvements, but it also revealed the starkly frightening conclusion that the organizational structure that had brought Duke to great prominence during its first sixty years was unsustainable going forward. In other words, in addition to the rigors of keeping the medical center operating efficiently, which was a task complicated and daunting enough on its own, we needed to deconstruct its operating model and replace it with one that could withstand the radical changes afoot in the external environment of American health care. Early on, we developed a long-range strategic plan that reflected two principles and related purposes: to set forth a coherent institutional vision, as opposed to what had evolved to be a hodgepodge of independent, nonintegrated departments; and to create an institutional vision and communicate that vision to all stakeholders so they would be committed to and thereby benefit from the plan they developed. The culmination of the first term was the deconstruction of the old uncoordinated formula. As is always the case when any human collectivity undertakes significant changes in organizational routines, there was some grousing and resistance. The pure ring of logic in such circumstances cannot dispel the emotions that churn with the disruption of comfortable and often self-interested ways of doing things. I admit to underestimating just how much churn there would be and with it how much resistance it would create. To survive as chancellor for a second term thus required some compromises on the part of myself and the institution, but those compromises in turn cleared the way for the development of a more coherent, centralized governance of the institution. That governance allowed the Duke University Medical Center to develop the comprehensive, integrated clinical network we needed to ensure the viability of the institution. Chapters 4 through 7 tell of the complex roller-coaster ride that composed the first five years of my tenure.

Chapter 8 continues the story into my second term, but it focuses mainly on the issues of management, the colleagues who aided me in my efforts, and what was learned about implementing change of the magnitude we undertook. During my second and third terms, we continued to raise the quality of the basic sciences as we enhanced the efficiency of management and operations throughout the system. The benefits of strategic and central planning became plain to see. It was as though we had created a central nervous system or brain within the organization that enabled it to parse the future. With the benefit of a broader cognitive horizon, we used the structures to solve the problems for which they were created and to envision solutions to problems that could not have been anticipated at the time the organizations developed.

The remainder of the book is largely thematic in describing major initiatives that spanned much of my tenure. Enhancing diversity, inclusion, and Duke's role in the community are discussed in chapter 9. As described in chapter 10, the Duke Clinical Research Institute proved to be a major success for academic medicine by demonstrating the power of translational and clinical research to facilitate the adoption of new technologies into clinical practice. The Duke University Health System, the subject of chapter 11, not only proved to be an exceptional accomplishment as a broadly distributed clinical operation but also provided revenues needed to sustain the organization, and it envisioned the broader understanding of the needs of patients that the health system served.

The next two chapters describe initiatives enabled by the more coherent organizational structure overseeing a vast clinical operation. The development of integrative medicine provided a compassionate, holistic, patient-centered approach far beyond treating molecular disease, to providing for patients' needs as human beings, and that is the subject of chapter 12. Moreover, with a far broader vision of the emerging discoveries in science and technology as a result of the genomic revolution, combined with the holistic needs of individuals, a new strategic approach to health care arose. The concepts of prospective health care, personalized health planning, and personalized medicine were articulated in the first part of my final term as chancellor, and by the end of that term, personalized health care was instituted for employees of Duke University. That is the subject of chapter 13.

Chapter 14 focuses on another key theme: fund-raising obligations and the powerful lessons they taught. Communication and media relations, reputation and crisis, and our efforts to create the proper balance between Duke's medical aspects and those of the rest of the university are the subjects of chapter 15.

This book concludes in chapter 16 with a focus on my exit in 2004 from three terms as chancellor, my reflections on my experience, and a synopsis of what I have been doing since stepping down. It also contains lessons I have learned in the hope that others may use them as a guide to navigate leadership roles in complex organizations.

A doctor's work is never really done, which is as it should be. There is no more important calling for me than advancing science and applying knowledge in the interest of humanity's health and well-being. Although I am no longer chancellor, I have not stopped thinking and caring about what is important to me—and that, beyond question, includes the progress, success, and high reputation of the Duke University Medical Center and all those who labor with dedication on its behalf. A brief epilogue serves as my proper exit and, dear reader, yours too if you make it that far.

I

THE JOURNEY

1

—

From Brooklyn to Duke

In January 1989, the Duke University Board of Trustees provided me with the awesome privilege and responsibility of being Duke's chancellor for health affairs. From the perspective of my humble beginnings in Bensonhurst, Brooklyn, the likelihood of my being offered this lofty position would have seemed so remote as to be considered impossible. Nonetheless, through a remarkable journey, highly convoluted and fraught with precarious turns, the story described in this book came to pass.

I was born in Brooklyn, New York, in 1940, the son of immigrants who fled the Ukraine at the time of the 1918 pogroms. My mother saw her father murdered at the hand of Cossacks. My father was a tough, persistent businessman who started with a push cart and worked his way up to owning a small but successful department store in the blue-collar section of Bensonhurst, Brooklyn.

Even when I attended public schools in Brooklyn in the 1950s, I knew I wanted to be a doctor, never mind the improbability posed by the foibles of life as the child of immigrant parents growing up in hardscrabble Bensonhurst. I attended tough neighborhood public schools in Bensonhurst and graduated from New Utrecht High School in 1957 at the lower rungs of the top quartile of my class. Most of my neighborhood friends were tough kids and had no intention of attending college, and even though I had a notion of a medical career, scholastics were not my highest priority as I was a product of the Brooklyn environment. With my parent's guidance, I made the unusual decision to go to Washington College, a small liberal arts school in Chestertown, Maryland. While there, I had my fun and flings, and while yet not truly focused on academics, I knew I would somehow become a doctor. Yet what we "know" about ourselves when we are in our twenties is a thin reed indeed, as most people discover to their eventual delight or dismay. Fortunately, graduating as a good but not outstanding student from Washington College gave me the opportunity to be admitted to an excellent state medical school.

On the first day of medical school at SUNY Downstate, I was so excited yet terrified at this momentous step toward fulfilling my life's dream that I could barely breathe. Fortunately, for the first time in my life, I deeply relished what I was learning, and study became my highest priority. I managed to graduate at the top of my class. When I came to Duke for my residency, I was closer still to living that dream, but like most of our dreams, it might have vanished in a waking moment as Duke's medical residency program was among the nation's most demanding. Certainly, it was then that my half-century love affair with Duke University began.

From that residency it was off to a research career at the National Institutes of Health (NIH), but it could have been to Vietnam had I not been awarded the highly sought after opportunity to become a research associate at the NIH. Soon after beginning my research there, I was fortunate to stumble onto seminal insights about the inflammatory process that enabled a basic understanding of how this complex system works. I stumbled in a fortunate way; I just as easily might have stumbled in vain and not pursued a career in academic medicine. From the NIH, I returned to Duke as an assistant professor and head of the Rheumatology Division at the Durham Veterans Affairs Hospital—the very place I had come to know so well during my residency. I worked my way up to being a successful physician-scientist, a Howard Hughes Medical Institute investigator, chief of the Rheumatology and Immunology Division at Duke, and Frederic M. Hanes Professor of Medicine. But in 1987, after a head-spinning ten-week sabbatical fellowship in Germany that allowed me to step away from Duke, I left the university for the burgeoning for-profit world of biotechnology at Genentech in San Francisco. No fellowship in Germany, most likely no Genentech.

Another career turn was soon to follow as on a brisk October afternoon in 1988, after less than two years at Genentech, I was driving back to San Francisco with David W. Martin, Jr, from a research retreat at Lake Tahoe. Dave, like me, was a senior vice president at Genentech. We had spent the previous three days in intense scientific discussions with our colleagues on the company's research team. Genentech was emerging as the number one biotech company at that time, employing some of the most innovative medical scientists in the country.

As Dave and I rounded a turn, in the distance I could see the San Francisco-Oakland Bay Bridge and, beyond it, the city of San Francisco. I was struck by the beauty of the surroundings and told Dave—who had been an undergraduate at Duke as well as a Duke medical school alumnus and resident—that finally, I felt as though I had left Duke and that San Francisco was now my home. Little did I appreciate the irony of that remark!

That afternoon I stopped by my office at Genentech before going home. As I approached my desk, I saw two pink telephone message slips. One was from my friend Dolph O. Adams, who at the time was a Duke professor of pathology; the other was from Robert J. Lefkowitz, a professor of medicine at Duke and my closest friend. I called Bob first. On hearing my voice he said, "Sit down and write the exact time and date on a piece of paper because once I give you this message, it will change your life forever." I was standing at the time and looked over at the clock, which read 4:35. It was set five minutes fast to help keep me on time, and I was a bit perplexed as to what time to write down. As I sat down at my desk, I wrote 4:35 and prepared to take notes. Bob told me that the search committee for Duke's chancellor for health affairs, of which he was a member, had chosen me to succeed William G. Anlyan. Bob said that Duke needed me and that it was *beshert*—"fated" in Yiddish, written in the Great Book, as it were—that I should return to Duke as its next chancellor for health affairs.

In many ways, the idea of leaving Genentech constituted a very difficult proposition. I loved my role in that company during my eighteen months there. I had the exhilarating experience of being transformed from an academic physician-scientist to a member of a new and exciting industry. I had had the challenging responsibility of leading the Food and Drug Administration (FDA) licensing of Activase, the first biotechnology blockbuster drug, and I had already been promoted to senior vice president. What's more, upon learning of Duke's offer, Genentech's chief operating officer and president, G. Kirk Raab, made me a most attractive offer to stay.

The idea of leaving Genentech was so difficult, and the temptation to stay was so compelling, that I almost did not accept the job at Duke. I temporized for what now seems to have been months, but which was in fact only days. In the end I felt I had no choice; deep emotional reasons drove me to accept the Duke offer to become its next chancellor for health affairs and dean of its School of Medicine.

I realized this job would involve tasks freighted with awesome responsibilities. My professional experience to that point had focused mainly on scientific research, teaching, and clinical practice, and what I knew beyond that I had learned outside of a university environment. To succeed at Duke, I understood that sound administration and foresightful management suited to university realities were required. Beyond this, neither the exact nature of the job nor a precise vision of what I wanted to achieve was yet clear to me.

But I took the job anyway because my experience had shown me that, with hard work, I could succeed. Up to that point, I had always taken the opportunity to assume a greater degree of responsibility and authority within the field of medicine when it availed itself, and I had never regretted doing so. I had the confidence that I would somehow do what needed to be done and that the institution and I would grow to success together. Put a bit differently, I was too unsure to be cocky, but I was too confident to be reticent. Things worked out, or so it seems to me now more than a decade after the end of my tenure. Duke and I did grow together, and we experienced the growing pains that inevitably accompany success.

As I have already suggested, the outcome of my tenure contrasts starkly with the inchoate vision I had at the outset. I confess to having little understanding of the nature of the job I had assumed, the complexity of the institution I would be leading, or the changes that would be needed to protect its viability in a rapidly evolving health care environment. Even to imply that at the beginning I understood, let alone planned for, the outcomes we achieved would be tendentious as well as plainly false. At the same time, my approach to my responsibilities was neither entirely incremental, opportunistic, nor in any sense random. What in retrospect might be understood as the result of a coherent plan was in reality something a good deal subtler.

Between master planning and reactive incrementalism lies another more flexible and realistic path to success—obeying fundamental underlying principles and applying them in steps to address needs, opportunities, and threats as they arise. John Maynard Keynes famously said that in the long run we are all dead, which is true enough. But failing to manage short-term challenges can be fatal, too, as all doctors understand. One must manage them, however, with a forward-leaning, integrated view of the future framed by clearly defined objectives.

Our underlying principle at Duke was to maximize the benefit to society of our core missions of education, research, and clinical care. This was not motherhood and apple pie; we really wanted to leverage the power of our academic missions to solve real-world health problems. Hence, principle-based decision making was coupled, when practical, with strategic planning to form a core for all we did. As we responded to pressing needs, we were able to anticipate and finally develop the means to synthesize a more coherent understanding of multiple complex issues and to create novel solutions based on a synthesis of our core capabilities.

So, while the outcome of fifteen and a half years of cumulative contingent judgments could not have been anticipated in 1989, the principles and processes underlying our approach ineluctably led to what we accomplished. In retrospect, I realize that the underlying principle of my life was to consistently choose a path that allowed me to have the broadest impact for good as a physician. Thus the path to medical school led me to be a physician, followed by the decision to pursue medical research so I could broadly expand medical knowledge. This steered me toward becoming an administrator to broaden my impact and to continue a logical progression not planned at the outset but made inevitable by adhering to principles.

I never thought of myself as a particularly religious person in the ritual sense, but I now understand how the underlying principles of always learning and seeking to do what is good, embedded in me from childhood, set a path through myriad contingencies that had what now seems an inevitable outcome.

2

—

History of the
Academic Medical Center

Medicine has been practiced in various forms since the earliest days
of human history, yet the ability of science to affect the profession
did not emerge in earnest until the latter part of the nineteenth
century. Until then, the prevalent theory of health and disease
was that both resulted from the relative imbalance of four puta-
tive bodily humors: yellow bile, black bile, blood, and phlegm. The
humoral theory had no scientific basis and the dominant therapies
it spawned; e.g., bloodletting, moxibustion, provided no effective
interventions. Toward the end of that century, however, emerging
sciences began impacting medicine. Rival microbiologists Robert Koch in Germany and Louis Pasteur in France unequivocally
identified microorganisms as causative agents of specific diseases.
Their demonstrations proving that infectious microbes caused
dreaded diseases such as tuberculosis and rabies had a profound
impact on physicians and the public alike. An external causative
agent was at work after all, not a mystical one: a microbe was directly responsible for many diseases. The findings, which came to
be called the "germ theory" of disease, clearly debunked previous
metaphysical theories and gave rise to the pathophysiological approach to disease.

Scientific progress accelerated in the new century as immunologists, such as Elie Metchnikoff and Paul Ehrlich, described innate and acquired mechanisms of resistance to infections (e.g., immunity), and others identified as "serum sickness" resulting from the administration of serum from immunized animals used as therapy for infections. Applying physics to medicine led to the use of X-rays for diagnostic imaging, and advances in chemistry allowed the synthesis of new specific therapeutic agents. Chemists such as Hermann E. Fischer in Germany developed capabilities to synthesize specific molecules to treat diseases, popularizing the concept of a "magic bullet" for the treatment of conditions such as syphilis. This added considerably to the excitement of the new era in medicine.

Thus, by the beginning of the twentieth century it had become clear that scientific research had the potential to transform the practice of medicine from an unscientific humoral imbalance model to one based on an understanding of the scientific basis of disease. However, medical practice at that time was virtually untouched by this new and expanding knowledge. Rather, it remained anecdotal, unscientific, and unregulated, with hundreds of "storefront" medical schools granting licenses with virtually no scientific training imparted.

Fortunately, the then young Carnegie Foundation commissioned a seminal study of medical education in the United States. It chose Abraham Flexner, the son of German-Jewish immigrants, to lead this effort. He published his book-length report, which became known as the Flexner Report, in 1910.[1] The report examined the status of medical education state by state and, to varying degrees, found much to criticize. Flexner's central point was that physician training was insufficiently enriched by science.

Flexner's findings crystallized widely felt dissatisfactions into a framework for a revolution in medical education and, ultimately, set the stage for the American century in medicine and research. His conclusions profoundly affected medical education and helped define the structure of the contemporary academic medical center, as the creation became known. In the arrangement he fostered, medical faculty responsible for teaching medical students were also involved in research and clinical care. Thus the faculty would be educators as well as physicians and scientists involved in creating new knowledge. The clinical practice of medicine would be taught to medical students and residents in training by the clinical faculty in a "teaching" hospital affiliated with the medical school. This institutional design caught on with alacrity in the United States due, ironically perhaps, to the then shallow roots of its institutional arrangements; it did not flourish as readily in Europe, despite the presence of great human capital, because institutional traditions were more rigidly entrenched.

The best early example of this vision was the "Johns Hopkins model," an outstanding school of medicine with its teaching faculty also involved in research while practicing in the Johns Hopkins Hospital in Baltimore, Maryland. In the Flexner model, students would be steeped in medicine based on science and would aim to master the pathophysiology of disease to the extent that current science would allow. Those aims would be the underlying paired goals of training and practice.

Flexner's new model provided a platform for substantial investments and progress in biomedical research. Shortly after World War II, the U.S. government began its historic and strong support of biomedical research, largely in academic medical centers. The national investment in those efforts, now well over $1 trillion and counting, was spearheaded after the war by enhanced funding for the NIH as a consequence of the influential Vannevar Bush report.[2]

The augmented funding that stimulated biomedical research performed in academic medical centers in turn spurred greater sophistication in our understanding of human diseases and the development of new technologies to diagnose and treat them. The explosion of knowledge about the complexity of human disease simultaneously drove the growth in clinical specialization. Academic medical centers, the nexus of medical education, research, and practice, became the primary drivers of clinical specialization. As a result, the number of medical schools in the United States fulfilling Flexnerian criteria grew from a dozen in 1910 to more than 140 today, and their size and complexity have increased as the potential for research and clinical application has expanded.[3] Academic medical centers not only have provided much of the research needed for the rapid developments of new diagnostics and therapeutics but also have become the sites to validate them clinically. Indeed, the pharmaceutical and biotechnology industries, among the greatest national economic drivers, would be unsustainable without academic biomedical research and clinical validation.

The impact of research and clinical practice on the growth and importance of academic medical centers cannot be overstated. By 1989, less than eighty years after Abraham Flexner's work, there were 126 medical schools and approximately four hundred affiliated primary teaching hospitals in the United States training some fifteen thousand new medical graduates per year. These were accompanied by ninety academic and professional societies enrolling seventy thousand faculty members.

Over the twentieth century, academic medical centers became increasingly important as foundational elements for the delivery of health care in the United States, in addition to being the primary forces in medical education and training of nurses and allied health care professionals. While constituting only 6 percent of the total number of hospitals in the United States, primary teaching hospitals delivered almost 50 percent of all charity care. Moreover, academic medical centers were generally the drivers of improving care, being the first to develop and embrace new medical technologies and therapeutic approaches. Beyond their disproportionate role in providing charity care, academic medical centers provided an essential safety net for emergency and urgent care through their fully staffed and technically advanced emergency rooms, trauma centers, intensive care units, and burn centers.

Academic medical centers thus became an increasingly important component of the nation's economy, with health care accounting for 17 percent of GNP at the turn of the twenty-first century. Beyond clinical care, academic medical centers' research has been absolutely essential to the creation and growth of the pharmaceutical and biotechnology industries in the United States and the world at large. As the business of health care delivery exploded, academic medical centers frequently became among the largest employers and biggest economic drivers in their communities. Durham, North Carolina, for example, changed its motto from "Bull City" to "City of Medicine" in 1998 as Duke University Medical Center (DUMC) became by far the largest employer in the region and among the top employers in the state.

What could not have been anticipated in 1910 was how academic medical centers would evolve into increasingly large and highly complex organizations. In his model, Flexner emphasized the education of physicians as well as the pedagogical importance of the school of medicine's clinical practices and research functions. These were obviously important for producing faculty who could teach future physicians the latest medical sciences and approaches to clinical practice. What also evolved, however, was an organization that, while continuing to train physicians, also developed astounding research and clinical capabilities that extended far beyond the need to educate medical students. During the second half of the twentieth century, research and clinical care rather than education became the overriding missions of most academic medical centers.

The pace and particulars of this transformation were idiosyncratic to each institution, but the pattern was set. While most medical schools moved from a primary focus on medical education to become academic medical centers focused on research and clinical care, the specific contours of change were shaped by economic and demographic factors. Given the need for practicing physicians, many states established medical schools specifically designed to train primary care doctors. For the research-intensive medical schools, reputational factors affected each institution's ability to recruit and retain the best faculty and students and to attract funding. The capacity to make research discoveries had a very high value and was supported by a massive infusion of government funding for biomedical research. The levels of research support and scientific discovery became currencies of reputation, both for individual faculty and for institutions.

Similarly, the process of clinical specialization became another characteristic of growth in size and organizational complexity; this process, too, was strongly influenced by the stature of individual institutions and their faculty, local needs, and opportunities. As a consequence of the alignment of research and practice, the rapid development of new insights into disease and treatment generated a far greater body of knowledge than generalist physicians could have been expected to master. This naturally led to a proliferation of clinical specialties. Moreover, the increasing revenues associated with clinical practice, particularly specialty practices, provided rich resources for growth—which tended to reinforce national reputations and local influence.

The resulting organizational size and complexity of academic medical centers were neither carefully planned nor centrally directed within institutions. Instead, development emerged incrementally as a consequence of opportunities for growth within the departments of each institution. This opportunistic approach had its advantages—speed, dexterity, and creativity— but it also piled up disadvantages over time, notably the displacement of strategic views of how best (or even whether) to organize or integrate the components of the institution to achieve a result that was greater than the sum of the parts.

Since Flexner's time, medical education has been broadly divided into learning the basic and clinical sciences. Given the specialized nature of the disciplines within these two groups, faculty was organized into departments. These departments grew in size and influence in keeping with the leadership of the chair, the productivity and growth of the faculty, and the availability of external funding to sustain their growth. In the basic sciences, the departments of biochemistry and microbiology were generally the most powerful, given their access to research funding, research advances, and thus their attendant stature within most institutions, which typically made their chairs the most dominant of the basic science departments.

The clinical faculty were also organized into departments. As research and clinical opportunities expanded, existing clinical departments grew and new departments arose. Medicine and surgery generally were the dominant clinical departments as a result of the breadth of their clinical practices and revenue production. Due to their wealth and ability to support departmental research, they tended to be the most powerful within the larger academic medical centers, exerting considerable influence and even control of academic medical centers' affairs. Thus, the chairs of medicine and surgery were often the most powerful leaders in most medical centers.

Seen together, the research and clinical missions clearly became more valued and better funded within academic medical centers than undergraduate medical education, which they began to dominate. Not surprisingly, most departments were highly autonomous, and the most powerful dominated the relatively weak and poorly organized central structures were putatively in charge of the academic medical centers. Departmental autonomy and the loose central control exerted by the academic medical centers were reinforced by the traditions of the universities of which academic medical centers were a part. A departmental structure characterized by numerous small units each having authority of its own fit naturally with the academic freedom and autonomy of the larger university's individual units and faculty members.

Thus, from the onset of the Johns Hopkins model and the 1910 Flexner Report, American medical schools evolved into the highly complex academic medical centers of the late twentieth century. They were alike in having been built by strong and largely independent departmental chairs who responded to national and local opportunities; they were alike, too, in that they evolved within the traditions of the academy. Despite their basic structural similarities, however, these institutions were also idiosyncratic expressions of individual traditions and cultures. Thus the oft-cited comment: "If you've seen one academic medical center . . . you've seen one academic medical center!"

Medical centers were alike also in that individuals and the individual parts dominated the overall organization. Many institutions achieved greatness, but unlike their constituent departmental units, they were not built to be nimble; they simply could not change course quickly because there was no mechanism to coordinate the actions of the individual departments. The best academic medical centers, those with strong national reputations for training physicians, performing highly regarded biomedical research, providing clinical training, and caring for a large number of patients, were highly complex organizational entities but with little ability to create central initiatives or to respond effectively to change in the external environment. One important power the chancellors (or deans) had was as the external voice of the institution and the lead fund-raiser. Through their bully pulpit, academic authority, and a limited number of financial resources, they could at times hold sway in exerting central authority, but, in general, the various departments set their own direction. In other words, a chancellor's direct authority was limited.

Virtually all the high-quality academic medical centers faced the same generic problem at the end of the 1980s: their capacity to do great research and deliver highly specialized care was rendered vulnerable by institutional slowness in responding to opportunities or threats. Each had long relied on income margins from clinical care to subsidize medical education and the portion of research costs not fully covered by external grants and contracts. In fact, neither the education, mission, nor the research core mission had been self-supporting for years at any major academic medical center. Medical school tuitions supported only a small fraction of the large faculty, while, in the case of research, external grants never covered all institutional costs. State institutions received state funding, but in most cases this amounted to a minority of their revenues. Historically, the best way to boost revenues had been for clinical chairs to add clinicians who would see more patients, perform more services, and thus produce more revenue according to the standard fee-for-service model.

This method had grown less reliable, however, as clinical margins began to shrink under pressure from cost containment efforts by insurance companies and health maintenance organization (HMO) entities. The pressure would only get worse, as I had seen firsthand in California in the late 1980s, where the managed care revolution began. This constituted a serious threat to the viability of almost every academic medical center in the United States. If growth, primarily in research, could not be sustained by shrinking margins from the clinical side, other sources of funds would be needed to "float the entire ship." Philanthropy and the commercialization of academic research discoveries were two potentially significant sources for revenue. Clearly, the academic medical center was approaching crisis, and Duke's medical center was certainly no exception.

3

—

Evolution of the Duke University
Medical Center

Duke University Medical Center (DUMC) was a child of James B. Duke's philanthropic vision, Carnegie's foresight, and Flexner's report, evident by the medical center's creation and structure. In 1924, when James B. Duke, one of the great philanthropists of the past century, developed the Duke Endowment Indenture of Trust and funded the development of Duke University's Medical School and Teaching Hospital, he used language that was clearly Flexnerian: "The advance in the science of medicine growing out of discoveries, such as in the field of bacteriology, chemistry and physics, and growing out of inventions such as the X-ray apparatus, make hospital facilities essential for obtaining the best results in the practice of medicine and surgery."[1]

Is it no accident that DUMC's founding dean, Wilburt C. Davison, and virtually the entire initial faculty came from Johns Hopkins Medical School. In July 1930, when the Duke University School of Medicine and Duke University Hospital (Duke Hospital) opened, medical students were trained by full-time faculty who were educators, researchers, and clinicians—serving the three core missions adopted by other "modern medical schools" pursuing the Flexner vision. By the 1960s, DUMC had earned an excellent reputation nationally. This was largely due to the leadership of Dean Davison and the recruitment of strong faculty, who had a dramatic impact on the institution locally and were recognized for their contributions nationally. In July 1960, Dean Davison took a sabbatical year; he continued as James B. Duke Professor of Pediatrics until September 1, 1961.

In February 1960, Arthur Hollis Edens, president of Duke University, resigned and was replaced by an interim president, J. Deryl Hart, who had been a professor of surgery in the School of Medicine. One of Hart's first decisions was to choose the next dean of the School of Medicine. For this position, he selected Barnes Woodall, a fellow surgeon who had previously been chief of neurosurgery at Duke. Woodall, like Dean Davison, attended medical school at Johns Hopkins University, receiving his medical degree in 1930. In 1937 he came to Duke, where as an assistant professor, he took the responsibility for organizing the initial neurosurgical service. Barnes Woodall proved to be a transitional medical school leader, relinquishing his deanship on June 30, 1964, to become the vice provost of Duke University. By that time, the president of Duke University was Douglas M. Knight, who appointed fellow Yalee William Anlyan as Duke School of Medicine's third dean. Bill, also a surgeon, had been associate dean of the School of Medicine under Barnes Woodall for the last year of Woodall's service.

Wilburt Davison deserves credit for the initial development and early maturation of Duke's School of Medicine and its medical center, and Barnes Woodall played a role in setting the stage for Bill Anlyan's twenty-five-year tenure from 1964 to 1989. Bill's title changed from dean to vice president for health affairs, Duke University in 1969, recognizing the medical center's increasing size, complexity, and importance to the university as well as the significance of this position in overseeing Duke Hospital. In 1983, the title changed once again to chancellor for health affairs of Duke University.

Under Bill's able leadership, the medical center grew considerably in size and stature; it became a regional power in academic medicine and was increasingly recognized nationally. In biochemistry, Philip Handler, Irwin Fridovich, and Robert L. Hill were known nationally for their important research. Phil Handler ultimately became president of the National Academy of Sciences, and Irwin Fridovich won high regard for his discovery of the enzyme superoxide dismutase. In immunology, D. Bernard Amos became a major leader in the emerging field of organ transplantation by defining the mechanisms of graft rejection. Eugene A. Stead, Jr. and James B. Wyngaarden created one of the nation's strongest departments of medicine. Groundbreaking research by Gene Stead (chair of medicine from 1947 to 1967) in cardiovascular physiology was widely published and helped change cardiovascular medicine from a largely anecdotally based practice to treatment based on clinical evidence. He also founded the nation's first physician assistant program at Duke in the 1960s. Jim Wyngaarden (chair of the Department of Medicine from 1967 to 1983), a superb physician-scientist in the field of purine metabolism, developed the Research Training Program that allowed medical students and emerging physician-scientists to train in outstanding research laboratories at Duke. Indeed, it was the reputation of the Research Training Program and Jim Wyngaarden that first brought me to Duke as a resident. As a cumulative result of these achievements, by 1983 Duke appeared regularly among the top ten recipients of NIH grants and ranked in the top ten medical schools by *U.S. News & World Report*.

Bill Anlyan was responsible for attracting international attention to Duke and was recognized for nurturing the careers of many students and colleagues. His relentless energy, high standards, ambition for Duke, and his love for people enabled him to create a vast philanthropic support for the institution. A factor in Bill's success was his outrageous determination to create and succeed. But what sustained him was his unflagging energy, persistence, and joy in being engaged with people.

In the spring of 1989 as Duke's new chancellor for health affairs, I was hosting my first major social event—the Emeriti Faculty Dinner. I was introduced by none other than Bill Anlyan. After a warm and generous introduction, Bill handed me a key—the "key to the kingdom." This act, on Bill's part, was very telling in that it revealed that his view of the chancellor's role was far more than overseer of a vast medical center, schools, hospitals, clinics—it was as the guardian of a kingdom—what an inspirational metaphor—a kingdom: vast, rich, capable of greatness but complex—needing compassion, understanding, and attention to its innumerable parts. Bill handed me a key—not a throne or crown—a key to its many rooms. It would be my choice as to which I'd enter, what I'd learn, and what I'd do. What profoundly valuable advice! Bill left this world on January 17, 2016. I will deeply miss my colleague and confidant, but most of all, I will miss my friend.

It was a daunting task and tremendous responsibility to follow in the steps of these giants in Duke Medicine as I assumed the reins of DUMC as chancellor for health affairs and the fourth dean of the School of Medicine in January 1989. To better appreciate what happened over my more than fifteen years as chancellor, it is important that I share my sense of what DUMC was like when I returned to campus. In 1989, DUMC could fairly be called a brilliant example of the post-Flexnerian academic medical center. It was highly regarded for the quality of its medical school, its hospital, its biomedical research, and particularly its clinical training programs in medicine and surgery. But how did this complex organization, made up of so many individual components, actually function? As a scientist, I naturally sought to understand the structure and function of this intricate entity for which I was assuming responsibility. How did it work? How was it organized? How was it financially sustained? And how did it respond to challenge and change? To lead DUMC successfully, I needed detailed answers to all these questions.

Like its academic medical center peers, DUMC had three well-identified core missions: education, research, and clinical care. Also like its peers, DUMC was composed of highly independent but ultimately interdependent entities subject to varying degrees of central authority or control. The looseness of the governance structure regarding the performance and coordination of the component entities of DUMC became significant impediments to generating change. As new external factors began to have an impact in the early 1990s, it became increasingly difficult for the institution to respond to threats or opportunities.

Further, with DUMC being part of a great parent university, decisions needed to be made in accord with the policies and will of the university as a whole. The university's views could be dominant. Although DUMC accounted for at least two-thirds of the entire university budget and certainly was the most complex operation within the institution, it was by no means a completely independent factor. These issues became important influences, for better or worse, over what I could and could not do as chancellor for health affairs.

To properly set the stage for the changes that occurred during my tenure, it makes sense to offer a brief description of the important functions of DUMC at the time.

Education
School of Medicine

The Duke University School of Medicine in 1989 was responsible for educating approximately 800 students pursuing various degrees and certificates. Of these, the School of Medicine had 452 students pursuing medical degrees (undergraduate medical education) and was busily admitting the entering class of 1990. In those days about 10 percent of each medical school class chose to study for a doctorate in a biological science as well as a medical degree. Enrollment in the prestigious combined MD/PhD program was 55. Smaller numbers chose other combined medical degrees: 7 in law and another 7 in science at the master's level. The remaining 348 students were enrolled in various graduate school programs pursuing PhDs or certification programs in Duke Hospital. In addition, about 8 percent of students pursuing PhDs in the Duke University graduate school were doing their thesis research in the basic science departments in the School of Medicine.

UNDERGRADUATE MEDICAL EDUCATION

The undergraduate dean of medical education oversaw the activities of the School of Medicine, which prepared students to achieve their medical degree, and was also responsible for all the educational programs of the School of Medicine as well as for developing and updating the medical school curriculum. The person in this position reported to the chancellor for health affairs, who was also the dean of the School of Medicine. Reporting to the undergraduate dean for medical education were associate deans assigned to coordinate the curriculum developed by the basic sciences and clinical sciences. Their functions integrated the courses in the respective areas, working with faculty in the basic science or clinical departments. An associate dean oversaw the admission process to the School of Medicine. Other assistant deans supervised core school functions such as financial aid and student affairs. To facilitate student mentoring and to deal with the inherent stresses of early medical education, each of three assistant deans was assigned one-third of the medical school class to render advice and nurture students as necessary over the course of their medical school training.

Financial support for the School of Medicine for all its functions, including the training of medical students, relied on medical school tuition, which at that time was about $13,000 per year. Revenues from medical school tuition provided approximately 6 percent of the total expenses of the School of Medicine. Thus, undergraduate medical education needed to be cross-subsidized via other revenues within the medical center.

GRADUATE MEDICAL EDUCATION

The largest overall education component of DUMC was its graduate medical programs. Clinical training positions, particularly in medicine and surgery, were highly sought after. These included internships, residencies, and clinical fellowships. Each clinical department offered training programs for medical school graduates leading to specialty certification. From internship through advanced fellowship training, Duke was renowned as a place to train following medical school graduation. Such training occurred at Duke Hospital, Duke outpatient clinics, and the Durham Veterans Affairs Hospital, a primary teaching hospital for Duke. In 1989, there were approximately 870 clinical trainees throughout the clinical departments.

ALLIED HEALTH PROGRAMS

Within Duke Hospital were training programs for physician assistants, physical therapists, and occupational therapists. The most significant enrollments were in physician assistant training (97), the allied health certificate program (103), and the health administration master's program (57). A director for each program reported to the undergraduate dean of medical education, who supervised all three programs. These programs were supported by tuition and funds from Duke Hospital and provided a rich source of individuals to provide services to Duke Hospital and elsewhere.

GRADUATE SCHOOL OF NURSING

The Duke Graduate School of Nursing was responsible for master's-level education in nursing (MSN). The dean of the School of Nursing reported directly to the chancellor. In 1989, the school had five faculty and fifty-four students; the undergraduate nursing program had been inactive for about a decade. Tuition revenue of $335,000 accounted for 46 percent of total educational and general expenditures of $730,000, requiring a cross-subsidy from the medical center to cover the remainder. In the subsequent years, the Graduate School of Nursing expanded dramatically.

Research

In 1989, the School of Medicine faculty consisted of 728 tenure-track individuals who had a primary appointment in one of the basic science or clinical departments. The faculty carried out one or more of the missions of the medical center: to teach, to do research, or to perform clinical care. Depending on the individual and his or her department, a faculty member likely would participate in at least two of the three core missions, with a major focus on one.

BASIC SCIENCE DEPARTMENTS

In the basic sciences, most of the faculty had their independent research that was their primary responsibility, along with securing external grants, generally from the NIH. In addition, many faculty members participated in undergraduate medical education, as well as mentoring doctoral and postdoctoral students in the graduate school. Basic science faculty, in coordination with the associate dean for the basic sciences, also assembled the basic science curriculum for undergraduate medical education.

CLINICAL DEPARTMENTS

Members of the clinical departments similarly participated in the core mission of the School of Medicine but focused predominantly on research or the practice of clinical medicine. They were responsible for clinical undergraduate medical education and the supervision of residents and fellows pursuing specialty training. In many departments, clinical faculty focused on laboratory-based research and spent perhaps 20 percent of their time practicing clinical medicine. The others generally devoted 80 percent of their effort to the clinical practice and 20 percent to supervising clinical trainees. In later years, as clinical-type research became more prominent, some faculty members spent half their time doing clinical research and the other half seeing patients.

GRADUATE RESEARCH EDUCATION

The graduate school of Duke University oversaw graduate research training leading to a master's degree or a doctorate of philosophy. In collaboration with the School of Medicine, particularly through the basic science departments, the graduate school provided graduate research education leading to a PhD with training occurring in each of the basic science departments. Postdoctoral research training also occurred in each of the basic science departments. Many clinical department faculty involved primarily in research had joint degrees in one and sometimes more of the basic science departments. Such faculty members participated in graduate resident training, but degrees were granted through the clinical science departments.

Research faculty in the clinical departments frequently trained graduate students as well as medical students pursuing research. Such faculty members generally had joint appointments in basic science departments, allowing them to participate in training graduate students.

Clinical Care

DUKE HOSPITAL AND CLINICS

Duke Hospital, wholly owned by Duke University, was the teaching hospital of the university and was licensed for 1,013 beds. Its operations were overseen by a CEO who reported to the chancellor for health affairs. The hospital's clinical faculty were full-time members of clinical departments in the School of Medicine as well as members of the Private Diagnostic Clinic (PDC) (described later), which was required in order to practice medicine at Duke Hospital.

In addition to inpatient facilities, the hospital had ambulatory (outpatient) facilities supported by faculty in the medical PDC and the surgical PDC divisions. Other ambulatory clinics, called "public clinics," served patients lacking sufficient insurance or financial means to be seen by faculty members. Those clinics also were organized in medical and surgical units and overseen by faculty members from the clinical departments (who also were, it bears repeating, members of the PDC). Patients in the public clinics were assigned a physician in training, either interns or residents. In 1989, the hospital generated $358 million in revenues and incurred $352 million in expenses, generating a margin of approximately $6 million.

PRIVATE DIAGNOSTIC CLINIC

The PDC was a separate for-profit partnership composed of members of the clinical faculty of Duke School of Medicine. The PDC, established in 1931, was incorporated as a limited liability company through the PDC Partnership Agreement with Duke University in 1972. This was the operational entity for the clinical faculty practice plan and consisted of two divisions: one medical and one surgical. The PDC was independent of Duke University in its operations and governance although, by the nature of its charter, its faculty and its leadership—the chairs of the clinical departments—had to be members of the clinical departments and thus reported to the chancellor. The PDC also maintained a contractual relationship with the university to "rent space in university-owned Duke Hospital clinics." In lieu of rent, a percentage of the PDC's total annual revenues flowed to DUMC's "Building Fund." This so-called 5(b) transfer formed an important source of revenue for the chancellor, who, in consultation with the leadership of the PDC, could draw on funds to support the greater clinical and academic needs of the medical center.

These main functions sat within an overarching structure, the DUMC, itself nested within another still-larger structure—Duke University. The chancellor for health affairs, who was also the dean of the School of Medicine, was responsible for the overall governance of DUMC, including the School of Medicine, its departments, the Graduate School of Nursing, and Duke Hospital. However, as my immediate predecessors well understood, these extensive responsibilities did not align well with the lesser actual authority of the position.

One of the chancellor's sources of authority related to his role as the chief academic officer of the medical center, which made him responsible for the appointment, promotion, and tenure (APT) of faculty. In the complicated process that regulated this function, proposals for faculty appointment or promotion originated in the departments, were then vetted through basic science or clinical science APT committees, and from there traveled on to the chancellor for health affairs. The chancellor sent his recommendations to the Duke University president "through" the office of the provost for approval by the Duke University Board of Trustees, which held the ultimate authority for all faculty APT decisions. Duke bylaws specifically stated that the chancellor for health affairs' recommendations went to the president "through," rather than "to," the provost, thereby indicating that the chancellor did not report to the provost but rather was subject to the rules established by his office. In practice, the provost's office oversaw the proposals from basic science faculty but left clinical proposals to the chancellor for health affairs. The chancellor was also responsible for the recruitment and retention of the department chairs, the dean of undergraduate medical education, the dean of the Graduate School of Nursing, and the CEO of Duke

Hospital. This was not an insignificant source of control, but it was one that could be but sparsely deployed.

The chancellor for health affairs oversaw various departmental budgets and institutional fund flows; though, in reality, his access to such funds for discretionary purposes was quite limited. Importantly, however, as head of the medical center, the chancellor had a highly visible platform that provided a means to influence overall directions and programs through logical and moral persuasion despite his limited financial resources.

There were, nevertheless, strong limitations to the chancellor's leadership authority. The academic rights of faculty and the culture of departments being nurtured by the chairs and faculty diminished the chancellor's influence. Historically, the chairs had exercised great autonomy over their departments. The clinical chairs controlled by far the greatest source of revenues derived from the practice of their faculty and played almost autonomous roles within their departments if they required no subsidization from the chancellor.

In particular, the chairs of the Departments of Medicine and Surgery, based on the departments' size and the strength of their reserves, played the dominant role in the leadership of the PDC, as well as their departments. They also controlled the directions of the clinical programs within the PDC as well as within Duke Hospital and clinics, since their clinical faculty were responsible for the majority of patient services. Limiting the authority of the chancellor was the independence of the PDC, whose members were the main driver of revenues for the clinical departments and Duke Hospital.

Several committees, all with somewhat murky origins as far as I could discern, existed to coordinate interactions among various entities—what in Washington would be called interagency groups within the executive branch bureaucracy. As is usually the case in Washington, too, these committees at Duke did not function as intended or hoped because the delegates felt more loyalty to their "home" departments than to the committee due to the ineluctable shape of budget lines.

In the aggregate, DUMC's governance could be described as a loose confederation of departments, their divisions, and faculty members, the School of Medicine, graduate medical training, the Graduate School of Nursing, allied health program, Duke Hospital, and the PDC. The chancellor had his own finance and administrative staff, development and communications offices, and an architect who supported his office, the medical center, and the university. In truth, there were no overall clear-cut lines of authority that unified these components. They functioned relatively autonomously under the leadership and guidance of the chancellor and numerous coordinating committees and through the intermittent goodwill of the chairs.

The organizational structure of what was becoming a nationally recognized medical center was not unique; indeed, it was typical of most academic medical centers. This structure worked well for the initial eighty years of academic medicine in the United States, but times were rapidly changing. Managed care was putting pressure on clinical practice margins and demanding the integration of clinical networks dominated by primary care physicians who were scarce in most specialty-oriented academic medical centers. Changes in clinical practice and its associated revenues were creating a crisis in academic medical centers in the United States as I took charge of DUMC.

4

—

Learning the Business

As of January 1989, I officially held principal responsibility for the progress and good reputation of the entire DUMC. I assumed my position with a deep sense of humility and considered my new role a very high honor for someone who was the son of poor immigrants from the Ukraine. Out of this commingled sense of humility and honor I committed myself to doing all I could to make Duke truly great.

But first I had to learn an entirely new job, and from January to the end of June, I'd be shuffling back and forth from California as I transitioned away from Genentech. I was only superficially familiar with administration and management as professional arts. I had acquired some on-the-job training in a for-profit environment but had no formal training in either. In many ways, it was "chutzpah" for me to accept this great responsibility given my dearth of administrative experience in an academic institution. Nonetheless, as I had done several times in my career, I threw myself into this great new challenge with a gut determination to do well.

I started from what I already knew, and what I knew told me that Duke was a very good but not an outstanding institution—at least not yet. As a faculty member in the Department of Medicine from 1972 to 1987, I had recognized many fine qualities within the institution, but its strengths did not extend across the board. Its greatest strengths were clinically oriented (a less-valued capability in academia) rather than in discovery or basic scientific research. Very few Duke faculty members could boast of national reputations for ground-breaking work in their fields. In the early 1980s, when industrialist and philanthropist Edwin C. "Jack" Whitehead, a Duke trustee, considered choosing Duke University as the site for his now-famous Whitehead Institute, his institute director advised him that it would be difficult to recruit outstanding people to Duke. So Jack set up shop at Massachusetts Institute of Technology (MIT) instead. When I began recruiting new faculty to Duke in 1989 and reached out to the great biomedical researchers I knew for advice, one bluntly said that no one he would recommend would consider coming to Duke, which he called a "backwater," somewhere in the South, far removed from the northeastern corridor of more prestigious institutions.

While most national leaders in medicine would have recognized Duke's medical center as a top ten institution in the 1980s, very few would have placed it in the very top tier along with Harvard, Johns Hopkins, Stanford, Yale, Washington University, or the University of California, San Francisco (UCSF). Duke had comparatively few members in the National Academy of Sciences or the Institute of Medicine. Although Duke was renowned for its Departments of Surgery and Medicine, there were few research areas in which the university played a leadership role. The institution had not re-cruited a new chair in any of its basic science departments for two decades. A particularly conspicuous deficit was in genetics, the most productive new field of research at that time. Harvard, UCSF, and Stanford were clear lead-ers in developing recombinant DNA technology, the basis of the success of Genentech and other emerging biotechnology companies. Duke was no-where to be seen in this important area of research.

Taking all this into account, I believed Duke could become a preemi-nent academic medical center, but to be among the very best would require developing and excelling in new directions. The metrics by which medi-cal centers were judged were heavily influenced by the size of their facul-ties, the ambit of their research facilities, the amount of research funding at their disposal, and their overall research productivity. Because of their sheer size advantages, it would have been foolhardy for Duke to follow the same path as Harvard or Hopkins and expect to catch up. Since Duke was in the top ten in nearly every area, despite being the best in none, our overall high quality would be part of our strength. But our greatest asset would be in the leadership of emerging areas of opportunity and need.

So I began to plot a way to leverage our current strength by developing agility and focus while creating new directions for academic medicine. We had significant resources and intensely loyal faculty and alumni. I envisioned that Duke could become what Stanford had been in the 1960s—the institution that had "taken off"—by developing its identity as an innovator in biotechnology. In the 1990s, Duke could become that innovative institution that others would want to emulate. Like the great Canadian ice hockey player Wayne Gretzky, I wanted Duke to be able to skate to where the puck was going to be, not where it was now.

I also sensed, in what was still a far less than fully formed vision, that Duke could be more than the sum of its parts by functioning better as an integrated whole. I believed, as well, that an academic medical center could build relevance in its core missions by meeting pressing societal needs. To this day I remain convinced that good science, common sense, and commitment, when joined together, can be a profoundly transformative force in human welfare if practiced with compassion and dedicated to meeting the needs of people. As I returned to Duke, given the recent and ongoing explosion in biomedical research, anything seemed possible. We could be proud of our capacity to make contributions to humanity in addition to the inherent importance of our research discoveries, training programs, and specialty care.

As a former Duke scientist and a committed Duke loyalist, I had been particularly embarrassed that my university had not been part of the development of recombinant DNA technology, the most exciting research breakthrough at that time. That feeling had sharpened during my time at Genentech, the giant pioneer in the field. Naturally, as I reflected on strategic goals and needs, I dedicated myself to the early recruitment of outstanding individuals in the basic sciences. The clinical operations were not my first priority, since they were stronger in reputation and, at that time, were generally generating sufficient clinical margins to account for all the cross-subsidization the medical center required. At least on the surface, the clinical side seemed to be running well. I was to learn otherwise, however, within the first year of my return to Duke.

I felt strongly that Duke needed a more coherent mechanism for strategic planning so that as an institution it could lead in the emerging areas of research and development related to health care. I was determined that we would never again miss out on an exciting new field of research or medical care—at least not on my watch. We would catch up in biotechnology, and we would begin by rebuilding the basic sciences. Beyond that, I intended to take every opportunity to enhance quality and our reputation across the board, and to find new directions to pursue in order to signal a new leadership era. We therefore had to get a fast start on long-range planning because we had a lot of ground to cover. I intuitively sensed that we needed to approach opportunities and risks at an institutional level, as well as through the activities of individual departments and faculty. Big changes in health care were coming, and we had to prepare ourselves for them.

Although I did not return to Durham with a detailed blueprint for DUMC's future, I knew I wanted to make a real and lasting positive difference. I was committed to doing all I could, and while I sensed the magnitude of the challenge, I never considered failure a possibility. This was not hubris; it was simply the way I approached new challenges—head down, persistent, and yet adaptable based on what I was learning. My greatest ambition was to lead the medical center in its next big jump in quality and recognition. I envisioned another leap of the sort Duke had made in the 1960s thanks to the infusion of outstanding physician-scientists and the ascension of a remarkable generation of departmental chairs.

Consequently, I turned my attention first to understanding the "business," learning how the medical center worked financially, reinvigorating the faculty, and engaging the chairs to establish an institutional focus. My first priority, as noted, was the basic sciences, and my method was to create an infusion of new chairs and outstanding faculty who were leaders or emerging leaders in cutting-edge research. I wanted to "hit the ground running," as the saying goes, but this turned out to be more complicated than I ever imagined. The ground, after all, can be a lot harder and rockier than it first appears.

— — —

Beginning in January and lasting until July 1989, I was on campus approximately two weeks each month, with the remainder of my time spent at Genentech. My family remained in California until we all relocated in late June after my son finished high school in San Mateo. For my Duke weeks, I flew to Durham each Sunday and returned to San Francisco late the following Friday. While being recruited as chancellor, I had stayed in the master suite of the president's house, but beginning in January, I stayed at the Washington Duke Inn as I began my term. My predecessor, Bill Anlyan, graciously provided space for me in the chancellor's suite, along with his senior management team and his excellent assistant, Joyce Ruark, who kindly helped me organize my schedule. Concurrently, I worked to complete my last major assignments at Genentech, which involved completing a long-range plan for research and development and helping with the transitions across my areas of responsibility.

Critical to my performance as chancellor for health affairs was gaining a deeper understanding of my responsibilities. In President H. Keith Brodie's appointment letter to me of November 10, 1988, he stated that my role was to "assume responsibility for the administration of our medical center—this is to include the medical school, Duke Hospital, our School of Nursing, and all of our allied health programs." I needed to identify and understand the workings of the component parts. I needed to learn how things actually worked in practice as opposed to theory or boxes on an organizational chart.

One of my major operational roles was to make sure that the finances of the medical center were well managed and were in the black, while ensuring that each unit was, to the extent possible, supporting itself. This was one of my most complex responsibilities, since most of the organizational units were expected to be "tubs on their own bottom," which is to say, paying their way through the revenues that they generated or had allocated to them. While this remained the expectation, the tubs varied widely in terms of their abilities to meet their bottom line; some were wealthy and some were losing money, but all were essential to the health and quality of the medical center as a whole.

At Genentech, I was responsible for the Departments of Pharmacology, Clinical Research, and Regulatory Affairs, with approximately three hundred staff reporting to me. As chancellor, I was ultimately responsible for the operations and quality of each DUMC entity and—a point worth stressing—for ensuring that they operated synergistically. The success of the medical center depended not only on the quality of its many parts but also on their ability and willingness to work together. At DUMC, there were sixteen departments, two schools, a hospital, a large clinical practice, and more than twelve thousand employees. While Genentech was a complex institution, it paled in comparison to an academic medical center as large as

Duke's. So I knew from the outset that this would be the most challenging management assignment I had ever taken on.

I had an additional and important responsibility as one of four senior officers of Duke University: President Brodie, Executive Vice President Eugene J. McDonald, Provost Phillip A. Griffith, and me as chancellor for health affairs. I began attending Keith Brodie's weekly senior officer meetings in the Allen Building.

The first five months were a deep dive into the multiple components of the medical center. I began to gain an understanding of each unit's function, its leadership, and its strengths and weaknesses. Many of these operations were totally new to me, and I wanted to understand them in sufficient depth. In that spirit, I adopted a fast-start approach, pouring myself into the job with total commitment. I talked to everyone, held open office hours, did weekly walk-around tours of the hospital, clinics, and labs—the proverbial drinking-from-the-fire-hydrant approach.

I immediately established my closest working team, choosing as my staff assistant Jodi Telander, who had worked with me in my laboratory at Duke between 1980 and 1987. A major initial decision, and by then a natural one, was appointing William J. Donelan, who had been the chief operating officer of Duke Hospital, as vice chancellor for medical center administration and chief financial officer. I had come to know and trust Bill when I was chief of rheumatology and immunology in the Department of Medicine, where Bill was the business director. He became my closest partner in the early development and operations of the medical center.

I spent a great deal of time with my principal direct reports, particularly with Bill Donelan; Andrew G. Wallace, MD, vice president for health affairs and CEO of Duke Hospital; Robert G. Winfree, associate vice president for health affairs (who had been Bill Anlyan's chief operating officer, as Donelan was mine); Bernard (Barney) McGinty, director of medical center financial management; and James L. "Pete" Bennett Jr., director of administration, who had been Bill Anlyan's chief of staff. I worked with Raymond C. "Bucky" Waters, Duke's former men's basketball coach and vice chancellor for medical center development, to understand the workings and needs of an operation for which I had responsibility but virtually no experience; with Doyle G. Graham, the pathologist and former chair at Vanderbilt who became dean of medical education, to learn about the needs of the school of medicine and the medical curriculum; and with Larry Nelson, the medical center's architect and assistant vice chancellor for health affairs.

Every member of the administration submitted to me a concise report describing their positions, the nature of their responsibilities, and what they perceived to be their major opportunities and challenges. I met with as many of the institution's key members as possible, thus enabling me to tour medical center operations and gain familiarity with many of its facilities. I left time, as I moved about campus, to talk to people where they worked. To get a better idea of issues within the institution, I opened up my appointment book to individuals who wanted to speak to me one-on-one in confidence.

I was inundated with reams of reading material, appointment after appointment with leaders and administrators of the institution, disgruntled faculty, and members of the university leadership. I found the experience almost overwhelming intellectually; there was so much to learn, yet many important things needed to be done at the same time. I took solace from the fact that I had had a similar experience when I started at Genentech, where, over the course of a year, I went from feeling overwhelmed to gaining perspective and some sense of confidence about what needed to be accomplished and how to do it.

Of all the components of the medical center, the area with which I was the least familiar was the hospital. Running a major teaching hospital is a complex operation, and I had no prior experience. One could learn a great deal from speaking with members of the hospital's leadership team, which of course I did. But I wanted to understand the nature of the operation in more detail. How did the food services run? How did the clinical units work beyond the actual care of patients?

I embarked on gaining a firsthand understanding of actual hospital operations. I developed a program for myself that I called "follow the sheet." It started with the bedsheet on one of the clinical unit's beds. I followed its path from a patient's bed to the laundry and back again to learn all the steps along the way, and thereby to see parts of the hospital and meet groups of individuals I would not normally have encountered.

One day I followed soiled patient linens to Duke Hospital's laundry facility off of Campus Drive, between east and west campus. As a frequent jogger along Campus Drive, I had long noticed a building barely visible from the street that looked vaguely like an industrial plant. That turned out to be Duke Hospital's laundry facility. What I found inside was that the building was not air-conditioned; the ambient temperature inside was well over 110 degrees, and virtually all the employees were African American, except for the individuals in charge, who were white. I was taken aback; this place looked like a sweatshop, not a place befitting Duke University. I ordered a change in our laundry operations to provide air-conditioning as well as a number of employee benefit programs, including courses to teach reading and writing skills to those who needed and wanted them. Seeing the laundry facility made me more aware of the plight of African American employees at Duke who occupied a great deal of the entry-level positions. I would need to confront a far greater impact from these inequities when we were forced to consider a hospital workforce reduction in later years (see chapter 9).

I had a similar sort of learning experience by following a patient's food tray. By doing this, I met individuals who taught me about many otherwise invisible responsibilities within the hospital. I learned about issues related to keeping patients' food warm until it was served at their bedside. I discovered one of the reasons hospital food is generally so tasteless is that it must be microwaved prior to being served, and as everyone knows, a microwave is not a chef's best friend.

By following the sheet and the tray and a few other odds and ends, I began learning how the medical center actually operated, how the units related to each other, how decisions were made (or not made, as the case may be), and, eventually and importantly, how its finances were administered. I slowly came to understand what the chancellor for health affairs and dean of the School of Medicine did and did not do. I also slowly grasped that the chancellor's portfolio, which had operated the institution very well for nearly six decades, might not be adequate for the future.

Above all, I was surprised by the extent to which the medical center was decentralized. The institution was departmentally oriented, and the chairs were not eager to give up their power. Resistance to any move to empower the institutional center had to be expected. Yet it was not immediately clear to me how to move; specifically, it was not obvious where I would find funds and how I would influence institutional directions. Early on I asked Bill Donelan on the spur of the moment, "What about the chancellor's discretionary fund?" He quickly scribbled on a sheet of notepaper all the budget lines that could be tapped—a grand total of about $4 million a year from the Building Fund *if* I could convince the clinical chairs to agree with the expenditures. Nowhere in sight was any budget line that might be reasonably described as a discretionary fund. I had negotiated the creation of a $10 million discretionary fund with President Brodie as part of my start-up package but learned later on that this commitment was not for funds I actually could use but only for the permission for me to raise them. This was an early signal, from my point of view, that dealing with Keith Brodie would not always be straightforward.

Having realized that Duke lacked both a centralized planning operation and significant discretionary funds for the chancellor, I asked myself a simple but critical question: Where was I going to get the money to provide traction for new initiatives? And, of course, there was the flip side of the budgetary coin, the power held by the chairs of the clinical departments, mainly in medicine and surgery. They effectively controlled the revenues created by operations in the Private Diagnostic Clinic, which amounted to about $110 million in 1989–1990.

As I set upon my goal of learning the business, I remembered a television interview from my youth in which Carl Furillo, the great outfielder for the Brooklyn Dodgers, said something that has stuck with me all these years. I was, and still am, a devout New York Yankees fan, but I admired Furillo and his terrific throwing arm; he could throw out runners from the right field wall. He was talking about the value of a big reputation, especially as he got older. What he did at the start of each new season, he explained, was to put everything he had into throwing out the first runner to challenge him—even if he knew his arm would be sore for a week from the exertion. That early success discouraged others from testing his arm, so he figured the pain was worth it.

Like Furillo, I was on the lookout for an important early accomplishment, and I saw the opportunity to address a major problem that had been festering within the institution the year before I arrived: the "B72.3 litigation." A patient, Ms. Betty Eldreth, alleged that she underwent unnecessary treatment for cancer due to a false positive diagnosis from a cancer test known as B72.3. This test was developed and run by a member of the Department of Pathology, and there were allegations of fraud against the developer, William Johnson, chief of cytology and cytogenetics. These were serious allegations, of course, and when they became public knowledge they generated a lot of local and even national attention. There were allegations of cover-ups, as well.

Andy Wallace, vice president for health affairs, handled the issue. He diligently investigated the allegations through several impartial university committees. Nonetheless, the controversy continued to simmer, and frustration with the inability to resolve the issue grew within the medical center. David B. Adcock, university counsel, indicated his displeasure with the lack of strong medical center leadership in making tough decisions to solve the problem. Meanwhile, the pathology faculty were sharply divided between a group of accusers and a group of defenders of both the test and its developer. No one in a senior position seemed willing to enter the fray under such conditions of stalemate. But I was willing.

One of my first actions was to call a leading medical ethicist, Arthur H. Rubenstein, who at that time was chair of medicine at the Pritzker School of Medicine at the University of Chicago, to ask his counsel and assistance. With his guidance, we assembled a blue-ribbon external review committee composed of highly esteemed leaders of medicine from throughout the United States. They were given total access to all the information we had and were free to write their own report, which, we announced from the outset, would be made public, whatever its findings turned out to be. The committee found no evidence of misconduct, only some indication of sloppy record keeping. The case was settled reasonably, and the matter finally was put behind us.

— — —

During the initial six months of 1989, I also faced the task of locating and securing a family residence. Judith, my wife until my final year as chancellor, led this search, and after visiting many homes, we chose a place between Durham and Chapel Hill, on the same street where we had lived prior to moving to San Francisco. Our new house, situated on a five-acre wooded lot abutting Duke Forest, was suitable for entertaining large numbers of people. Judith and our son, Ted, then eighteen years old, moved back to Durham in June; we spent the first several days at the Washington Duke Inn while our belongings arrived from California. Being fully relocated at Duke allowed me to focus more intensely on the immediate tasks at hand.

Thus, by July 1, 1989, when I was finally free to devote my full attention to the duties as chancellor, I had learned a great deal about the workings of the institution. Little did I know how much more was to come as I became engaged in its day-to-day operations.

5

—

Getting Down to Business

An onrushing crisis in academic medical centers in the United States was becoming fact number one as I joined the medical center full-time in July 1989. Much of this situation was a consequence of the need of these institutions to rapidly adapt to changes in health care delivery that, if not met, could lead to their financial collapse (described more fully in chapter 11). I soon discovered that Duke's highly complex entity that I held in great esteem, while beautiful on the outside, was rapidly moving toward unsustainability, was rife with inequities and inefficiencies in governance and, worst of all, was perhaps unable to change sufficiently to survive the looming threats to its viability.

I ramped up my efforts to understand all the working parts of the medical center and how they meshed, or did not mesh, together. I was developing a sense of the leadership cadres and assessing which positions probably needed to be changed. At the same time, I was proceeding with obvious key initiatives while developing action plans for improvements, especially in the basic sciences. We were pursuing long-range planning, which I had set in motion during my first month in office, and which would include features aimed at better organization of operations such as finance and budgeting.

Long-range planning became a high priority. Although Duke had developed the capacity to do good research and deliver exquisite clinical care, no grand design had ever been devised to maximize the institution's capabilities as a whole. This view grew from my previous experience on the faculty; like most of my colleagues, I was provincial—narrowly focused on my own activity. I knew most about my own laboratory and was acquainted with many people in the Sands Building where my laboratory was housed. I certainly knew a lot about the Division of Rheumatology and Immunology, where I was division chief. I knew the Department of Medicine well and appreciated its extremely strong programs, particularly on the clinical training side. I was aware of other prominent department leaders, and I had met Chancellor Bill Anlyan on several occasions. But I had virtually no feel for or interest in the medical center as such or in larger university politics. I was in business for myself, and Duke provided me the platform to be successful at it. My job, as I conceived it, was to fund my laboratory, be productive, and contribute to my division, department, and field of research. As far as I knew or heard, this was what Duke expected of me as well. And it was what Duke expected of others like me.

Over time, it was natural that some chairs, divisions, and departments would accrue more prestige, resources, and bureaucratic clout than others. When I took office as chancellor, this was certainly the case. In basic sciences the most powerful chairs were Robert L. Hill in biochemistry and Wolfgang K. (Bill) Joklik in microbiology and immunology. On the clinical side David C. Sabiston, Jr., then celebrating his twenty-fifth year as chair of surgery, and Joseph C. Greenfield, Jr., the chair of medicine since 1983, were clearly primus inter pares. The degree of departmental autonomy and the ability of these powerful personalities to dominate what happened throughout the medical center were formidable, and the seniority of most of these chairs contributed to their clout.

Drs. Sabiston and Greenfield also headed the surgery and medicine divisions of the PDC, which generated a hefty share of the medical center's revenues. According to Carl E. Ravin, chair of radiology, the legendary Dave Sabiston had pooh-poohed rumors that he wanted to succeed Bill Anlyan as chancellor, asking, "Why would I want to give up all my power?" It was Joe Greenfield, a distinguished cardiologist and Civil War buff from Georgia, with whom I would later disagree about several matters, who told me that being chancellor "is like being the pope, who doesn't have an army, either."

The PDC also suffered from issues with which I became more familiar over time. The clinical department chairs had sorted themselves out as the "giants" and the "dwarfs." The giants were the big moneymakers of medicine and surgery, and the dwarfs were every other department, some of which were actually losing money. Carl Ravin, a dwarf chairman with an attitude, told a wonderful story about what happened if a dwarf chair differed with a giant chair in a meeting: the dwarf chair would receive in the mail a T-shirt bearing the words "DWARF POWER." On the one hand, this was an example, harmless in itself, of amusing self-awareness; on the other hand, it was dismaying because it suggested a lower level of interdisciplinary cooperation and collegiality than was required to respond institutionally to opportunities or threats.

I had been vaguely aware of agitation within and among the basic science departments before leaving for Genentech in 1987. Between 1986 and 1988, several of my former colleagues in the basic sciences grew increasingly displeased with the direction the medical center was taking in research. They were dissatisfied with the de facto governance provided by the entrenched chairs; they wanted decision making to be more broadly shared among the faculty. So a group of faculty organized and brought forward to Bill Anlyan, and presumably to President Keith Brodie, several recommendations for change. Some people referred to this period as the "French Revolution." Brodie evidently supported this movement and appointed his close colleague Charles E. Putman as medical school dean over Bill Anlyan's objections. Charles resigned after a year, but Keith Brodie got Bill Anlyan to agree to move from chancellor for health affairs to a "promotion" as university chancellor, opening the way for new leadership of the medical center—me.

— — —

By the summer of 1989, it was time to transition from learning and planning to taking action on the tasks at hand. One of the features of the chancellor's job that attracted me was that three departments—neurobiology, cell biology, and pharmacology—had interim leaderships; the search for new leaders in these areas presented a golden opportunity to build quality and reputation and to create a bigger and better buzz about Duke. In my determination to elevate the quality and stature of our research programs in the basic sciences, it was essential that the first search for the founding chair of the new Department of Neurobiology result in the recruitment of an eminent researcher and thought leader in the field. My goal was to do the same with the other two chairs and thus make a strong statement that Duke would take its place among the leaders of biomedical research. This was extremely important, since research strength was the key to the national reputation of an academic medical center. Excellent patient care was certainly critical but was not as easily quantifiable as NIH research funding levels or the stature of the institution's faculty.

Those three searches, if done right, could also bring in creative new leaders who were established in their field and capable of gathering outstanding young talent around them. Choosing well was doubly important for neurobiology, which was emerging as an area of special opportunity, one likely to produce a great yield on investments in research and discovery. Convinced that the initial search must produce a stellar appointment (another Furillo moment), we would look for a luminary, a "name brand," who would add to Duke's luster and set a very high bar for future recruitments. We pulled together enough coin of the realm (space as well as dollars) we thought we needed to attract an outstanding candidate—and I was prepared to cobble together more support funds if necessary. We narrowed the search to three highly qualified candidates, including one from an Ivy League institution who had assembled a big research center but who might prove prohibitively expensive and perhaps had already peaked in his career.

We were blessed by good fortune. In 1990, we recruited our first choice, Dale Purves, who had been elected a member of the National Academy of Sciences the previous year and was known as a real thought leader. In addition, it seemed to me that of the candidates we considered, Dale was the most likely to continue to grow in his own career. Over the years, he has done so, gaining international fame for his theoretical and experimental work in visual and auditory perception. His impact on science and medicine, on his department, and on his students, colleagues, and Duke itself has been extraordinary; his tenure as chair lasted until 2002. Most recently he helped Duke launch its medical school "annex" in Singapore, and the fifth edition of his textbook *Neuroscience* was published in 2011.

We quickly moved forward on the other two searches to add depth and recognition of the quality of our basic sciences. David Botstein, a well-known geneticist and former colleague at Genentech, suggested Michael P. Sheetz. We recruited him in 1990 to chair the Department of Cell Biology, which he did for more than a decade before accepting the William R. Kenan, Jr. Professor of Cell Biology chair at Columbia University. Mike achieved distinction for describing the forces at work in cell structure and function. In 2012, he received the Albert Lasker Basic Medical Research Award for his work in cellular biology, work he now is pursuing in Singapore.

In 1991, we succeeded in attracting Anthony R. Means from the Baylor College of Medicine to take over the Department of Pharmacology and Cancer Biology. Currently, Tony is professor emeritus of Pharmacology and Cancer Biology in the department he chaired for more than a decade. He also serves as associate director for basic research emeritus of the Duke Cancer Center, the new and large (seven-story, 267,000-square-foot) center he created and codirected as Duke sought a permanent leader of this new facility.

In addition to these three recruits, we filled several other positions in the basic science departments between 1989 and 1994. John D. Shelburne became interim chair of the Department of Pathology in 1989. In 1991, Salvatore V. Pizzo became the department's permanent chair and remained so until the end of 2014. Sal was a Duke product, having received his MD and PhD from Duke in 1973 before joining the faculty and rising in 1985 to the rank of professor. An accomplished experimental pathologist and researcher, he is well known for his superb teaching ability and is a valued colleague. In addition to being chair, Sal was a strong advocate for and leader of our MD/PhD training program.

The list of basic science departments increased with the addition of the Department of Molecular Cancer Biology in 1993 and the Department of Genetics in 1994. The Department of Molecular Cancer Biology evolved from the Section of Cell Growth, Regulation, and Oncogenesis, which was created in 1988, and Robert M. Bell, James B. Duke Professor of Biochemistry, became its new chair in 1993. Bob remained chair until the department merged with the Department of Pharmacology to form the Department of Pharmacology and Cancer Biology in 1995. The Department of Genetics (previously the Section of Genetics) came into being in 1994, and Joseph R. Nevins, professor of microbiology, became its first chair. Joe had previously been the head of the Section of Genetics.

Christian R. H. Raetz, an MD and PhD, succeeded Bob Hill as chair of the Department of Biochemistry in 1993. Chris had been vice president for basic research at Merck Research Laboratories in New Jersey, where he had shepherded several drugs through the approval process of the FDA, including the cholesterol-lowering medicine Zocor.

Bill Joklik, who served as chair of the Department of Microbiology and Immunology from 1968, retired in 1994, and Jack D. Keene, a faculty member, became interim chair. In 1994, following a national search, Jack became permanent chair. In 1992, the department underwent reorganization, and as a result the Department of Immunology became a separate department. An outstanding young immunologist, Thomas F. Tedder, previously a faculty member at Dana-Farber Cancer Center and Harvard Medical School, agreed to come to Duke as the founding chair of the Department of Immunology.

— — —

Enhancing our research capability and renown provided the impetus for my first major foray in big-time fund-raising, described in greater detail in chapter 14. I hoped to gain the support of Jack Whitehead, who had made his fortune through Technicon, a firm founded by his father in 1939. Technicon made bioanalytical laboratory equipment and developed an instrument to perform a new clinical laboratory assay by measuring eighteen determinants from a single sample, the famed "Chem 18." Much of the validation of the test occurred at the Durham VA Hospital, and Jack's interest in and loyalty to Duke made it his original choice for the location of the Whitehead Institute. When this failed to come about, Jack instead pledged a $10 million gift to be paid over ten years. For his gift mechanism, he chose an endowment that would provide about $50,000 in income annually to support three of the strongest recruits in academic biomedicine. Jack truly appreciated and wanted to help Duke, especially after deeply disappointing people at the university when he chose to locate his institute at MIT. Despite this, he had paid only about $2.3 million toward his pledge by the time I arrived on the scene, and there was scant, if any, indication of more to come.

Bucky Waters, vice chancellor of medical center development, suggested that I meet with Jack and reestablish the financial commitment he had made to Duke. Bucky warned me that this would not be an easy negotiation; Jack seemingly had lost interest in Duke and was focused intently on the newly formed Whitehead Institute in Cambridge. He also described Jack as a gruff guy and a hard negotiator. I agreed to meet with Jack but feared the prospect. I knew I had to directly ask a tough man to change his mind again about making a major contribution to the medical center. If I failed, I would turn the Carl Furillo rule upside down, and that would not make for a good optic. I visited Jack Whitehead in his office in Greenwich, Connecticut. After a very short time with him, I realized with a sigh of relief that his reputation for being brusque, crusty, and a tough negotiator was nothing more than nonnatives' failure to appreciate the standard-issue New Yorker personality. Moreover, shortly after we met, Jack told me that his original family name was Weiskopf (a precise Germanic-Yiddish reverse translation of Whitehead) and that he was not just a New Yorker but a Jewish New Yorker, like me.

We hit it off extremely well, and I came not only to admire but to truly care for Jack Whitehead. Judith and I became regular guests at Jack's magnificent ski lodge in Vail, Colorado, where each year he would assemble small parties of interesting people, mostly notables in medicine, for a full week of skiing in one of the most wonderful places in the world. During these trips, I had the opportunity to ski with and get to know fascinating individuals like David Baltimore, the Nobel laureate and director of the Whitehead Institute, and Alain C. Enthoven, the highly regarded health care economist from Stanford.

Ski trips aside, I was successful in resuming the flow of Whitehead money to Duke. Jack not only agreed to recommit to his gift but agreed to increase it and focus it in a way that enabled us to leverage his contribution to markedly improve our basic science research faculty. Our goal then and throughout my tenure was to recruit the next great generation of scholars—to find the best, bring them in, and provide them with financial, administrative, and collegial support as they were beginning to organize laboratories and were not yet able to be self-supporting through external funding. The agreement between the Whitehead Charitable Foundation and Duke University dated July 31, 1991, outlined the vehicle we designed: the Whitehead Scholars Program.

Basically, we persuaded Jack that the existing program of relying on endowment income was not well suited to recruiting a strong cadre of new faculty and doing so reasonably quickly. Our idea was to supply more upfront resources by spending down the funds over about ten years rather than spending only the income from an endowment. We signed new agreements that provided an initial balance of $12.7 million, including gifts to date, their income, and capital appreciation; an additional $1 million also was committed. The revamped program allowed us to adapt to the financial realities of increasingly expensive start-up funds for new researchers. With it, we provided $500,000 over five years to each of the thirty-six Whitehead Scholars recruited over the nine-year life of the program. We brought in great young researchers and, at the time this book is being written, all but a couple of them remain on the faculty and continue to strengthen Duke's reputation.

Without question, a major factor in the program's success was Jack Whitehead's willingness to use his name and contacts to create a phenomenal selection committee. Because the Whitehead Institute was already gaining national prominence, Whitehead's association with a Duke faculty recruitment program, along with a generous stipend, gave us a strong competitive edge to bring the best and brightest to our medical center. Jack and I agreed that these appointments should be staged nationally to signal highly prestigious appointments. To achieve this, we developed an absolutely first-rate selection committee that not only lent luster to the program but provided access to the stream of the best young talent through its members' own contacts and colleagues.

While choosing the selection committee, I had in mind the comment of David Botstein, the man who had predicted that the best and the brightest would not come to the Duke "backwater." I sought to offset that perception by using internationally known researchers to recruit the most promising prospects, allaying any concerns that highly regarded candidates might have. The selection committee included David Baltimore, Philip A. Sharp, and Tortsen N. Wiesel, each of whom had won a Nobel Prize; Jim Wyngaarden, former chair of the Department of Medicine at Duke and director of the NIH; and Bob Lefkowitz, who would win the Nobel Prize in Chemistry in 2012. This outstanding group not only played a key role in evaluating candidates but also spread the word that Duke was an up-and-coming place to be.

— — —

Breathing new life and vigor into the clinical departments turned out to be more complicated and ultimately more problematic than doing so for the basic sciences. Historically, clinical department chairs had great authority within their departments and long seniority as chairs. As is often the case in the U.S. Supreme Court, they were replaced only upon extraordinary circumstances such as retirement, the decision of the chair to leave the institution, or death. Each department was expected to be self-sufficient in regard to its funding and to choose its own direction regarding the nature of its clinical practice and areas of research. Moreover, because research required subsidization from other sources—not from clinical margins—the clinical departments best situated to create those margins had the strongest research programs and usually became the most important departments by national reputation and influence within the medical center.

Such was the standing tradition, but it was a tradition whose raison d'être was eroding by the late 1980s at Duke and nationally. Clinical margins were narrowing; subsidies from those departments for other functions of the medical center were shrinking. This was of profound importance because, for decades, the internal finances of clinical departments had determined the size of their clinical activities. For example, Jim Wyngaarden, chair of medicine from 1967 to 1983, could invest in recruiting a promising new researcher until he or she was fully funded by grant support because Jim knew his department had sufficient financial reserves for the purpose, and, if necessary, it could raise more money. He had a group of creative researchers in his department who were getting grants, writing papers, and making discoveries. In fact, I was recruited through this process in 1972, as was Bob Lefkowitz in 1973. Jim Wyngaarden also had assembled talented physicians in the clinical trenches who were seeing patients in the PDC and creating healthy clinical margins—"margin" being a not-for-profit institutional synonym for "profit." Jim counted on them to generate a surplus to support his research faculty recruitments. If the research group needed more money, Jim knew that a few more clinicians would earn that margin because, in those days, clinical activities were performed on a cost-plus basis.

A key concern when I arrived was the Department of Pediatrics, which had been losing money for several years. Psychiatry, too, faced strong financial problems as reimbursement for office-based psychiatry generated little to no margin. On the horizon, it was clear that the Department of Obstetrics and Gynecology (OB/GYN) would be soon losing money too, as reimbursement for obstetrics could not sustain itself. As clinical reimbursement margins continued to shrink throughout the system, the cross-subsidization structure of the clinical department enterprise would become increasingly difficult to sustain.

What was even more worrisome to me was that the burgeoning competition among some departments for shrinking clinical revenues was happening in a way similar to what the uniformed armed services do when the defense budget pie shrinks—they try to poach on each other's budgetary turf to secure a larger percentage of a smaller total. In particular, the Department of Medicine, generally tied with the Department of Surgery as the department that produced the highest margins, was feeling the pressure of low reimbursement from many of its noninvasive services. As invasive diagnostic imaging became more important and lucrative, the Department of Radiology became increasingly important. The Department of Anesthesiology, as an integral underpinning for the Department of Surgery along with associated revenue from surgical procedures, had a sound financial basis. Similarly, the Department of Pathology, running the hospital diagnostic laboratories and autopsy services, managed to remain financially sound. Although there were differences in their size, prestige, and influence, they could all pretty much go their own way. Other departments did not enjoy as comfortable and stable a financial circumstance. Usually, these were the departments that, because of their nature, involved clinicians spending more time with patients but doing fewer procedures.

On the other hand, imaging by invasive means such as coronary arteriography performed in the Department of Medicine produced generous reimbursements. Joe Greenfield, the aggressive and entrepreneurial chair, saw opportunities for the Department of Medicine to move beyond the imaging of the coronary arteries into the imaging of distal sites such as the renal arteries and peripheral vasculature, a function historically within the purview of the Department of Radiology. This generated a great deal of animosity between the two departments.

Within the first year of my return to Duke, recognition gradually emerged that the clinical department model had come under great financial pressure, and that pressure was leading to institutional distress and dissension. A helpful analogy may be to think of clinical departments as businesses in a shopping mall owned by the medical center; it follows that the viability of the enterprise depended on the success of each as well as the aggregate of the individual stores. When business began to slow down, stores suffered in general, but fierce competition among the stores in the same mall was not a good recipe for the success of the whole.

It was also becoming apparent that the strength of the clinical departments, individually and as a whole, depended on a high volume of patient referrals to Duke. These referrals depended in turn on the provision of high-quality service to the patients and physicians, as well as an appropriate distribution of physicians to meet the needs of the patients being referred. The operation of the overall clinical practice was a responsibility of the PDC, but the PDC was not structured to oversee an integrated clinical practice. Moreover, the PDC, as an independent entity with a contract to provide clinical service to Duke, excluded the chancellor from any direct role in its oversight. There was no central means to ensure ease of access for patient appointments; indeed, most faculty insisted that only they and their assistants be authorized to schedule appointments.

No general oversight existed to ensure the overall quality of services, nor was there any central means of organizing the practice so that it was maximally responsive to the needs of referring physicians. This was of critical importance in the long run, since Duke's clinical practice was heavily dependent on referrals from physicians throughout North Carolina. Yet the PDC lacked any strong incentive to build a primary care capacity: primary care lost money, and everyone knew it. Thus, Duke's departmentally based clinical practice model was not well structured to meet the needs of a changing environment where service and efficiency mattered more than ever. The incentives for outside physicians to refer patients to Duke were shifting as a consequence of managed care, which increasingly stressed the need for primary care.

Alleviating the financial problems within the clinical departments clearly required a more robust and efficient clinical operation, yet the independence of the clinical departments and the PDC obstructed this goal. This led us to conclude that for Duke's viability, let alone success in becoming a national leader in academic medicine, we needed to be a more coherent organization that used resources efficiently from the perspective of the whole institution. We required a level of strategic and operational planning that the legacy of Duke's first six decades did not provide.

This situation reminded me of an anatomical metaphor: DUMC, a complex living institution with independently moving parts, lacked a central nervous system (a brain to coordinate them). With some management ganglia here and some administrative ganglia there, it lacked the institutional coordination needed to generate full situational awareness. We needed to sustain the viability of the independent parts while creating the capability of making the whole greater than the sum of the individual parts. We needed an overall strategic plan to address our institutional health, including growth in the basic sciences and, when possible, in the clinical departments; financial sustainability; development of a coherent clinical practice organization; and overall institutional goals to attain a position of national leadership

To begin doing this, we needed to strengthen the function of the CEO of Duke Hospital so that it supported the clinical practice but was not dominated by the individual clinical department chairs. Prior to 1989, the Duke Hospital CEO was largely a position that emphasized running the hospital operation and keeping the clinical chairs satisfied. As the need for a more cost-effective, coordinated delivery system developed, the desire for the hospital CEO to be a more powerful and strategically oriented change agent became a priority. This being the case, Andy Wallace, a superb and innovative cardiologist and an academician who was serving as Duke Hospital's CEO, agreed to move to the position of vice chancellor for academic affairs in 1990. A high-energy, business-oriented CEO from Toronto, W. Vickery Stoughton, a fast mover and highly independent individual, became our preferred change agent to replace Andy.

— — —

Beyond the organization of the basic sciences and clinical enterprise, urgent but often unpredictable decision points sometimes pop up that require concentrated attention, and how these decision points are handled can color an entire new administration's effort. In my case, an urgent early decision point concerned the future of the Graduate School of Nursing, whose status posed important challenges and opportunities. In an effort to enhance the finances of Duke University, A. Kenneth Pye (chancellor of the university in 1979) had recommended closing the Duke University School of Nursing. Despite protests from many areas, the university's Board of Trustees had voted to do this, and the school graduated its last bachelor of science in nursing class in 1984. The then chancellor for health affairs, Bill Anlyan, did, however, allow the continuation of a small master's program, and thus the Graduate School of Nursing was born. By the time I arrived in 1989, the school's existing faculty had dwindled to fewer than ten. Dorothy J. Brundage, dean of the School of Nursing, was doing her best to keep this below-critical-mass program in operation.

I faced the decision of letting the school continue to dwindle and ultimately go extinct, or revitalizing it so it could develop programs consistent with evolving models of health care. A school of Duke's size could not aspire to be the best at everything, so we needed to select priorities and opportunities with surgical precision. After turning the matter over in my mind for several weeks and consulting informally with a series of wise colleagues, I decided to go all in: Duke would have a Graduate School of Nursing that would rank among the nation's best, and that graduate school would be designed for health care models on the leading edge of twenty-first-century medicine. We launched a national search for a new dean of nursing in 1991 and chose Mary T. Champagne, from the University of North Carolina, for the post. I was impressed with Mary's energy, freshness of vision, and unstinting belief that Duke's Graduate School of Nursing could develop into a leading institution. Indeed, she infused the school with a new sense of direction and purpose, and its achievements ultimately exceeded our wildest dreams.

During my first year, I learned a lot about the operations of this complex medical center, but more importantly, I began to develop a strong sense about what needed to be done to preserve and improve it. By early 1991, it was clear that what I needed to do would be far more challenging than my initial, simplistic ideas of what the position entailed.

6

—

Reconstruction

During the fall of 1989, an event occurred that had an important impact early in my first term and profoundly affected the development of the medical center's first long-range strategic plan. At a dinner in Washington, DC, I found myself sitting next to Daniel C. Tosteson, dean of the Harvard School of Medicine and a member of Duke's Board of Trustees. On Dan's other side was Willian N. Kelley, the newly appointed executive vice president of the University of Pennsylvania Medical Center. Bill had been head of Duke's Division of Rheumatology and Genetics when Jim Wyngaarden recruited me, and Bill and I had developed an enduring friendship. I told Dan almost as a jest that, now that I had made the plunge into assuming the role as chancellor for health affairs at Duke, it was his responsibility as a former Duke faculty member, a member of its board, and a nationally preeminent dean, to help me succeed. Without missing a step, Dan took out a pen and on my napkin wrote the name and telephone number of Steven J. Ruma—his trusted and valuable consultant. Dan claimed that he could not run the Harvard School of Medicine without Steve and suggested I call him to see if I could enlist him to be my consultant as well. Bill Kelley, being no fool, also jotted down Steve's number.

I called Steve Ruma soon thereafter, and he agreed to visit Duke, at which time we decided that he would also be my consultant. We agreed on a contract that had great consequence for me and for the institution. Steve was a clinical psychologist who had wandered into academic consulting. At that time, he directed a deans' advisory program for the Association of American Medical Colleges (AAMC). Virtually all new deans spent a week with Steve at "dean's school," held once a year, usually in Florida. In addition to me, Steve worked with a small, select group of deans on an ongoing basis. The group included Dan Tosteson, Bill Kelley, Michael M.E. Johns, III, dean at Johns Hopkins; William Peck, dean at Washington University; and Gerard N. Burrow, dean at Yale.

Steve and I developed an intense professional and personal relationship. He was a highly engaging individual, proud of his Sicilian heritage and fiercely committed to his clients. Steve was my strategic and operational adviser as well as friend and, as a clinical psychologist, was an excellent source of counseling. He once told me to "hold your friends close but your enemies closer." With his contacts at the AAMC and his close professional relations with the deans of some of the nation's best medical schools, Steve had a broad and deep understanding of the role of the dean. Moreover, he was a keen observer of individuals and quickly identified the strengths and weaknesses of those he encountered. He sized me up quickly and suggested that I needed more guile!

Steve visited Duke about every six weeks. We would meet for dinner at the Washington Duke Inn; then, over the next day or two, Steve would meet key leaders of the medical center and university. He spent time with me assessing the strength of my team, analyzing what was going on outside my office suite, and, importantly, laying the groundwork for our first long-range strategic plan. His counsel proved invaluable.

— — —

Shortly after the conclusion of my first year as chancellor, President Keith Brodie gave me the opportunity to share my view of Duke's medical center and its future with the Board of Trustees. On October 5, 1990, I presented a detailed evaluation of what I had learned thus far, along with an assessment of future risks and opportunities. (Excerpts from the October 5, 1990, presentation to the Board of Trustees are included in appendix 2.) Suffice it to say that while this maiden assessment proved in some ways an optimistic document, in other ways it understated what we would accomplish over the next fourteen years. In an odd way it confirmed both my interpersonal naïveté—my dearth of guile, I suppose—and my relentless determination to succeed. When I read it now, nearly a quarter century later, I alternatively cringe and smile.

My presentation on the state of DUMC generated a great deal of enthusiasm, and the board encouraged us to identify the needs and opportunities the institution would face. So in the latter part of 1990, along with my senior leadership team and with the help of Steve Ruma, we began laying the groundwork for the further development of the institution's first institution-wide long-range plan.

Our principal goal was to generate a detailed assessment of the needs and opportunities, as well as an agreement on goals for each department and major center in the institution. Importantly, we would also identify interdepartmental goals and objectives that transcended individual organizational structures and represented an institution-wide approach to solving problems and creating opportunities. On January 28, 1991, I sent a letter to each chair and center head, asking these individuals to work closely with their faculty to create a document that addressed the following areas:

1. Status of your field
2. Status of your department within the field
3. Current programs in your department that should be expanded or strengthened
4. Programs that are likely to be downsized or redirected
5. New programs that should be initiated

The letter emphasized the importance of a broad buy-in on the part of departmental faculty and division chiefs. I asked that a first draft be submitted by no later than March 29, 1991. To help organize this effort, Duncan Yaggy, director and chief planning officer of Duke Hospital, met with the chairs and their key faculty. Bill Donelan, Bob Winfree, Larry Nelson, Barney McGinty, and my staff assistant worked with Duncan to coordinate the efforts into a single, integrated plan. The departmental plans would be essential components of the budgeting process for future years.

In addition, we formed a steering committee to advise the chancellor and to deal with issues that transcended departmental boundaries. We provided a full description of the process and what was expected from each department to each chair. The purpose was to facilitate decisions concerning the following:

- The assessment of existing programs
- The creation and allocation of new research space
- The development of core research support facilities and shared technologies
- The uses and development of newly acquired land north of Erwin Road
- The selection and recruitment of new chairs and faculty
- The creation and funding of proposed interdisciplinary research efforts (e.g., gene therapy, developmental biology, structural biology)
- The development of new clinical facilities and services
- The magnitude and strategy of development efforts essential to the implementation of new programs

Following the completion of the departmental planning process, key members of my senior management team and I met with all departmental and center chairs on multiple occasions to refine their individual plans. We proceeded based on a broader institutional understanding of the other departments' plans, as well as the availability of resources. Interdepartmental groups were assembled to evaluate opportunities and needs in education, research, and clinical areas. These were in turn refined, quantified insofar as possible, and discussed with numerous interdepartmental committees and ultimately with the Medical Center Policy Advisory Committee (MedPAC), a committee composed of the chancellor for health affairs, dean of undergraduate medical education, dean of the School of Nursing, the chairs of the medical school departments, key center directors, and a medical student (usually the president of the Davison Society) as an observer. Representatives of the Basic Sciences Faculty Steering Committee and the Clinical Sciences Faculty Council on Academic Affairs also participated as observers. MedPAC met at least four times a year, usually prior to meetings of the Duke University Board of Trustees.

By September 1991, the Duke University Medical Center Long Range Plan (Long Range Plan hereafter) was complete. The five-year plan identified priorities in educational programs, including changes in the undergraduate medical curriculum and in residency and fellowship training, expansion of continuing medical education, and a commitment to strengthen programs in nursing education as well as opportunities in graduate education and allied health. An important outcome of the planning process was the identification of interdisciplinary research programs to be emphasized. These included genetics, with a decision to create a section of genetics with up to ten new faculty; strengthening efforts in signal transduction, the neurosciences, immunology, and structural biology; and investment in core technologies to support research in multiple areas. For the first time, institution-wide interdisciplinary clinical programs were identified, including aging, cardiovascular health, oncology, transplantation, musculoskeletal disease, and children's health. We also identified clinical service initiatives to address the following areas:

- Improved patient satisfaction through hospital/PDC reorganization
- Programs in quality assurance and cost-effectiveness
- Strengthening of outreach programs
- Programs designed to enhance managed care
- Planning for and commitment to a new ambulatory facility

The Long Range Plan outlined recruitment targets for leadership in the major academic areas for 1991–1996, including new chairs for the Departments of Biochemistry, Community and Family Medicine, Human Genetics, Medicine, Microbiology and Immunology, Ophthalmology, Psychiatry, and Surgery. Our goal was to add seventy-four new research-oriented faculty in the basic sciences and clinical departments over five years and, moreover, to specify the expertise foci of such recruits. Furthermore, the plan identified specific resources, in both finances and space, required for all recruits and program expansions. For example, it identified the need for approximately $300 million for buildings and facilities during the first five years of the plan, including new research buildings, as well as $30 million to renovate existing facilities. Our efforts defined sources and uses of funds for each component of the plan. We also specified the development of new clinical technologies, an office of technology transfer, and the strengthening and expansion of the medical center's development efforts. We estimated a need for an additional $70 million in development pledges by June 30, 1996, to support the growth projected within the plan.

It would be hard to overstate the importance of the Long Range Plan to the eventual success, or lack thereof, of the institution during my tenure.

Certainly, it was absolutely formative to my first term. The plan set out a comprehensive analysis of threats and opportunities within all the areas of the medical center. Importantly, it identified several new investment opportunities, set expectations for performance, and developed priorities for the utilization of resources that transcended the interest of any single department or entity within the institution. It demonstrated the need for central leadership to create an institutional focus, and by identifying priorities for the entire medical center, it constituted the first formal planning process by any major entity within the university. It therefore demonstrated to the university leadership and its Board of Trustees the level of discipline with which the medical center would bind itself in attempting to achieve its goals of excellence.

Perhaps most important, the Long Range Plan clearly established DUMC's overarching mission to create societal benefits through our core missions of education, research, and clinical care to create new and better models of health care delivery. At that time, this overarching mission was unique for academic medical centers. The plan was prescient in envisioning a direction for the medical center that remains relevant today. The Long Range Plan was widely distributed within the medical center, presented to the university leadership, and formally presented to the Board of Trustees in 1991.

— — —

With the initial planning process behind us, the blueprint for the remainder of my first term became clearer. Initiatives were undertaken according to the plan in all the core missions of the medical center involving education, research, and clinical activities.

New personnel made a difference, too. I wanted to bring to Duke a name-brand leader of academic administration and an individual who still had "fire in the belly" to do something important. The recruitment of Gordon G. Hammes as the institution's first vice chancellor for academic affairs in 1991 filled both of these needs and was essential to putting the Long Range Plan effectively into practice. Gordon had been chair of the Department of Chemistry and Chemical Biology at Cornell University and developer and head of the university's Biotechnology Program. He had left Cornell to take the position of vice chancellor of academic affairs at the University of California at Santa Barbara prior to coming to Duke in 1991. Gordon was an outstanding researcher in the field of enzyme kinetics and a member of the National Academy of Sciences. It was clear that the recruitment of a highly recognized individual as our vice chancellor for academic affairs not only would be helpful internally but also would signal that Duke was aspiring to be the very best. Gordon played an essential role in setting extremely high standards for everything he was involved in. We designated the school of medicine, the basic science departments, and the research components of the clinical departments as Gordon's responsibilities. Given Gordon's lack of a medical degree, we devised a dotted-line reporting relationship of the clinical chairs and the dean for undergraduate medical education to me as well as to Gordon.

Based on the Long Range Plan, the revised curriculum for undergraduate teaching in the school of medicine led to basic changes in teaching methods. Within the first year the staff introduced a far greater use of small-group, problem-based teams and provided new educational technologies, including computers. By the third year, scholarly activities broadened from basic science research to include clinical research, health policy, health law, health administration, public health, medical history, and medical ethics. We decided that, where appropriate, students would be enabled to pursue completion of master's degrees. We also placed an increased emphasis on continuing medical education and decided that nursing education at the graduate level would remain a high priority.

We strengthened graduate education within the basic science departments of the medical center through increased collaboration with the graduate school of Duke University. In that arrangement, we collaborated with the university to reorganize biomedical graduate programs. We evaluated training in allied health programs and very much liked what we found—this training turned out to be an underappreciated institutional strength, and we saw immediately the export potential of this program. In other words, we depended on it to train individuals not only for DUMC but also for the growing needs in allied health throughout the United States.

The Long Range Plan enabled the medical center administration to work with all its component entities in a collaborative way. We did this both to meet the needs of the individual parts and to bring them together wherever it would advance higher-order goals. That latter effort was multifaceted. We wanted to lend validity to the involvement of medical center administration in matters from which it had heretofore been largely absent; that included, where appropriate, intrusion into the affairs of schools and departments to enhance cost-effectiveness, rationally allocate resources, develop institutional understanding of levels of performance, and create new programs. In the basic sciences, for example, the plan identified key research areas and specified the number and nature of new faculty to be recruited over the next five years. Identifying specific areas for research of new faculty and central resources for their recruitment enabled Gordon and me to be involved in new faculty recruitment within the departments. Previously, the chair and faculty of each department determined the nature of the research of any new departmental faculty. With the Long Range Plan in hand, department chairs and their faculty would be authorized to recruit one or more new faculty members specifically working in an area identified as a high priority. We expected that such faculty would be recruited as a result of a national search, with the understanding that the person selected must be recognized as being among the top two individuals in the United States in their field.

We understood how the traditional "old boys" network of senior chairs and their apprentices worked to generate new faculty appointments. It functioned the same way in the rest of the university as well, and in other universities, too. It worked well enough when change in the basic sciences, clinical practice, and technologies was reasonably slow; when institutional priorities trumped broader outcomes; and when recruiting women and minorities into the medical profession was little more than an afterthought. But times had changed, and a good-enough system of recruitment depending on informal networks was no longer adequate for an institution seeking top-tier performance and status.

We fully expected that new faculty appointments requiring institutional oversight would initially generate resistance, at least within "nondwarf" departments; we were not disappointed. For example, the Biochemistry Department suspected that these "gifts of new faculty" were actually Trojan horses ultimately designed to impinge on heretofore sacrosanct core principles of departmental independence. There was some truth to this suspicion; but, we considered it necessary to break the stronghold of departmental chairs in setting their own directions, especially when those directions did not mesh with the strategic needs of the medical center as a whole. Once the faculty understood that we were not pursuing the unforgivable sin of greater centralization for its own sake, that we were not madcap, power-hungry bureaucrats, the newly mandated arrangements for additional faculty coming with central resources won acceptance by the chairs. Along with new initiatives, such as the Whitehead Scholars Program, we launched a robust expansion of the basic sciences in key areas of new opportunities.

Another important emphasis within the basic sciences was to improve the efficiency of their operations and the clarity of their resource management procedures. Unlike clinical departments, where funds from the practice of medicine created the bulk of their revenues, basic science departments had no such revenues. They had to rely instead on external research grants plus internal budget allocations. Historically, departments were assigned research space centrally, with the allocation of space determined by the department chair. Each basic science department was allocated central funding resources to cover a portion of its tenured faculty's salary as well as other administrative infrastructure costs with the understanding that grant support and reserves would support the rest of the department's activity. The financial underpinning of basic science departments had been quite subjective and varied widely among departments.

We decided on a new procedure in which the medical center would fund half of each basic science department's tenured faculty salary, plus a specific amount for administrative and infrastructure needs. If departments brought in more external funds or spent less, they would build departmental reserves. To better understand and manage departmental research space, an allocation for each faculty member would be identified. Their funding from external grant support would be calculated to determine cost recovery per square foot for each investigator. The development of these metrics helped create a transparency of research funding productivity to minimize misallocation of space.

The development of more objective budgeting for the basic sciences and the transparency metrics of resource allocation did not win unanimous, enthusiastic support. Some initially described the creation of space allocation related to external research support as a demoralizing landlord-renter environment. Nonetheless, a more objective and transparent budgeting process made management and, indeed, leadership of the basic sciences much more effective. Of course it reduced the arbitrary power of the chairs, but even the most turf-conscious among them ultimately found it hard to argue with the rationale for reform.

In research, the Long Range Plan helped identify key emerging areas of biomedical research most likely to affect the basic understanding of health and disease. Strengthening the chairs of the basic science departments was always among my highest priorities, as was the recruitment of outstanding junior investigators. Creating efficiencies in the research infrastructure was also critical, since externally funded research (including grants from the NIH) always required additional subsidization from the recipient institution. Prior to the early 1990s, no meaningful oversight existed at Duke as to the cost-effective utilization of research resources and the allocation of expensive research space based on the needs and productivity of the independent investigators. The utilization of research resources was evaluated across the medical center and the information shared with departmental chairs, who were the assigners of research space allocated to their departments. These studies showed occasionally large inefficiencies in utilization of research space based on historic assignments of space to investigators who no longer needed it or were not using it effectively. The development of oversight of biomedical research allowed department chairs to reassign space more equitably within their departments on an objective basis. Moreover, it allowed the identification of needed core facilities to enhance research capabilities across departments. As a consequence, basic science departments developed stronger financial foundations, enabling cross-subsidization of these departments by clinical surpluses to be used more cost-effectively to recruit faculty and purchase laboratory equipment.

Gordon Hammes, with his exquisite standards, also led a major reorganization of the appointment, promotion, and tenure (APT) process. He created a strong basic science APT committee and encouraged the creation of high standards for appointment and promotion. He led an effort that, for the first time, created objective standards for the clinical departments, as well.

We also elevated the criteria for achieving tenure in the basic sciences. Faculty soon learned to take the new procedures seriously. In one painful and difficult decision, a very popular and moderately successful individual in the Department of Microbiology and Immunology was denied tenure after being at Duke for five years. This decision ultimately diminished the immunology department's support for my first reappointment, but we were determined that key tenure appointments should no longer lean so hard on popularity and other "soft" evaluative factors subject to emotional considerations. In due course it became clear that the APT process within the medical center had been entirely reset and established at a very high and far more objective standard.

From 1991 to 1994, we recruited excellent faculty into the basic science departments, all of them in the areas identified in the Long Range Plan. When Nannerl O. (Nan) Keohane became Duke University president in 1993, she charged the university provost to see that such rigor became a university-wide standard. This would not be the last time the medical center paved the way for university-wide reform.

— — —

Among the many things I learned at Genentech was the value of basic discovery research in providing opportunities to create groundbreaking therapeutics. Genentech focused on the emerging field of recombinant DNA technology and had recruited outstanding scientists whose discovery of specific genes enabled the development of a new field of therapeutics based on artificially synthesized proteins. Genentech's discovery research created highly valuable products, making the company one of the darlings of Wall Street. It deserved to be: in 1987 Genentech invested roughly $6 million in basic research, and its revenues were exceeding several hundred million per year. That is quite a handsome investment-to-margin ratio.

Thus, discovery research, when commercialized, had the potential to create substantial revenues. When I was head of Genentech's medical research and development, we pursued outstanding basic research within the company. For the biopharmaceutical industry to be even more successful, however, I believed it needed synergistic relationships with academia. I pursued these at Genentech, and most other biopharma companies did as well. When I arrived as chancellor, I realized immediately that we had vastly more research capabilities than any private sector company, even a successful one like Genentech. That was in part because academic institutions benefited from large infusions of government funding. While companies reached out to academic medicine, academic medical centers rarely thought in terms of commercial applications. Despite its enormous commercial potential, and despite the critical importance of our research to the understanding of life processes and disease, DUMC was certainly not providing revenue for the university.

One of my goals, therefore, in returning to Duke was to create mechanisms within the institution that allowed basic research to continue in an unfettered way and, when appropriate, to collaborate with outside entities capable of commercializing such discoveries for the public good. Knowing that our colleagues in the biopharmaceutical industry desired strategic relationships with academic research institutions, I sought to develop a culture within Duke that recognized the importance and appropriateness of collaborations between academia and industry.

Creating a revenue stream from the commercialization of academic initiatives made a great deal of sense to me in the early 1990s as academic medical centers increasingly suffered from decreased margins from clinical practice and decreased relative funding from the NIH. Obviously, we needed to pay close attention to protect the culture of independence within academia so that it continued to be a major source of unfettered investigator-initiated research. We also had to be mindful to protect against conflicts of interest; no serious university could allow the behavior of faculty to be overly influenced by commercial interests.

So, in 1991, we established the Office of Science and Technology. The office had several functions: to facilitate the transfer of medical and non-medical discoveries into commercial application by advising faculty as to the potential commercial value of their discoveries; to facilitate patenting research discoveries; and to act as a front door to the medical center and university for any industry interested in Duke's intellectual property or in collaborating with Duke investigators. Its goal was to provide "one-stop shopping" for commercial enterprises wanting to leverage the intellectual and physical resources of Duke's research while facilitating initiatives by faculty to commercialize their research. We embraced the importance of protecting the university's objectivity and independence while attempting to create value for its research. We established strong oversight groups of faculty and administrators with an eye toward deepening research integrity and avoiding conflicts of interest. We also set up strict means to preserve the rights of faculty to control their research and to publish their work.

Thomas Glenn became the first head of the Office of Science and Technology. I recruited Tom from Genentech, where he was vice president for pharmaceutical sciences. Tom helped establish the function but soon was recruited away. A search began for Tom's replacement and, fortunately, the committee identified Robert L. Taber who was recruited in late 1992 as associate vice chancellor to assume responsibility for patent and licensing activities for the entire university. Over the next few years he acquired additional responsibility for new venture development, international initiatives, commercial agreements, and selected vending relationships and was promoted to vice chancellor in 1998.

Bob was the perfect person to head this function. After earning his PhD from the University of Pittsburgh School of Medicine, he had done a post-doctoral fellowship at MIT with the Nobel laureate David Baltimore. Bob not only had performed independent research but also had studied in the laboratory of a superb and accomplished scientist. He had held a number of academic appointments, but in 1981 he decided to participate in the founding of a company called Integrated Genetics, Inc. In 1985, he became president and CEO of EG&G MRI based in Worcester, Massachusetts, a division of what is now PerkinElmer. In 1990, Bob had become the founder, president, and CEO of One Cell Systems, an analytic device company based at MIT.

Clearly, Bob understood both academia and industry and the opportunities to synergize the strengths of both worlds. Importantly, too, he was a creative, upbeat, and affable man with a great sense of humor. Under his leadership, the Office of Science and Technology helped promote an entrepreneurial spirit throughout Duke. Bob played an instrumental role in conceiving and developing the operational structure of the Duke Clinical Research Institute (DCRI) and served on its board. Under his leadership, in addition to dramatically increasing the number of patents filed for Duke discoveries and licensing funds from research commercialization, Duke developed a strategic relationship with the Targan Corporation to develop anticancer drugs. Bob also helped create the Duke Center for Genetic and Cell Therapeutics, enabled by funding from Rhone-Poulenc Rohr. Likewise, he helped establish a Duke collaboration with Glaxo in cancer research and the development of the Duke Center for Genetics with a major grant from Glaxo Wellcome. What is more, he created a nexus between the medical center and the government of Singapore to found the Duke–National University of Singapore (Duke-NUS) Graduate Medical School, a critical development that likely would not have occurred without Bob's interest in exploring collaborations with Singapore, a hub for biomedical research.

Importantly, all these related developments—the Office of Science and Technology; the appreciation of the importance of academic-industrial collaborations and synergies; the development of the DCRI, which is discussed in chapter 10; and numerous strategic relationships with industry—brought about, in my view, a balanced understanding of the contemporary academic health system as one with an overarching mission to contribute broadly to societal good while maintaining its viability in an ever more challenging financial world. From the time of its inception through 2004, the Office of Science and Technology completed almost 5,400 research agreements, saw more than 390 U.S. patents issued, received ongoing royalty income of nearly $4 million per year, and, in collaboration with the DCRI, brought in over $900 million of corporate-sponsored research, by far, the most of any academic medical center anywhere.

— — —

When I was a Department of Medicine faculty member at Duke from 1972 to 1987, the chairs of medicine, Jim Wyngaarden and then Joe Greenfield, were my bosses. Dave Sabiston, chair of surgery, was a legendary icon I greatly admired. I viewed the other clinical departments' chairs with great respect as well due to the lofty stature of their positions. As chancellor, I retained a sense of reverence for the clinical chair as a generic category, and I admit to feeling a bit odd when I first realized that they all now reported to me. In particular, Joe had been my attending physician when I was an intern and my boss when he assumed the chair of medicine in 1983, so I felt particular deference toward him. Of all the challenges I faced in taking on the highest administrative and academic role in DUMC, the change in my status relative to the chairs was among the most difficult to parse. To better coordinate the activities of clinical departments and to develop an open line of communication between the chancellor's office and the clinical chairs, soon after July 1989, I established a monthly meeting with the clinical chairs, with myself as chair of the chairs. I always felt a bit uneasy walking into that meeting, seeing everyone wearing their starched white coats, staring at me, and awaiting my initial words to them, a great many of them no doubt thinking that they had better things to do than to attend another damned meeting.

Perhaps the only thing worse for busy people than having to attend "yet another" meeting is to show up for one in vain. On one Monday morning early in the fall of 1989, while I was taking a shower and getting ready to start my week, Judith barged into the bathroom with a message that all the clinical chairs were in my conference room awaiting the start of the meeting. Somehow, I had forgotten that this early morning meeting was on my calendar. It was one of the most uncomfortable moments of my first year as chancellor. I pondered what excuse I might give for missing this meeting as

I visualized them sitting there in the conference room and wondered what they might be saying as I was five, ten, and then many more minutes late. I had my office reschedule the meeting, and at that rescheduled occasion, I offered no invented excuse. I simply said, "Gentlemen, my apologies; I will never again be late for another clinical chairs meeting." And I never was.

As 1989 turned into the new decade, I became more comfortable with the reality of my new relationship with the clinical chairs. More important, as I learned about the true status of each clinical department and the departments' relationships to each other and to the PDC, I realized that important changes needed to be made and that, in making them, I'd often set myself at odds with some, if not most, of these capable and experienced professionals.

As noted, each clinical department was expected to be fully self-supporting from clinical and external research revenues. Moreover, the departments' clinical practice revenues as well as the revenues of Duke Hospital depended, to a degree, on their coordinated functions. For example, the Department of Surgery needed a close collaborative relationship with the Department of Anesthesiology. It also relied heavily on referrals from the Department of Medicine and support from the Department of Pathology for diagnostic procedures. The clinical practice of all the departments was operated by the PDC, whose success was vital for the success of the departments, Duke Hospital, and the medical center—and thus for the university itself. Therefore, the relationships among the clinical chairs, as the leaders of the PDC, were critical to the success of clinical operations and all that depended on them.

It was abundantly clear that there were serious problems on the clinical side of the medical center. The first and most obvious sign was the severe financial pressure facing many departments, some of which were losing money for the first time. At clinical chair meetings, the tension was sometimes palpable. The Departments of Medicine and Surgery were economically strong (at least at that time) and large, so they had little patience or sympathy for money-losing departments. They believed their own success was evidence of the hard work of their faculty, but in truth it was due more to the nature of their practices. At numerous clinical chair meetings, the moneymakers lectured their peers that "slothfulness should not be tolerated," implying inaccurately that a substandard work ethic accounted for the trouble in, say, the Departments of Pediatrics, Psychiatry, or OB/GYN.

Tension between the chairs of medicine and radiology began to mount, driven in part by Carl Ravin's resistance to the uncontested leadership of

Joe Greenfield, who expected never to be challenged openly by other chairs. At one meeting in February 1990, the animosity between Carl and Joe became, let us say, inappropriately expressed. Appalled by the tone of their exchange, I indicated that I expected all chairs to work together collegially and respectfully, without delay or reserve. I followed up with letters to Joe and Carl.

It thus became painfully obvious by my second year in office that we needed to make changes in the leadership of some clinical departments. By 1990, Dave Sabiston made clear to me his disappointment with the chair of anesthesiology, W. David Watkins, who had come to Duke in 1983 from Brigham and Women's Hospital in Boston. Watkins had a strong reputation as a researcher and academician, but he was not a well-trained clinician. He did not practice anesthesiology at Duke, and Sabiston believed that the anesthesiology department's clinical capabilities suffered as a consequence. But the truth was that Dave Sabiston found it appalling that Watkins walked around in surgical scrubs as though he was a clinician despite the fact that he never participated clinically. This, of course, affected the Department of Surgery, where functions are highly dependent on the anesthesiologists, so Sabiston had an undeniable right to express his view. While Dave Sabiston was the ultimate gentleman in public, he expressed to me privately his strong desire that I replace Watkins as chair. It was Sabiston's first, and by far the most important, request he made of me early on.

Other advice I received regarding the chairs came from the university's president, Keith Brodie, who was also former chair of the Department of Psychiatry. While on the surface Keith was warm, friendly, engaging, and outgoing, with me he was at times surprisingly critical of others whom he supported in public. One such issue related to none other than the institutional icon, Dave Sabiston. Keith felt Dave was beyond retirement age and needed to be replaced as quickly as possible. Another was Bernard J. Carroll, chair of psychiatry. Keith made it clear that he expected me to replace him as well. Another chair who evoked concerns from other clinical chairs was Charles B. Hammond, head of OB/GYN. Joe Greenfield told me that Chuck was allowing his department to sink into debtor status.

There is nothing new about faculty members in university departments being resentful, jealous, whiny, and petty. Even Woodrow Wilson, when he was president of Princeton University, observed that in academic settings the more petty a peeve is, the more bitterly it is fought over. But most people think that because medicine is inherently *not* petty, the backbiting, scheming, bad-mouthing, and "positioning" so common among arts and science faculties do not take place. Alas, they do—and as chancellor, it was often my job to do necessary things that put me in the cross fire.

Thus, I knew by 1990 that I would need to act decisively, yet thoughtfully, to better organize the clinical departments and to improve the quality and collegiality of their leadership. The planning process and the Long Range Plan opened a logical pathway to review and improve the clinical enterprise, but I knew there was no painless or animosity-free path to do this. There was no pleasing everyone, and doing that was not compatible with my role. I was beginning to learn firsthand that someone who makes no enemies has never done anything consequential.

As I interpreted the need to change leadership in the clinical departments, I saw the most immediate problems being anesthesiology, psychiatry, followed by OB/GYN. Dave Sabiston was a strong and highly respected chair at Duke and nationally. He was also as an individual I knew I could count on to support rational initiatives. I admired Dave and knew that he respected me as his superior, almost in a military sense. Dave would need to retire soon no matter what I did or President Brodie wanted me to do; age dictated that. But this could be put off for the time being.

Joe Greenfield posed another major issue. He was by nature a heroic loner. He prided himself on his rural southern roots and seemed to relish being brilliant yet selectively asocial. Joe attracted intense loyalty from his colleagues in the Department of Medicine as well as in the Division of Cardiology. As a faculty member in the Department of Medicine in my prior Duke incarnation, I personally admired Joe and his unusual style of leadership because he got things done. He strongly supported his team and belligerently dismissed outsiders. Within my first year, I knew Joe was going to be a big problem; his behavior and personality were increasingly creating dissension. Joe resisted anything that would diminish his dictatorial power as the leader of the Department of Medicine, the PDC, and thus the medical center. In his previous communications with Bill Anlyan, he indicated that he intended to serve only ten years as chair. Thus, the math said that Joe had agreed to step down in 1993. I thought I could tolerate two and half more years of Joe by managing around him. So I began initiating changes elsewhere.

— — —

Prior to 1990, no formal length of appointment existed for chairs, and, as already mentioned, most chairmen served long terms, often until retirement or, in a few cases, until death in office. There had never been any expectation, let alone a formal process, to review chairs until Bill Anlyan established the need for such a process in 1988. Prior to this, DUMC department chairs served theoretically at the behest of the chancellor, but there was no precedent for a chancellor to remove a chair at will. I thus initiated the process for the evaluation of the departments and the performance of chairs on a five-year basis. This mirrored the length of time for review of high university administrators at Duke outside the medical complex.

I set the order of the external reviews to begin with anesthesiology and proceed to psychiatry, OB/GYN, and radiology. Pediatrics became an additional important focus for leadership change, but here the circumstances were different. So in 1990 the chairs of the Departments of Anesthesiology, Psychiatry, OB/GYN, and Pediatrics were either under review or about to come under review, and plans for changes in the Departments of Medicine and Surgery were not far behind.

One of the most difficult and onerous responsibilities of anyone in an administrative role is dismissing an individual who reports to them. In my career, I have had to do this perhaps a dozen or more times. Knowing that a decision to dismiss would change an individual's career and life and that I would be responsible for conveying this to the person was always very painful to me. The fact that I had grown up within the academic medical hierarchy, and that chairs were among the very apex, made any dismissal of a chair all the more difficult.

The reviews of the Departments of Anesthesiology and Psychiatry raised very serious concerns about the performance of those two departmental chairs, and along with what I had already learned and seen personally, I was faced with the need to replace those two chairs. In both instances, the individuals responded to the news graciously and with understanding.

David Watkins, of the Department of Anesthesiology, was the first chair whose department was reviewed. In October 1990, I indicated to him that he would not be renewed as chair. David left Duke before the end of his term, and I appointed Joseph G. (Jerry) Reves, then chief of the Division of Cardiology and Thoracic Anesthesiology, as interim chair. We undertook a national search for the next chair of anesthesiology and found the best choice was someone already at Duke: Jerry Reves. Jerry was as good as anyone identified externally, and I sensed that I could work with him to strengthen the department. Further, I knew that he was respected by Drs. Sabiston and Greenfield as an honest broker who would mediate issues among the chairs in an institutionally responsible way.

The review of the Department of Psychiatry revealed widespread concerns, making it clear to me that Barney Carroll needed to be replaced. Barney, a tall, impressive, and distinguished individual, had a reputation for being brusque and, at times, confrontational. I was therefore not looking forward to the conversation in which I had to tell him he would not be reappointed. But when we spoke, he couldn't have been more gentlemanly and understanding of the decision. He made my task as easy as it could be, and we subsequently retained our collegial relationship as he moved to Central Regional Hospital in Butner, North Carolina. Dan G. Blazer, then dean of medical education, served as interim chair of the Department of Psychiatry while we conducted a national search for a replacement. I saw the opportunity here to recruit a nationally recognized individual whom I believed would be not only an excellent chair but also a strong advocate for collaboration. Allen J. Francis, previously professor of psychiatry at Columbia and a nationally respected figure as chair of the task force that compiled the *Diagnostic and Statistical Manual* (DSM-IV), which defines the nature of the entire field of psychiatry, agreed to come to Duke in 1992. I personally liked Allen; but, more important, I was certain that he would be strong enough to navigate the power dynamics among the chairs at that time. To be an effective departmental chair at DUMC, it was not enough to be a superb medical professional; one also had to have a personality suited to the interpersonal dynamics at play. Allen proved adept at this, and at critical moments during my struggle for reappointment, he proved to be a loyal and effective supporter.

The third clinical department review concerned OB/GYN. Given the fact that the first two reviews had led to the dismissal of the chairs, and that OB/GYN was facing increasing economic difficulties, the scuttlebutt among the clinical chairs was that "Snyderman had a plan" to use the departmental reviews as a pretext or subterfuge to replace all of the chairs. This was at best partially true: the reviews were not at all a pretext, and I had not prejudged their outcomes or tried to manipulate them to arrive at particular judgments. At the same time, given my increasingly intimate knowledge of how things were, it wasn't rocket science to guess some of the outcomes.

The review of the Department of OB/GYN rendered a clear description of the strengths and weaknesses of the department as well as its leader, Chuck Hammond. After pondering the desirability of retaining or replacing Chuck, I decided to keep him in his position; I articulated my expectations for his performance going forward, and he agreed to meet them. The problems we were experiencing at Duke were common throughout the country, given the difficulties of reimbursement for obstetrics. I found Chuck to be a competent chair who was willing to implement changes we agreed would strengthen the department.

Samuel L. Katz, a warm, endearing person who was much loved by his Department of Pediatrics colleagues and who was internationally recognized for his work in vaccines, had already announced his desire to retire in 1989. Given the terrible financial status of his department and the fact that the titans, Greenfield and Sabiston, did not respect him as a leader, it was clear that pediatrics would need a new chair even independent of an external review. Nonetheless, because I needed to sequence the clinical chairs' turnover, and I needed time to conduct a national search for this position, I asked Sam to remain until we could find a suitable replacement. Being a Duke loyalist, he agreed and stayed until 1990, when we recruited Michael M. Frank to Duke from the NIH. I had known Mike to be an excellent researcher in a field related to my own when I was at the NIH. He was a pragmatic, intelligent, and determined individual. Although he had had no prior administrative experience in an academic institution, I believed Mike was the best among the candidates identified in a national search. Duke was fortunate to get him to function in that capacity.

The external review of the Department of Radiology indicated considerable strengths but also some weaknesses, particularly in the area of research, and provided important information about how to strengthen the department. Based on it, and on my respect for Carl Ravin as an individual and as a leader with the fortitude to stand up to the assaults of the Department of Medicine and Joe Greenfield, I decided to reappoint Carl as well. This proved to be a good decision as Carl assumed increasing leadership among the clinical departments and later became a collaborative and effective first president of the PDC.

Robert Machemer, chair of ophthalmology when I arrived, was scheduled to retire in 1991. W. Banks Anderson, Jr. a highly respected member of the Ophthalmology Department served as interim chair in 1991–1992 while a national search for the new chair was underway. As a result of the search, David L. Epstein from UCSF, a nationally recognized expert in the field of glaucoma treatment, was recruited in 1992.

Prior to 1991, radiation oncology, a specialty focused on treating cancer using radiation technologies, was situated within the Department of Radiology. This seemed to make sense administratively when the program was very small, but the responsibilities of this activity had little in common with radiology other than the name. The primary function of radiology is imaging, whereas radiation oncology is devoted to therapy for cancer. There was a strong movement nationally and within Duke to separate the two departments, a direction I applauded and encouraged. We soon created a new department, with Leonard R. Prosnitz, a professor in the Department of Radiology and a nationally recognized figure in Radiation Oncology, as its first chair. Len served one five-year term; Edward C. Halperin, a strong internal candidate, succeeded him in 1996.

In late 1992, George R. Parkerson, Jr., announced that he would be retiring as chair of Department of Community and Family Medicine. After a national search, J. Lloyd Michener, who had been a resident in family medicine at Duke from 1978 to 1981 and a Kellogg Fellow in Family Medicine during 1981–1982, became the next chair of the department in 1994.

What was abundantly clear by 1991 as these chair reviews and assignments were playing out was that the leadership of the individual clinical departments was of great importance and a high priority to sustain or improve. Even more important, however, was the need to alleviate the dissension among some of the department chairs and to address the historical dominance of the Departments of Medicine and Surgery at a time when better coordination of the clinical enterprise as a whole was so vital. The unusually combative chair of the Department of Medicine and the resulting lack of collegiality and respect among the clinical chairs had created an environment in which the cross-departmental coordination of activities so necessary to deliver coherent clinical care was difficult and becoming more so. Thus, while we needed to ensure that each department functioned as well as it could, the greater challenge was to develop a coherent collaborative spirit among the clinical departments.

7

—

Fighting for Renewal

The five-year review of senior officers, now standard at Duke, was a novel requirement in 1993, when I became the first university officer to go through a formal process for reappointment. It was only right that I be subjected to it, since I was the one who introduced the idea within the medical center. As at peer institutions, the practice was intended to help administrators enhance their job performance by identifying areas for improvement and deserving of further investment. Of course, regular five-year reviews also were designed to facilitate changes in leadership when they became necessary, or merely desirable, since reappointment was no longer a certainty.

The timing of my review followed from my original employment agreement in 1989; thus, the review would occur in 1993. My offer letter from President Keith Brodie indicated that deans were expected to serve at least two five-year terms. Indeed, my predecessor, Bill Anlyan, had been in place for twenty-five years. Thus, I had no reason to think the review would be determinative of my tenure as chancellor. My review was led by the president and involved several constituencies, particularly the faculty. The final decision regarding my reappointment rested with the Board of Trustees. On January 25, 1993, President Brodie sent a letter to Richard M. Burton, chair of the Academic Council, requesting that a review committee be formed with appropriate faculty representation. He expected that the faculty review committee would be deliberate and would forward a recommendation to him for his decision, to be acted upon at the May 1993 meeting of the Board of Trustees. Roger C. Barr, professor of biomedical engineering, chaired the review committee. The other members were Dani P. Bolognesi, surgery; Pamela B. Gann, dean of the School of Law; Annabel M. Patterson, English; James N. Siedow, botany; Robert E. Webster, biochemistry; and Jim Wyngaarden, medicine. The committee went to work in mid-March, broadly soliciting comments, conducting interviews (two with me), and sometimes, I was told, engaging in animated internal discussions.

The timing of my review proved to be exquisitely problematic in several ways. The review committee solicited opinions from any and all interested parties, signed or anonymous, at a period when a confluence of initiatives I had begun was creating stress in various components of the medical center. As a consequence, as the time of my reappointment decision was nearing, various individuals and constituencies perceived a rare opportunity to voice confidential objections to my reappointment and thereby block the new directions set forth by medical center leadership. The period from late-March to May 15, 1993, proved to be a tumultuous and difficult time for many, especially for my wife, Judith, our son, Ted (a Duke undergraduate at the time), and me.

The position of chancellor for health affairs at Duke, unlike any other position on campus, is as much corporate as it is academic. It asks a lot of an academic committee with no clinical faculty, health administrators, health care experts, or business leaders to weigh in on the performance of someone who must be an academic leader, a businessman, an agent of institutional change, and a manager responsible for a major clinical enterprise constituting two-thirds of the university's total budget. The controversial changes I had put into place were concerned largely with rationalizing clinical structures, boosting the efficiency of operations, and streamlining the business of health care delivery. It was clear that the chancellor's capacity to make needed organizational changes would at times be unpopular. But having this occur in the face of an academic review that would determine my tenure was something I had not anticipated.

The voices of disquiet coming primarily from a small minority of faculty from one clinical department were accorded a great deal of weight by the review committee, which, I assume, erroneously presumed that these voices expressed the feelings of the entire medical complex. As a consequence, I found myself in an unexpectedly precarious position. The committee had a hard time understanding that the strongest critics of my performance were motivated by what became an orchestrated effort on the part of members of the Department of Medicine to block my decision to remove their chair.

The review process brought into focus the changes my team and I were implementing in the medical center. Context, as they say, is everything (or nearly so), and 1993 was a time of significant change at Duke. The university itself was undergoing a change of leadership at the top, with Keith Brodie retiring after having served less than two terms to make way for Nan Keohane, president of Wellesley College, who was slated to take office at Duke on July 1, 1993. The leadership of the Board of Trustees also was changing; Philip J. (Jack) Baugh's term as chair was ending, and John W. Chandler, who had led the search to bring Nan to Duke, would take over on July 1.

— — —

It is important to revisit the environment at DUMC from August 1992 through my first reappointment by Duke's Board of Trustees on May 15, 1993. Changes occurring at DUMC in late 1992, were in my view necessary for the institution's viability, yet undoubtedly caused anxiety for many. My colleagues and I were just two years into the institution's first five-year comprehensive strategic plan. Reductions in clinical revenue necessitated painful budget cuts, which were just getting under way or being planned. This involved the first reduction in employment levels that, while relatively small in number and mostly to be accomplished by attrition, created an understandable source of apprehension among employees, particularly hospital staff. It also was a time of heightened tensions surrounding race and gender in a socially conservative and historically white male–dominated institution that just happened to be the biggest employer in the area, and thus important in one way or another to nearly everyone. Another source of apprehension constituted an irony that arose as a result of our initiatives to improve employee morale. I was deeply committed to creating a better and more equitable workplace and to improving performance and patient services, but to do that, change was necessary. In 1992, I had initiated a series of open forums in the hospital and elsewhere in an effort to better understand employee issues and to improve communications throughout the institution. Those sessions told us a lot about what employees thought about working on the "Duke Plantation," a term expressed often by many members of our African American workforce who held disproportionately lower-paid positions. These issues are discussed more extensively in chapter 9.

In a comprehensive effort with the Gallup Organization, we undertook an opinion survey designed to help us understand what employees were thinking and to set a reference point by which we could judge our efforts to improve employee morale. The project proved very useful in identifying the roots of deep employee dissatisfaction within, primarily, the hospital workforce.

The top five factors needing change related to employees' desire for respect from their supervisors, respect for the importance of their jobs, constructive criticism, being listened to, and policies that were fair and consistently applied. Surprising to me, compensation was the last of the major issues of importance to our workforce. Dignity and respect trumped money, just as they had in the lab environment I had nurtured many years earlier at Duke.

The bureaucratic hierarchy that had developed in Duke Hospital over its sixty years had created an environment that was increasingly untenable for its employees. While I was committed to changing it, the process of self-analysis and reflection allowed long-standing animosities to surface. We needed greater efficiencies in operations while reorganizing administratively to provide better service. But, just as our lower-paid positions needed an infusion of dignity and respect, those were the positions most vulnerable to workforce reductions.

Some medical center faculty were on edge because of the focus on productivity and efficiency, as well as the centralizing initiatives—such as creating offices for planning and marketing—which appeared bureaucratic and would inevitably increase the authority of the central administration. It may be difficult for many members of the Duke medicine family today to imagine that in 1989, the medical center was essentially decentralized, with each of the nearly one thousand practicing physicians within the PDC operating more or less independently, with their own secretaries keeping their schedules and making their appointments. The lack of centralization and the questionable reliability of getting an appointment with Duke's physicians made it difficult for referring physicians or patients to engage with our institution. They could call a central telephone number, but there wasn't a lot of useful information that we could give them once a connection was established. Further, DUMC central had but a fragmentary knowledge of what its PDC doctors were actually doing on any given day or week and could not, in any case, schedule appointments for them. From my perspective, the problem at the time was not the present situation so much as the future. It was going to become impossible to sustain such a clinical system financially in the face of managed care.

The autonomy and power of the PDC, which was essentially controlled by Joe Greenfield as head of medicine and Dave Sabiston as head of surgery, limited our ability to initiate and manage change. Joe, in particular, resisted my involvement. Dave, in contrast, while a strong leader of his department and the PDC, respected and supported the unique position of the chancellor as the integrating force for the medical center.

The process of reviewing the departmental chairs for reappointment was perhaps my most important tool in modernizing the medical center, but, naturally enough, it also was the source of much of the anxiety. From the time I took office to the time of my first review, we appointed eleven chairs, for the Departments of Cell Biology, Microbiology, Neurobiology, Pathology, Pharmacology, Anesthesiology, OB/GYN, Ophthalmology, Pediatrics, Psychiatry, and Radiology. Many of these were a consequence of retirement, but of the eleven, only two (radiology and OB/GYN) won reappointment. The numbers seemed to speak for themselves.

— — —

Of all the issues we were dealing with during the early years of my first term, the most troublesome concerned the scheduled retirements of Dave Sabiston and Joe Greenfield, which were announced during the same year as my review. Dave's legendary term as the chair of surgery already had been extended well beyond the customary retirement age of sixty-five, and, as already noted, President Brodie had pressured me to replace him. Joe had promised to step down in 1993, but he subsequently sought an extension until 1996. I wished to replace Joe by 1994 at the latest, and this led to a confrontation between us. The juxtaposition of the replacement of Drs. Sabiston and Greenfield, the chairs of the two most important clinical departments, generated a huge problem at a time when other important changes were contributing to the ambient stress, particularly among the faculty in the Department of Medicine. In retrospect, it was a critical error of judgment on my part not to realize the magnitude of the anxiety that the confluence of all these changes would create. Nor did I anticipate the consequences that this anxiety would have on my own reappointment review.

Until 1991, chairs served pretty much at their own discretion. For this reason, I had taken pains to reaffirm Joe Greenfield's retirement date early in my tenure. I met with him on December 9, 1990, at which time he asked that the agreed upon date of July 1, 1993, be moved back, in order to stage in successive years the searches for Dave Sabiston's and his own replacement. I reflected on his request and, in a letter of January 28, 1991, said that if we did move back the date, "it would be difficult for me to extend the date beyond July of 1994," noting it would be "advantageous" to have the next chair of medicine assign space for the department in the new Medical Sciences Research Building (MSRB), which was to be completed in 1994. "I greatly value your views, your support, and your leadership of the Department of Medicine at Duke," I told him. "Since we both have the interests of the Department and the Medical Center as among our highest priorities, I am sure we can work together to determine the optimal timing for your succession."

Alas, we were not able to do that. A series of exchanges and meetings I had with Joe in August 1992, the summer before my review began, failed to resolve our differences. We reached a crisis point on August 10, when Joe wrote a "Dear Ralph" letter ostensibly designed to "clarify the issue" of his retirement as chair. He noted that his understanding with Chancellor Anlyan had been that he would submit his resignation in the spring of 1993, assuming that new leadership was in place in the Department of Surgery and that the Department of Medicine "was in good shape." That, he made clear to me, was the sticking point. "At this juncture, I feel that this is not an appropriate action. Therefore, I plan to retire (according to the university's policy) after I reach 65 years of age on July 20, 1996. I assume that you will concur with this decision, if not, please contact me immediately."

Joe and I met to discuss this issue and, whereas previous meetings had been civil and polite, our meeting of August 12, 1992, turned out to be anything but. "You can't fire me," he said, but "I'm giving you the opportunity to resign." Unless I resigned from office, Joe said, he would stay as chair two more years and oppose my initiatives for reform. I had no intention of being intimidated. Later that same day I wrote a "Dear Joe" letter in which I stated, "I have decided that it would be best that you vacate the chair no later than June 30, 1994."

The timing of my review provided a major boost to Joe's effort to deny my reappointment. Joe was obviously emboldened by the loyal and increasingly vocal support he got from the cardiology faculty in the Department of Medicine, and by the accompanying public attention. This strengthened his wholehearted determination to save the Department of Medicine by having me replaced as chancellor. Joe's open antagonism toward me since 1992 aggravated tensions throughout the institution. Joe had staunch support in components of the Department of Medicine, my former department, especially in the Cardiology Division, of which he was previously the chief. He and his supporters actively opposed my reappointment as chancellor, the most obvious manifestation of which was a coordinated letter-writing campaign to the Barr Committee. At its worst moments, the battle over my appointment became deeply personal.

As discontent became more visible in the medical center, the media became attentive. This was natural because DUMC was the region's largest employer, and so the potential sacking of its leader provided a novel and interesting story. In September 1992, the Duke student newspaper, the *Chronicle*, picked up on the diverse reactions to change expressed by medical center staff. According to the article, entitled "Bad Blood?," relations between medical center employees and administrators "may be the best or worst in years, depending on whom you speak to." Wrenching articles and blazing headlines about my first reappointment were frequent. Years later, I still find it emotionally difficult to review the very public examination of the twists and turns of the battle. The ordeal lasted barely a month in the spring of 1993, but at the time it seemed to grind on without end.

— — —

For all the intensity of the events in the spring of 1993, the year of my review had begun quietly, with positive feedback from the Board of Trustees. On January 15, 1993, I had presented a report to the Board of Trustee's Executive Committee, the essence of which was that we were on target and moving forward in our strategic plan. Then, on March 17, 1993, tensions at DUMC became the stuff of an editorial cartoon in Durham's *Herald-Sun* newspaper that depicted a patient lying in a hospital bed hooked up to an IV. Surrounded by demoralized staff beating on walls or committing suicide by gun or hanging, the patient says, "Well . . . I suppose it could be worse. I could be working here." The basis of the cartoon was in part related to hospital employees' discontent as a result of the efforts to identify areas in need of change. Previously, employees weren't asked their views or told of any impending decisions. In addition, the threat of a workforce reduction and changes initiated in the clinical practices heightened concerns.

The Barr Committee began its work in March 1993. What my team and I had accomplished or put into action up to that time was a natural and appropriate subject for review. Because sources of tension within the medical center related to changes designed to increase performance and to prepare for both the possibility of national health care reform and the certain onslaught of managed care, it was important for me to describe to the committee the forces necessitating such changes, so that its members would be able to grasp the larger context. The financial problems that began to appear in our clinical departments, especially the Department of Medicine, the largest and historically the biggest revenue producer, resulted from changes in clinical reimbursement, patient referrals, inefficient management, and resistance to collaboration with other departments. Changes related to managed care began to stress hospital revenues as well.

Within a few years—a fact worth keeping in mind—all academic health centers came under heavy financial pressure, and some, such as the University of Pennsylvania, suffered huge losses and were forced to reorganize. The year 1993 was a time when the old order in health care was changing, and it was clear that Duke had to get in front of change or risk ruin. Thus, in meetings with committee staff and interviews with committee principals, I laid this out in detail. Given that opportunity, I welcomed the work of the Barr Committee because I believed it would focus everyone's attention on our potential for future success. As I told the *Chronicle* and other media in March, "I want to take the full power of this institution and turn it into a magnificent engine for social change in the health care arena." I did my best to communicate both the challenges and the opportunities we faced to anyone who would listen, inside Duke and outside in the broader community.

A very unfortunate event then occurred on April 27, 1993, which proved to be a focal point in the objections to my reappointment. It began while I was away from Duke at a meeting of the AAMC Council of Deans in Arizona. Although it was known within the medical center that both Drs. Sabiston and Greenfield were to be replaced by the end of June 1994, this information was not generally known outside the medical center. A reporter from the *Herald-Sun* called my office to find out if t his was true and, as I was away, was referred to Vicki Y. Saito, our newly recruited director of communications. Rather than calling me, Vicki confirmed the truth of the story and, in her comments, described the replacements in a manner that, some thought, failed to pay proper respect to the major contributions that Drs. Sabiston and Greenfield had made to the medical center. The subsequent article turned out to be a harmful flash point because it suggested that the medical center administration (me in particular) was determined to replace foundational pillars of the medical center without appreciating or honoring their worth. The publication of this story touched off a firestorm of anger within the medical center, one particularly suited to the waging of Joe Greenfield's "civil war." When I learned of the situation, I immediately flew back to Durham in an attempt to correct the distorted impression created by Vicki's unfortunate comments.

The unintended slight to both Drs. Greenfield and Sabiston echoed well beyond the medical center and university. I was deeply troubled by the impression given in the article that I was blasé about replacing Joe and Dave and that I personally did not value their seminal contributions to the institution. The day after my return, I attended the Durham Rotary Club luncheon and, although not scheduled to speak, took the stage and delivered an extemporaneous and heartfelt tribute to Joe and Dave. I also indicated that the newspaper story neither reflected the situation at Duke nor communicated my high regard for the contributions of these two medical center leaders.

Worried about the increasingly negative tone and adverse impacts of internal strife on the medical center, I reached out to Joe on April 30, 1993. My handwritten two-page letter was a personal and confidential appeal that also was heartfelt. "Dear Joe," I began,

> Since returning to Duke from a meeting, I've tried to meet with you to apologize for the awful article in Tuesday's Durham *Herald-Sun*. I was mortified by the story and accept responsibility for not having had a press

release handy in case such a situation arose. I was hoping (wrongly) that the search would not be a big issue for the press so that we could go on running things smoothly as we had discussed. Joe, I am very distressed by the events of the past week. Like you, I love the Department of Medicine and want to minimize anxiety and uncertainty. Unless you and I stand together in this as much as possible, the entire institution will lose. You and I had an agreement which I accepted as a bond. If you feel I broke it, please, let's talk since I didn't intend to do so. For the good of the department, the medical center and Duke, let's get back on the same team. I want to work with you! I'll call you after the clinical meeting for an appointment.

I signed it, "As always, Ralph."

The intensity of the faculty revolt against my leadership, while essentially limited to one division within one department, grew in subsequent weeks. On May 2, 1993, the broad public learned of the battle to force my resignation. "Movement to Oust Head of Medical Center Growing," headlined the *Herald-Sun*, with a subhead that read, "Employee Morale Sinks." The article began ominously, "A movement is quietly building among Duke University Medical Center staff to oust Ralph Snyderman as the head of the center, according to several Duke sources." It said some interesting things about me, such as the following comment from an anonymous source in relation to the results of chair reviews: "He's choosing people who will say 'yes' to him. . . . He's the king and he wants lieutenants who will say 'yes.'" The article pointed out that, during the previous year, Vick Stoughton had left his post as vice chancellor for health affairs and CEO of Duke Hospital after just one year in office, saying that I had not given him the promised degree of autonomy. Vick and I had our differences, and I had indeed pushed him to consult more closely with me on major decisions after having been surprised more than a few times by them. But his decision to leave had surprised me even more.

I continued my efforts to put our internal conflict into a meaningful national context while reaching out to Dave and especially Joe, who understandably felt publicly slighted and insulted. It is worth noting, however, that both Dave and Joe had joined me in a written statement, issued May 4, 1993, deploring the *Herald-Sun* article of April 27 that "inappropriately and inaccurately announced" their planned retirements. "The article led to confusion and anxiety on the part of some faculty, and we are working together in a very positive way to dispel any misconceptions or misunderstandings," the statement read. "We furthermore do not believe that any useful purpose will be served through a continued dialogue in the press."

Another measure was an opinion piece I wrote entitled, "Changes at Duke Medical Center Will Improve Health Care," which appeared in the May 5, 1993, *Herald-Sun*. I focused on the fact that the American health care system was entering "a period of enormous change" and reaffirmed my belief in Duke's ability to play a leadership role. I explained that my confidence was rooted in history and specifically in the tradition of great leadership at Duke's medical center. I took pains to place Dave Sabiston and Joe Greenfield as among the succession of "giants in their fields" who had led Duke to greatness, writing, "It is regrettable in recent news articles about the long-planned retirements . . . that insufficient attention was paid to the extraordinary achievements of these physician-scientists. . . . They have contributed much to Duke University Medical Center's current stature, and it is a source of embarrassment to the medical center and to me that their achievements were slighted."

My efforts achieved no noticeable success in the Department of Medicine. On that same day, May 5, the Durham paper reported, "Duke Rift Widens between Physicians and Chancellor." Further reporting of the fight to deny my renewal was published on May 6, 1993, when the *Raleigh News & Observer* reported that the previous day two hundred members of the Department of Medicine had sent a petition demanding my resignation to Keith Brodie, Nan Keohane, and Jack Baugh, the chair of the University Board, who was an attentive mentor and an astute political adviser as I dealt with the rebellion. "Duke Doctors Angry over Job Shuffling," the headline read. As recorded in that article, I again defended my action, noting that discontent was confined to one division (cardiology) of one department (medicine). "I don't think there is a broad feeling among clinical faculty that I have not been responsive to them," I said. I again denied that Joe Greenfield was being forced to resign, noting once more that he agreed to serve ten years when he was appointed in 1983 and that I had met with him in March to confirm his plans. The May 6, 1993, story referenced the

Department of Medicine meetings as well as a second meeting attended by some one hundred faculty from various departments, who essentially applauded my report on the status of the Long Range Plan. The contrast between the meetings could not have been more stark.

— — —

By this time, running with my closest friend and colleague Bob Lefkowitz had become an essential sustainer of my mental as well as physical health. We met at the Seeley Mudd Building off Science Drive each morning and ran down University Drive, down Buchanan Boulevard, across East Campus, and then back. One day, while talking about the reappointment trials and the hits that I was taking in the press, I shared with Bob how it all felt to me: "I visualize myself as a large elephant charging through the dense jungle. From the shadows, spears are being thrown at me and some of them are sticking. But I have this thick hide and I'm still thundering through." I remember wondering if there would eventually be enough spears to take me down. But I never seriously thought that would happen.

But it was a walk, not a run that provided one of the most healing experiences during that troubled time. Joel L. Fleishman, a Duke University Law School acquaintance, saw my distress and, Orthodox rabbi that he also is, felt an obligation to perform a deed of loving-kindness—*hesed* in Hebrew. He reached out to me even though we were not close friends at that time. I knew Joel, as did almost everyone else, because of his successful fund-raising efforts on behalf of the university. He suggested we take a walk, and I gratefully accepted. We headed out along Flowers Drive; I just talked, and in the course of talking things out over what became a somewhat surprisingly long walk—well over an hour in duration—I came to feel a comfort I had sorely lacked. Like Bob Lefkowitz and like a good psychiatrist, Joel had the capacity to listen and question thoughtfully without making judgments. I needed to sort out the issues and my emotions along with them. He helped put me at ease, and I have been his grateful friend ever since.

My membership in Durham's Beth El congregation also provided me comfort and strength. Although being a largely secular Jew, I regularly attended services at High Holy days and during difficult times, would pay particular attention to parts of the prayer service asking G_d to protect us from those speaking evil of us and intending to do us harm.

On May 8, I received some welcome public support, this time from a Duke legend whose advice and encouragement had sustained me more than once over the years. In a letter to the editor of the *Herald-Sun*, Mary Duke Biddle Trent Semans (granddaughter of Benjamin N. Duke and the great-granddaughter of Washington Duke), a highly esteemed and influential member of the Duke community, defended me and Duke and disputed the version of events detailed in the April 27 article ("Duke Medical Center Shakeup Continues"), which had first publicized the revolt. "There is an implication of some sort of mysterious design to replace Drs. David Sabiston and Joseph Greenfield, both revered chairmen and both of international reputation," Mary wrote. "In fact, the usual protocol is being followed. The retirement age for chairmen has been 65. . . . This system has been in force since Duke Hospital opened."

A welcome bit of encouragement in the press also came from board chairman Jack Baugh, who showed reporters a letter to me from all but one of the clinical chairs (that one being Greenfield) expressing support for my reappointment. "I don't know how much more I need," Jack said.

But there also was criticism from Gene Stead, then eighty-four, one of the Duke greats who had inspired me as an intern. Gene (like Joe Greenfield, also from Georgia) told the *Herald-Sun* that my Greenfield decision was a "tragedy because he really built that department." In his opinion, personal dislike had triggered my decision. Gene also indicated his view that I should not be reappointed. That verdict was painful to hear from a man I admired and who had been chair of medicine during my residency years at Duke.

While the aforementioned events were ongoing, a number of the chairs wrote individually on my behalf to the Barr Committee. I particularly enjoyed a letter from Carl Ravin, chair of radiology, and his colleagues, who sent copies to Jack Baugh, Keith Brodie, and Nan Keohane as well. "The alleged outpouring of dissatisfaction with Dr. Snyderman's performance clearly seems to us to be a resistance to change and a desire to remain with traditional approaches," Ravin et al. wrote. "Unfortunately, the external environment in which Duke Medical Center now finds itself has changed significantly and will continue to change at a very rapid pace."

Earlier, on May 4, Bob Bell, head of the Section of Cell Growth Regulation and Oncogenesis, and eight other chairs or heads, including Drs. Sheetz, Purves, Nevins, and Pizzo, sent their letters of support to the Barr

Committee. But May 4 was also the date when faculty in the Department of Medicine delivered a letter to Roger Barr and his committee, saying they were "gravely concerned by the escalating crisis in the Medical Center," fearful for the future of the department, lacking in "confidence and trust" in the medical center administration, and calling for "prompt and decisive" action by Brodie, Keohane, and the Board of Trustees. Copies went out to Nan Keohane, Jack Baugh, and John Chandler, and a supporting petition with some two hundred signatures found its way to Keith Brodie. The next day, May 5, 1993, ten chairs of clinical departments (all but Greenfield) issued a letter to the Barr Committee strongly supporting me.

Thanks largely to the work of the clinical chairs, this flurry of letters supporting and condemning me settled down after May 7, when Joe and I finally reached an accord on his tenure. As stipulated, Joe agreed to "work in a collegial and cooperative fashion," and I agreed that the appointment of a new medicine chair would take place six months to a year after the surgery chair search was completed. There was collective agreement for Joe to engage in clinical efforts with the hospital to help medicine balance its departmental budget. Jack Baugh's letter of May 10 to his board colleagues described this accord as "a workable and more than fair agreement at this time," noting that it extended Joe Greenfield's tenure by one year. He also lauded Keith Brodie's diligence, saying Keith "deserves a great deal of credit for bringing all factions together for the best interests of Duke University."

As the accord demonstrated, I had relented by one year on the Greenfield tenure issue. I believed doing so was best for the institution. On May 10, 1993, the *Herald-Sun* reported on page 1: "Chancellor Changes Mind: Duke Hospital Chairman's Replacement to Be Delayed." Doing so cleared the way for the peace treaty governing future relations between Joe Greenfield and me, under which we conducted searches for chairs in surgery and medicine over the next two years. At the same time, and most important to me personally, changing my stance on Joe removed the one major obstacle to my reappointment.

— — —

On May 10, the Barr Committee submitted its report to Keith Brodie, noting its unanimous recommendation that I be reappointed for a term of two years (1994–1996), with a "comprehensive review" to be conducted in spring 1995. The report cited the "nearly unanimous support of Dr. Snyderman" from clinical and basic science chairs, noting parenthetically, "A special exception exits in medicine." There were references to numerous complaints about ideas, projects, and requests stalled in the "green zone," meaning my office, and the view held by some that clinical faculty "are not in the loop of governance." The driving points boiled down to a criticism of leadership style, inadequate communication, and insufficient progress in addressing concerns of minority and women employees:

> The review committee sees its recommendation as a pragmatic action, compatible with the accord worked out in the last few days in the President's office. In the spirit of that accord, it also recommends a candid statement to the faculty of the period of reappointment and an unambiguous statement that changes will be expected in the problem areas identified in the review. By the same token, the committee thinks that the Medical Center can move forward under Dr. Snyderman's leadership and that current major searches can proceed and be successful. The committee further believes that the present problems may be resolved, with effort and good will from all directions, and that success in resolving them would be a basis for Dr. Snyderman's possible reappointment for a third term.

I was surprised the report was so negative. I had met with the committee twice, first in March and again in April, and enjoyed the opportunity to talk with the members. I particularly recall a fascinating discussion with a member from the English Department, who, for some reason, had reached the conclusion that I enjoyed taking risks and actively sought them out. What I was really doing was choosing the path that best *mitigated* risk and still got the job done. As a physician—and perhaps this is a key distinction between the academic and medical worlds—your mission is to identify risk and remove it. You are trained to choose the therapy that is least risky for the patient, but that choice virtually always involves doing *something*, and doing anything inherently runs *some* risk. When I was chancellor, there were all kinds of risks facing DUMC, so I didn't perceive myself as seeking risk; rather, risk was thrust at us, and I was trying to reduce it. Apparently, this was a tough concept for some on the committee to parse.

My main problem with the review's outcome was with the recommended reappointment of only two years. I viewed this as a slap in the face and would risk making me a lame duck—unable to push through necessary changes because those resisting the changes, particularly Joe Greenfield, could take heart that if they waited me out for only two years, they would essentially get their way. In that light, I couldn't understand what the committee members were thinking. Why would they want to reappoint a chancellor whose general direction they applauded if they put him in a situation where he could not do what they thought so laudable? Clearly, it seemed that they could not have understood the situation I had in dealing with Joe. I was especially offended by an innuendo of sexual indiscretion, which was raised by my adversaries but was abject bullshit (pardon the Brooklyn eruption). It may be hubris, but I was surprised that any members of the committee would oppose my reappointment.

Notwithstanding these wounds to both logic and pride, I immediately put the confidential report away and repressed thoughts about it, an ability that has allowed me to press on more than once in tough times. That same day I wrote the department chairs to thank them for their strong support in resolving the issue of searches for the chairs of surgery and medicine. I shared with them the statement I would issue to all faculty the next day:

> After discussions, and in agreement with all the clinical chairs, I have decided to stagger the succession of the chairs of Surgery and Medicine so that the new chair of Medicine will take office up to 12 months after Dr. Sabiston's successor is identified. Dr. Greenfield has agreed to the extension of his term and has indicated his enthusiasm for serving with his fellow chairs and the chancellor for health affairs during the remainder of his tenure as chairman. This will permit a smooth transition of leadership for these two large departments. I believe that this arrangement will allay concerns regarding the simultaneous searches for Surgery and Medicine chairs. I am very pleased by the strong leadership of the clinical chairs and the support of the faculty.

Only a short time elapsed between the release of the report to the appropriate individuals and the decision by the board regarding my reappointment. During this time, Nan Keohane had arrived on campus in advance of the board meeting to get acquainted with her new colleagues and to prepare for her first meeting before starting her presidency in July. She, of course, had consulted with Keith Brodie and was familiar with the Barr Committee report and the recommended two-year term. As noted, that term was certain to compromise my authority if I accepted it; Joe Greenfield would win because it would enable him to outlast such a short appointment. I therefore had a tremendous problem, which of course was also a problem for my new boss.

Nan and I met on a Thursday in early May 1993. Perhaps it is fair to say that she interrogated me rather than merely met with me as we sat down together in the Allen Building to discuss the reappointment. We met in the room adjoining the president's office, and she was sitting in a higher chair than mine and thus was looking down at me. The rumor of sexual misbehavior on my part—despite having been found to be malicious and wholly without merit in an internal investigation conducted by university counsel David Adcock many months earlier—had surfaced indirectly in the Barr Committee report, much to my dismay and anger. Worse, Nan had evidently heard another rumor suggesting a different sexual impropriety—from what source I could not possibly know, since the alleged impropriety never took place. She surprised me by asking about it directly, looking me straight in the eye. While taken aback, I looked directly into her eyes and, without ambiguity, denied it totally; it was, after all, untrue. This issue never came up between us again.

The next night, a Friday, after a dinner meeting with the board's Executive Committee, Nan and I resumed discussion of the term of my reappointment. She proposed that I postpone a decision to accept reappointment until the next Executive Committee meeting in June. Nan suggested that I spend several weeks with her at Wellesley College during June. She felt that this would give us time to become better acquainted. She did not explain any other reason for this, but indicated that once she got to know me, she would be fully prepared to weigh in with the board. I listened to her but did not respond; maybe I was stunned by the idea and needed time to consider it. Maybe I did not quite grasp the essence of what she was proposing. But in retrospect, because I hadn't protested, she may have thought I had agreed to her suggestion. I don't believe I had, and I certainly didn't mean to do so. In any case, I reached my decision early Saturday morning, May 15, while getting ready for the full board meeting. I was standing at the kitchen sink looking out the window. I saw Judith walking back to the house with the *Herald-Sun*, open in her hands. The look on her face as she read the headlines was one of the saddest, most touching things I'd ever seen. At that moment I knew, here on the morning of the board meeting, that another bad story loomed. She handed me the newspaper without saying anything—she tended to keep these kinds of feelings hidden. Indeed, I was the headliner again, with a story indicating that I could be out that very day.

I made the decision right then and there that in no way was I going to postpone a decision and spend weeks at Wellesley. We couldn't keep this going for another month, and I could not afford to be out of town for such an extended period; it would be irresponsible to do so at any time, and it would certainly be so now. I knew that Joe Greenfield would be empowered by anything other than a reappointment that provided me with sufficient time to do what needed doing. I came up with a proposed solution: a compromise three-year reappointment that would allow sufficient time to be effective in my job. That term would give me until July 1997, two years beyond Joe's retirement. That, I believe would be enough, since his internal support was already beginning to splinter.

I hoped the three-year reappointment would be a compromise satisfactory to everybody. I mentioned the idea to Jack Baugh, the board chair, before the meeting started, and he reminded me that I had his full support for a full five-year term if I wanted it. While Keith Brodie was problematic to me during the renewal battle, Jack was a steady source of good advice and support. He was a politician and a successful one. "I know how to count votes," he assured me. I could have, according to him, forced it through for the full five years. When I told Nan, in contrast, she looked me in the eye, pursed her lips, and said, "Don't fight me on this." She still wanted to hold off a month.

Nevertheless, when I got up in front of the board, with Nan sitting there looking at me, I said I wanted three years. My new boss was upset with me, but in my view, I offered the ideal compromise to resolve a terrible situation. Getting a full five-year term would have put the board and the administration in direct opposition to a faculty committee. It also would have naturally posed a difficulty for the committee, and the Academic Council. On the other hand, a two-year term would have been a clear defeat that would have undermined my authority at a critical juncture in the medical center's history. At that moment, personal issues also weighed heavily: I didn't want to put my wife and son through further trauma.

On May 15, the Board of Trustees unanimously approved my reappointment, an action documented by the *News & Observer* with this headline: "Snyderman to Remain at Duke: President Keith Brodie and Incoming

Chief Nan Keohane Praise the Hospital Director, Who Is Reappointed to an Unusual 3-Year Term." Unusual, indeed. To her credit, Nan never mentioned the matter to me again.

— — —

In the following days and weeks, I took steps to address the major thrust of the Barr Committee's criticisms: a lack of transparency in operations and inadequate communication. I was determined to develop a more open and interactive administration. We moved quickly to create committees that allowed me to spend more time with larger groups of faculty in both the clinical and basic sciences. We introduced open forums and town hall meetings which focused on the most pressing health care and clinical issues. We planned new institutional publications, set up drop-in visit opportunities on my calendar, and planned new "walk-around" time devoted to meeting people in their medical center settings. I particularly enjoyed evening meetings at my home, where, for two and a half hours every month or so, members of the various constituencies and I could talk about issues candidly and informally.

One of the harshest criticisms I faced, which I believed was unjustified, was that I was indifferent to issues concerning women and minorities. Nonetheless, this criticism sharpened my focus and quickened my efforts at greater minority advancement. Consequently, the medical center moved away from the inherent bias of the "best person for the job" dictum in choosing new hires and toward a broader contextual understanding of what constitutes "best" and created an engaged, effective, diverse workforce and organization as discussed in chapter 9.

The agreement that led to my reappointment had other repercussions. One was the loss of a good friendship and a close working relationship with Steve Ruma. He had been with me as a friend and adviser for almost three years. One of the conditions for reappointment was that I would, at least for a period of time, have Steve essentially disappear from campus. It seems he had become a kind of a lightning rod with some chairs who believed he was too negative about people whose operations he was reviewing on my behalf. They felt that I gave his opinions too much weight. Jerry Reves, head of anesthesiology and for many years a Greenfield colleague, had first advised me, candidly and helpfully, on how much Steve's involvement was resented.

Given such strong opinions voiced by people whose judgment I valued, I acceded to the request.

At our next meeting on campus, I informed Steve that I wanted to hold off on an extension of his contract, which ended June 30, for six months or so to let things settle down. "Ralph, you're firing me," he replied. "No way am I firing you," I protested, but he picked up his coat and went out the door. A couple of years later I called to see if we could restart our friendship. "It's not time for that," he said. A few years later, he died tragically in a crash of his private plane.

Nan returned to campus as president in July, and we got along very well. A few months later, at her request, I had lunch with a writer for a notable magazine that was doing a piece on Nan as the first woman to head a major American university. I described Nan as "intriguing" and talked of my respect for her brightness and objectivity. "As Snyderman well should," I recall the writer's comment, pointing out that my future rested in Nan's hands. Certainly we had a bad start over the reappointment matter, but over the next year our working relationship, one of mutual trust and respect, couldn't have been more positive. Following a year of working together, Nan surprised me in June 1994 when she told me that she was recommending my full five-year second term at the Executive Committee meeting of Duke's board. I did not ask her to do that, so her decision surprised and gratified me. My term now extended out to its normal length after all, without need for an interim review.

— — —

As I reflect on the period from August 1992 through my first reappointment by Duke's Board of Trustees on May 15, 1993, I appreciate better the magnitude of the challenges and difficulties I experienced and, in particular, the vulnerability I faced in nearly being removed from the position I had crossed the country from San Francisco to assume. In retrospect, I am impressed not only by the degree of my vulnerability but by my dogmatic tenacity, which all but blinded me to how tenuous the situation had become. I am mindful that many of the difficulties were simply part and parcel of the magnitude of change I sought, but I was frankly out of my depth in being able to estimate the institutional support I would need to succeed. Clearly, as I assumed the position of chancellor for health affairs, I was long on determination, cold logic, and maybe vision, but I was supremely naive, if not to say utterly oblivious, regarding the difficulties involved in fundamentally changing the direction of an academic institution. On the other hand, without my naïveté, as well as my inability to even entertain the possibility of failure, I might well have failed to be reappointed.

At times during the chaos and turmoil of the reappointment process, particularly from the appointment of the Barr Committee to its concluding report, several individuals had a profound impact on me and, to an extent, on the outcome. Keith Brodie is a prime case in point. Keith recruited me warmly, enthusiastically, and effectively; if not for him, I would not have left Genentech to return to Duke in 1989. Keith's personality, reflected in his choice to be a psychiatrist, was one of surface warmth, engagement, enthusiasm, and encouragement. During my early years as chancellor, I saw nothing but this side of him. At the time of my reappointment battle, however, Keith's lack of support surprised and disappointed me, especially because that is when I needed it most. It led me to believe that Keith, indeed, did *not* want me to be reappointed.

Jack Baugh, chair of the Board of Trustees and a former marine fighter pilot and intelligence officer, was one of the most stalwart individuals I have ever met. Jack and I developed a trusting relationship in the year before my reappointment. I met with him frequently to seek his advice on matters of leadership. I greatly respected Jack and valued his honesty, loyalty, integrity, and love for Duke University. I believe Jack saw my total commitment to Duke, my honesty and integrity, and probably also my naïveté and occasional lack of emotional intelligence. When I was most vulnerable, Jack remained a loyal and trusted supporter, making clear that he would do all that was appropriate and in his power to retain me in office. I could not have survived the process without him. Perhaps more important than his backing of my reappointment was the encouragement he gave me through our personal interactions, which increased in intensity during May 1993. My appreciation and admiration for him have continued to grow over all these many years.

I came to know Dani Bolognese, a member of the Barr Committee, in the early 1970s when both of us had laboratories in the Sands Basic Research Building. Dani, a professor of surgery and prominent virologist, ultimately did seminal research in the area of HIV. Early in our careers, we would often meet coming in from the parking lot to the Sands Building and talk about our sons, about research, about life in general. In short, Dani and I had bonded early on, and I liked and trusted him; I believed, too, that the feeling was mutual. When Dani was appointed to the Barr Committee, he called me and indicated that he would remain a loyal supporter. At several times during the review process, Dani and I spoke late at night, during which conversations he warned me about the degree of resistance the committee was getting from DUMC faculty. His calls were not meant to alarm me but to indicate the magnitude of the problem, and he did so in a totally appropriate manner. Dani's participation, I believe, was a key factor in the committee's movement away from a "no reappointment" position to the compromise two-year term. Dani gave me a sense of strength and support, and he will always be one of my true and loyal friends. Mary Semans also proved to be a strong supporter of the medical center and my leadership. Over the years, we developed a close friendship and I came to increasingly value her as a remarkable leader and the remaining tie to the will of the Duke family.

Over the years, too, I have reflected on the "civil war" that Joe Greenfield launched against me. On one level, it may seem silly and grandiose, but Joe was a student of the Civil War and an accomplished hunter who had written books on his sport. Joe at least won a battle, since he kept the chairmanship a year longer than I wanted. However, it was a Pyrrhic victory because, thankfully for Duke, he lost the war in that following my reappointment, the role and the power of the department chairs were made more compatible with the needs of the institution as well as the departments. In addition, following Joe's retirement, the PDC, under new leadership, became an increasingly effective partner and a strategic component of the evolving health system.

However one views any struggle or any war, there are always losers and casualties. My family, close friends, and colleagues were traumatized. A campaign of rumor and innuendo embarrassed me as did my having such a difficult time being reappointed. Despite the pain and turmoil, I came out wiser, far more humble, yet tougher and more attentive to listening and to learning from others. I believe I emerged a stronger and better leader, even more committed to helping focus the multifold resources at Duke toward creating the nation's leading academic health enterprise. For this, I am grateful.

8

—

A New Beginning

On reflection, I consider my first term as having been a combined trial by fire and on-the-job training that, ultimately and thankfully, allowed me to devote the next eleven years to the real job at hand: helping to create a contemporary academic health system that could succeed and lead in an environment threatening its very existence. When I was an intern at Duke, my colleagues and I used to quip, "If it doesn't kill you, it's a learning experience." In a way, that described my first four years as chancellor. It often hurt, but it didn't kill me, so I learned through the experiences.

By 1993, I had detailed knowledge and understanding of how the medical center was structured, how it functioned, and how it related to the university as a whole. I had a good idea of the strengths and weaknesses of its various components, as well as those of its leadership and many of the faculty. I had spent considerable time meeting with each department and learning about the medical center directly from the faculty. I also knew many of the faculty members personally and felt close to and engaged with what they were doing as both scientists and clinicians. I learned the detailed workings of the clinical operations, as well as the functioning of a complicated hospital and the operations of Duke University itself. I now grasped its politics—how things actually got done. Importantly, too, I learned that the once glorious Flexner model of the academic medical center had been rendered unviable as a consequence of changes in health care delivery and funding. And, I came to believe that a restructured academic medical institution could contribute far more to meeting the health needs of society.

Aside from learning a great deal about Duke's medical center, I also learned something about myself. My initial approach to the job was heavily derivative of my time as a physician-scientist, and it proved inadequate to leading a complex, multifunctioning organization undergoing dramatic change. As a scientist and researcher, it was second nature to me, in approaching any question, to develop a hypothesis and then test that hypothesis in an experiment in order to disprove or support its "truth." As a scientist, envisioning what the "right answer" might be was integral to the process, and it was also the greatest challenge to solving the problem. Without realizing it, I assumed the same process applied to being Duke's chancellor for health affairs. I considered that my job was to unravel and understand the complexity of the institution and, when I saw problems or issues requiring change in organizational routines, to envision the best end state and devise a means to achieve it.

Unlike in scientific research however, I learned that defining what seemed to be the right answer was but a small fraction of the job of chancellor. The rest was being sure the answer was correct while being able to convince others that the proposed solution was indeed the most appropriate one, not just in a narrow sense but in connection with the myriad moving parts of a complex culture. That put a premium on being able to convince many others that a proposed solution was indeed the most appropriate one. Listening to many constituencies and modifying the approach accordingly were expected parts of the process.

I wish that when I was an undergraduate someone had made me read and understand Karl Popper's distinction between open and closed systems—between, as he put it, "clouds and clocks." All human institutions are open systems—clouds—because human beings have volition and are capable of independent action, meaning that a system will change and grow, and not always in predictable ways. This is not like science, a closed system, where bacteria or molecules could never imagine trying to outsmart a researcher or act differently tomorrow than today under identical physical conditions just because they "feel like it." Humans do that sort of thing all the time.

I also learned a closely related lesson: the need for clear and frequent communication with all constituencies in the medical center and the university. I had imagined that saying something clearly and precisely, several times and even face-to-face, eyeball-to-eyeball, was sufficient for people to understand my message. This turned out to be a grossly inadequate and unreasonable expectation. People often hear what they expect or want to hear, not what is actually being said to them, particularly if it differs qualitatively from anything they have heard before. As the leader of a large, complex institution, I realized but slowly that I needed to communicate more effectively on an ongoing basis, repeating, listening, and refining messages again and again and again, and doing so in a way tailored to many separate groups that made up the medical center, the university, and the community. The faculty, students, administration, staff, alumni, patients, university administration, Board of Trustees, donors, and community constituents all needed to be considered, listened to, and supported, each in their own way.

The first four years not only educated me and greatly challenged my intellect but also toughened me and hopefully made me wiser. They certainly made me far more humble, a trait necessary to any manager if he or she is to effectively listen, learn, and embrace different ideas and attitudes. I came to understand that my role as chancellor for health affairs was less a personal achievement and more a privilege and responsibility through which I subsumed myself to the greater needs of a magnificent institution.

— — —

My second term began with the transition of Dave Sabiston and Joe Greenfield out of their roles as chairs of the two most powerful departments of the School of Medicine, a development that shifted the locus of de facto decision making within the medical center to the "green zone." This color designation related to a way-finding initiative in the hospital and clinics, instituted earlier in the 1980s, to help patients (and others) navigate the vast, complex indoor geography of the medical center. The green zone housed the offices of the chancellor, but the term was often used in a slightly derogatory way to refer to where the top administration resided.

The intimation was that the guys who ran things constituted a kind of monkey-in-the-machine-room phenomenon, interlopers and power-hungry centralizers who did not understand the "way things worked." A key challenge still facing my team beyond 1993 was how to develop an organizational structure that could enable the medical center and hospital to act more coherently, cost-effectively, and strategically to accomplish its core missions. No doubt we sometimes did act like monkeys in the machine room, but that was because the "way things worked" wasn't working very well anymore, and it was impossible to always know what modifications would work, and what second- and third-order implications even positive changes might have. Managing a complex open system is not a science as much as a craft. But we had no choice but to try new approaches, because idling along with the status quo was not an option in the face of impending change.

Among the highest priorities we set to enable orderly and constructive change was the recruitment of a new generation of chairs and, in particular, replacements for Dave Sabiston and Joe Greenfield. After Dave formally announced his retirement in March 1993, a national search ensued to find and entice a replacement to come to Duke. The stature of the Department of Surgery as the best in the nation and the iconic nature of Dave made this chair position perhaps the most desirable at that time. Some of the best individuals in the country clearly wanted the job. In one of the very rare instances that Dave asked me for anything, he indicated his desire that I appoint a loyal trainee of his: Robert W. Anderson, then chair of surgery at Evanston Hospital and chief of cardiothoracic surgery at Northwestern University Medical School in Chicago. Bob received his undergraduate degree at Duke and his advanced surgical training under Dave, and he also served on the surgery faculty from 1972 to 1977. Because Bob was among the group conveyed to me by the search committee, I chose him for the job. He assumed the chair in the summer of 1994.

Once his appointment was announced, I initiated the search for Joe's replacement in April 1994. A national search identified several suitable candidates, including Barton F. Haynes, a member of our own faculty. I had, along with Jim Wyngaarden, recruited Bart to Duke as a member of the Division of Rheumatology and Immunology in 1980. Bart was a superb clinician, educator, researcher, and a true Duke loyalist. The medicine faculty thought highly of him, and he fully embraced the need for collaboration among the departments and the medical center administration. Although Bart was reluctant to accept the position, at a dinner we had alone at the Washington Duke Inn, I told him, simply and directly, that we needed him. He agreed to accept the job and began as chair of medicine effective July 1995. Thus, the stage was nearly set to address the larger issues careening out of the changing world of academic medicine.

In July 1998, Allen Francis, chair of the Department of Psychiatry, indicated that he would retire to spend more time with his wife, who tragically was succumbing to cancer. We replaced Allen with Ranga R. Krishnan, an esteemed member of the department. Ranga proved to be an effective and creative chair of a department whose clinical practice model was rapidly changing. In 2008, he was appointed dean of the Duke-NUS Graduate Medical School in Singapore, where he played a major role in assuring the success of that institution.

— — —

Another daunting challenge—this one new to my second term—lay in establishing an effective and collegial relationship with my new boss, Nan Keohane, and the senior officers she selected, including executive vice president Tallman Trask, III and provost Peter Lange. My initial relationship with Nan had commenced at the most stressful time of my reappointment battle, and the only way to sum it up at that point was as enigmatic. I think we both were a bit unsure what the other was up to, and I had rejected her advice at a critical moment over the duration of my reappointment as chancellor. Fortunately, both of us approached our relationship with mutual respect and the will to make it work well. I clearly needed to get to know, learn from, and inform Nan and her team about the workings of the medical center and to establish a close and productive working relationship with them. This was critical to me because, as the second phase of my tenure began, I started to contemplate what I expected would probably be my last term. As it happened, I ended up continuing on for an additional eleven years, but my first reappointment process gave me few expectations that I would want to serve such a lengthy tenure. All I knew in July 1993 was that a big job stood before me, and I probably had just five more years to accomplish most of it. I realized too that I could not master the challenge without a productive relationship with Nan.

Nannerl Overholser Keohane proved to be both a respected colleague and a challenge for me. Born on September 18, 1940, in Blytheville, Arkansas, she was the daughter of Grace and James Overholser, a Presbyterian minister. When she was a child, her family relocated several times, living in Texas and South Carolina before returning in 1952 to Arkansas, where she graduated as valedictorian from Hot Springs High School, prior to attending Wellesley

College on a scholarship. She then studied at Oxford on a Marshall Scholarship and subsequently earned a PhD in political science from Yale.

In stark contrast, I was born and raised in the tough neighborhood of Bensonhurst, Brooklyn, by immigrant Jewish parents from Eastern Europe. I was educated predominantly in public schools. While I experienced the prejudice sometimes directed toward me as a Jew, I did not consciously think of being Jewish as an important component of my approach to my job. I understood the nature of the biases, but I steered a path so they would not get in my way or particularly bother me. My boss at Genentech, Kirk Raab, once told me that his greatest desire was to gain membership in the exclusive Burlingame Country Club. He quipped that despite all my accomplishments, I'd never be a member because Jews were strictly excluded and, what's more, as far as he could tell, I didn't give a damn. That was so true: I couldn't have cared less about membership in a private club that excluded Jews. That, it seemed to me, was the club's problem. Nonetheless, I am Jewish, I was raised Jewish, and I was educated in public schools where most everyone was either Jewish or Italian.

Nan and I were cast in different molds, and one could not have expected a more unlikely pair in the two highest positions at Duke University. I found Nan to be a highly articulate, intelligent, thoughtful, and focused individual; it would not be accurate to describe her as warm and fuzzy. While our initial relationship did not start well, following her assumption as president our interactions became collegial and mutually respectful for most of the time we served our respective terms. The exceptions came later in our tenures, when the strains of the relationships between Duke University and its health system, crises within the medical center, and differences in leadership styles created tension and, at times, disagreements between us. Although the differences were occasionally severe, they did not diminish our abilities to get our respective jobs done and, for me at least, to retain my respect and high professional regard for her.

Beginning in the summer of 1993, I often strolled through various portions of the medical center with Nan, detailing the component parts of the medical center and how they all functioned together. Nan appreciated learning about the medical center, and I enjoyed having the opportunity to teach her. I considered it essential for us to have a close working relationship and for that relationship to be so perceived by the leadership and rank and file throughout the medical enterprise. To have Nan better appreciate the role of a physician and the nature of medical education, I invited her to attend medical teaching rounds on numerous occasions. She enjoyed this; she would wear a long white coat on rounds as would any attending physician. We always indicated to patients that Nan was not a physician but rather president of Duke University; otherwise, Nan was just like the rest of the team in white on the clinical units of Duke Hospital, reviewing the status of patients being treated there.

As Nan learned about DUMC and me, I learned about her and her leadership style. She was among the nation's leading academic administrators and scholars. Both her upbringing and her path to Duke were very different than mine. Nan was very conscious of the difficulties women experienced achieving prominence in a male-dominated world, and she was keenly aware of the active, passive, and unconscious discrimination toward women and underrepresented minorities. Nan was at heart a feminist; she prominently displayed a portrait of her heroine, Virginia Woolf, in her office. Nan led by open engagement, interchanges, and debate among groups while seeking consensus for important decisions. She was composed, precise, and careful in her communication; she was not given to small talk.

Growing up in a tough neighborhood in Brooklyn, I, conversely, became self-reliant, toughened, and thick-skinned. I preferred to independently reason out solutions to problems before engaging others. I didn't think of myself as being inflexible; I just was more comfortable developing an approach to a problem without prior vetting by a focus group. Nan was, if anything, overly inclusive in decision making; she in turn viewed me as exclusive and hierarchical. I understood but did not share her views of my leadership style.

Nan and I would meet weekly in her office for an hour, at which time I would do my best to keep her informed of the current issues within my area of responsibility. In addition, we held weekly senior officers meetings in her office, where a small group of university officers discussed matters of interest. I generally looked forward to both of these meetings because they were both productive and unfailingly collegial.

Consequently, when in 1996 we were formulating the basic concepts for the development of the Duke University Health System (DUHS), I kept Nan apprised as our thoughts evolved. As detailed in chapter 11, we decided on a model for a corporate entity, specifying that the health enterprise would be an independent operating unit but would be overseen and owned by Duke University. To Nan's credit, she understood the reasons for such a hybrid entity: a corporate health system owned by the university. She supported this bold endeavor in principle, and I give her great credit for her bravery and objectivity in supporting this initiative, the first of its kind in American academics. During the creation of DUHS, however, Nan all but obsessed about keeping the health system from spinning away from the university. Because so much of Duke's economic structure relied on a viable medical complex, her concerns were clearly justified, again in principle.

I never tried to keep anything from Nan or the Board of Trustees. Typically, in the morning before our weekly meeting, I would make a list of agenda items. I didn't always give this task the diligence I should have. On one occasion, for example, the medical center was enmeshed in a negotiation with the PDC that required a vote of its membership. While my favored outcome won a substantial majority of the votes cast, the PDC leadership determined that the vote failed because not enough members voted to constitute an absolute majority. For some reason, I forgot to mention this to Nan during our one-on-one, but as soon as I got back to my office, I realized the omission and called her immediately. She was furious that I had withheld the information and felt I was not being forthcoming with her. She probably knew about that vote already because David Adcock, who was university counsel and a senior officer, would often inform Nan of events in the medical center prior to my meeting with her. David probably presented the matter as more serious and final than I thought it was. Thus, Nan was waiting for me to relate the disappointing PDC vote to her; when I did not do so, she concluded that I was withholding negative information intentionally.

Despite incidents such as these, I believe we continued to function as a good working team throughout most of our tenures. Alas, however, even good relationships often erode from the rough edges of onrushing reality and underlying differences in perceptions of them. Over time, our mutual trust became strained as challenges and occasional crises, large and small, followed in the normal course of events.

— — —

Matters of high university politics aside, as I began my second term I was determined to oversee more diligently the continued improvement of the basic science and clinical departments and to enhance the efficiency of their operations. We needed to continuously foster improvements in all our educational programs and ensure the efficient operation of the medical center and hospital. Most important, we needed to create the vision and then the reality of a health care delivery system that could respond on the curve of change to the rapid dislocation of the health care environment brought about by the emergence of managed care and insurance company efforts to reduce costs.

In medicine, we often say that form follows function, which means that a part of the body looks as it does because of what it is there to do. To fulfill a given function, one needs to have the appropriate form or structure to enable it. In 1989, DUMC was structured as a semifeudal kingdom, with strong quasi-independent component parts and a weak center. That center did provide infrastructure support in the form of financial oversight, regulatory compliance, alumni support, and fund-raising. But despite the Long Range Plan and all we had accomplished in the first term, we still needed a far more coherent and integrated capability to act as a single entity in response to the needs and opportunities of a rapidly changing environment. We had to modernize the medical center educational capabilities and develop new programs; we had to focus on important interdisciplinary areas and acquire the human capital and financial resources needed for the purpose; and we had to develop new and more effective models of health care delivery.

To do this we needed a central nervous system—a brain that integrated the functions of all the component parts of the medical center. We needed an ability to perceive, think, create ideas, and then act as a single decision system. During the early years of my second term, my team and I expanded the organizational structure to include offices of planning, communications, and development and alumni affairs. Within Duke Hospital, we recruited individuals to deal with managed care, strategic relationships, and network development. The combination of new functions, new capabilities, and new means to communicate among them created an evolving governing structure and generated the central nervous system we needed. In 1993, my senior leadership team consisted of the following individuals:

William J. Donelan, vice chancellor for administration, CFO
Gordon G. Hammes, vice chancellor for medical center academic affairs
Mark C. Rogers, executive director, vice chancellor for health affairs
    and CEO of Duke Hospital
Raymond C. "Bucky" Waters, vice chancellor for development
Dan G. Blazer, dean of medical education, School of Medicine

Mary T. Champagne, dean, School of Nursing

Bernard McGinty, director, medical center financial management

Vicki Y. Saito, assistant vice chancellor/director of medical center
communications

Larry Nelson, assistant vice president for health affairs, planning, and
university architect

Steven G. Sloate, associate vice chancellor for planning

Paul M. Rosenberg, associate vice chancellor and chief operating
officer, Duke health network

To bridge the activities of the various components, we developed committees to integrate all aspects of clinical delivery at the highest executive level,
including the hospital, the office of the chancellor, the leadership of the PDC,
and representatives of the clinical faculty. The design for a more corporate
structure within the medical center focused on the inadequate oversight
and integration of clinical operations. Prior to my appointment, each of the
more than nine hundred clinical faculty members of the PDC functioned independently, keeping their own appointment schedules and accounts. The
PDC's ability to coordinate care was limited by its department-driven operational structure, which remained in place until 1995. (I describe the situation more fully in chapter 11, which deals with the creation of the health
system.)

The individual clinical chairs, faculty, and the hospital's CEO determined
the number of beds available for admission for each speciality. Clinical volumes, rather than any strategic plans, determined the assignment of beds.
Neither patients nor their primary care physicians outside of the Duke system could make an appointment for the patient except by directly engaging
with a Duke physician's office. The system worked thanks to the high reputation of Duke and the individual physicians within it. Referring physicians
had preferred specialists within Duke for different needs and knew specifically whom within Duke they wanted their patients to see. It was virtually
unheard of for a patient to self-refer to Duke, since no centralized system
existed through which to make an appointment. Moreover, if a Duke physician's schedule got overloaded, there was no mechanism in place to refer
patients to another equally competent physician within the Duke medical
community. This system worked before the existence of managed care or
local competition, but it was starkly vulnerable to the rise of both.

To better coordinate care, we needed, among other things, a strong, strategic-minded CEO of Duke Hospital. We sought someone capable of maximizing cost-effectiveness while envisioning the creation of the new Duke University health network we were trying to build. The clinical practices, controlled by the clinical department chairs, needed to be better integrated into the operations of the hospital. We also needed to build a strong capability for a health services network development, strategic planning, business development, marketing of clinical services, and developing a culture supportive of excellence in patient care and service.

As noted in chapter 5, we brought in Vick Stoughton as CEO of Duke Hospital in 1991. Within a year, his initiatives in cost-cutting and efficiency enhancement caused great anxiety among the chairs. Moreover, he often acted without engaging me. When I tried to rein him in by insisting that he work more closely with the senior leadership, he resigned. I chose Mark C. Rogers, an associate dean at Johns Hopkins University and chair of the Department of Anesthesiology, as Vick's replacement. Both Mark and his wife, Elizabeth, trained at Duke, and Mark was increasingly eager to take on new leadership responsibilities. He had a master's degree in business from Wharton, a strong entrepreneurial bent, and, importantly, an understanding of how to succeed in a managed care environment.

Mark recruited a first-rate administrative team with a strong strategic and business acumen. He selected Michael D. Israel as the chief operating officer of Duke Hospital. Mike had previously served as chief operating officer at St. Luke's Hospital in Houston, Texas. Paul M. Rosenberg, an attorney with experience in building clinical networks, became chief operating officer of the Duke health network to enhance services for patients and referring physicians and to develop a plan for integrating clinical services throughout the network.

Mark saw the need to substantially trim hospital expenses because all the financial forecasts indicated that, given projections of increasing pressure on hospital margins and a large, inefficient workforce, the hospital would be losing money within two years. To avoid predicted deficits, we needed not only to expand revenues but also to drastically cut expenses. To bring expenses in line with revenues, Mark and his team recommended a workforce reduction of 1,040 positions, which amounted to almost 10 percent of the hospital workforce. To justify these draconian cuts, I showed Nan Keohane and our university board the projected crossing of revenue and expense lines within two years if we stood pat. Reluctantly, we agreed that work-force reductions had to happen.

Mark and his team studied in great detail how to make the reductions and mitigate their impact; all of us were conscious that Duke was by far Durham's largest employer. As discussed in more detail in chapter 9, we carefully planned the announcement of the layoffs, but that failed to pre-vent resentment, particularly in the African American community, which felt it would be unfairly burdened by the brunt of the layoffs. Fortunately, virtually all of the workforce reduction was accomplished through volun-teer retirement programs, attrition, and position elimination.

Mark served as Duke Hospital's CEO for five years and proved to be the right person for the job at that time. Mark was extremely bright, and his experiences as head of a clinical department in building physician net-works at Hopkins and his training as a Wharton MBA prepared him well to understand the dysfunctional nature of Duke's clinical enterprise, and to envision ways to create a new model of health care delivery. Mark liked to describe himself as an orthogonal thinker, that is, one who sees things dif-ferently from others and is untethered by conventional mental habits. He also spoke frankly about whatever was on his mind and did not worry about the consequences. His frankness in dealing with the entrenched powers, such as departmental chairs and even the university administration itself, made his leadership style unusual at best. Patience was also not among his strong suits. He frequently would get up and leave meetings after having been there for only a few minutes. If he thought the meeting was wasting his time, he made no effort to hide his assessment from others.

Still, Mark was an outstanding strategic thinker and someone who actually said and took the boot for things I only dared to think. Similar to Vick Stoughton, however, Mark sometimes acted without consulting me, causing me to be blindsided more often that I appreciated. This led to episodic friction between us. On one occasion, for example, he devel-oped a strategic alliance with a large pharmaceutical company, but I only learned of it through an announcement in a front-page *Wall Street Journal* article that a colleague pointed out to me during a meeting away from the Duke campus. Furious, I phoned Mark to take him to task for not telling me what he was doing. I was astonished by his sincere amazement that I wasn't proud of him for getting Duke Hospital on the front page of the *Wall Street Journal*.

Nonetheless, Mark and his team played an important role in helping me envision the creation of a broader Duke health system. He helped break down the walls between the medical center administration and the clinical chairs. His brusqueness often allowed me to be the more reasoned, compassionate diplomat in reconciling tensions between hospital administration and the clinical practice. By the end of Mark's first five-year term, much of the needed modernization of the clinical infrastructure was in place, as well as a better understanding of the type of network Duke would need to remain viable in the rapidly changing health care market. Mark and I were effective colleagues and became lasting friends.

Five years of dealing with the Duke bureaucracy, including the university president's office, was enough for Mark. Rather than endure a bruising review for another five-year appointment, Mark leapt to the commercial world, accepting a high position at PerkinElmer. He subsequently built a successful career in venture capital. Mike Israel succeeded Mark as vice chancellor for health affairs and CEO of Duke Hospital in 1996.

— — —

The complexity of DUHS required an outstanding senior management team in order to be successful, and we were fortunate to develop such a group. In 1996, we recruited Alvis R. Swinney as vice chancellor for business development and marketing from Baylor Health System in Dallas to lead our efforts in developing clinical marketing capabilities. Gordon D. Williams came to Duke to be vice dean for finance and administration in the School of Medicine in 1999. Gordon was a savvy and experienced administrator who served previously at the University of Pennsylvania and as director of the private practice plan at Northwestern Medical Center. He became a prominent member of the medical center's administrative team. We appointed Kenneth C. Morris as chief financial officer of the DUHS, also in 1999. Ken had been senior vice president of finance for Mission and St. Joseph's Health System in Asheville, North Carolina. He played a pivotal role as the health system's first chief financial officer and became one of my most valued partners as he crisply analyzed the impact of our ideas or decision on the health system's finances.

Gary L. Stiles, someone I had known from his time as a fellow in Bob Lefkowitz's lab and through his leadership of the Duke Cardiology Division in the Department of Medicine, became DUHS's first chief medical officer in 1999. Gary's appointment occurred despite the fact that in 1993 he was one of the leaders in the Department of Medicine who sought to oust me as chancellor for health affairs. I tend not to hold grudges, and I credit my upbringing with that virtue. If you held grudges growing up in hard-knock Brooklyn, pretty soon you would have no one but your shadow to talk to. I always liked Gary, so after a frank conversation with him, during which we discussed whether he could indeed be loyal to me, I became convinced that he could. And he was: Gary proved to be an outstanding, effective, and creative chief medical officer. He deserves singular credit for rolling out the first version of Duke prospective health care, a transformational model of care and the subject of chapter 13.

By 2001, we needed new leadership in the position of CEO of Duke Hospital. Mike Israel was ready to move on after many years of excellent service, and I envisioned his successor as a leader who was highly respected by our physicians, an excellent physician, and capable of leading the emerging health system. We chose William J. Fulkerson, Jr., a leading pulmonary specialist we had been grooming for years to assume greater responsibility for administration within the clinical services at Duke. Having already served as executive medical director of the PDC, he enjoyed the trust and admiration of our clinical faculty and clinical leadership. So in April 2002 we appointed Bill as chief executive officer at Duke Hospital, and he became an important member of the senior leadership team.

As the complexity of the health system grew, information technology became more important. Prior to 2003, the focus had been on computers, computer systems, and technology. The health system needed a senior-level officer to lead the efforts to harness technology to provide the needed information to operationally and strategically link the multiple components of the health system. I reasoned that the chief informational officer, akin to a chief medical officer and chief financial officer, should be a member of my senior leadership team. For this position, Asif Ahmad, previously chief information officer/chief technology officer at The Ohio State University Health System and Medical Center, was chosen. Asif was the right person for the job and viewed his role as providing strategic solutions to meet the information and operational needs of the health system. I found him to be a valuable colleague and a refreshing voice among my senior leadership team.

In medical education, our goals going forward were to grow capabilities to analyze the curriculum of our medical school so that the physicians we trained were capable of envisioning and leading in medicine as it would be practiced after they graduated. We continued our focus on excellence, creativity, leadership, competence, and compassion, but most important, we tried to envision the rapidly changing capabilities and roles that physicians would need in the twenty-first century. Hence, in 1994 Duke became the nation's first school to offer medical school students training in cost-effectiveness in medical care. In 1996, we expanded the physician's assistant program, and in 1998, we created the degree of doctorate in physical therapy, making our institution among a few that granted such a degree.

We also reorganized the medical school curriculum, particularly in the basic science year, to focus on three overarching topics: molecules and cells, the normal body, and the body and disease. Students for the first time received training in the importance of mindfulness and meditation, including an understanding of the need for caring and compassion and the need to involve and engage patients in their own care.

A unique aspect of the "new" medical school curriculum launched in 1966 was the establishment of the third year as a largely elective period. The idea was to compress the basic science years from two years to one, allowing the second year for intense clinical exposure and the third year for time to delve deeply into areas in which the students were most interested. Most students chose to work in the research laboratories of medical school faculty. For those pursuing the MD/PhD degree, this saved them a year in obtaining their PhD. By the late 1990s, it was clear that students were interested in more diverse opportunities than research alone. After intense discussions at MedPAC it was agreed that third-year students could pursue either a master's degree in public health in collaboration with the University of North Carolina, a master's of science in clinical research with the DCRI, or a master's in business administration with the Fuqua School of Business. This option proved to be increasingly popular and in 2004, 30 percent of our students were pursing the master's degree option.

In 1998, Duke's School of Medicine partnered with the NIH (described fully in chapter 10) to create a training program leading to a master's degree in clinical research. This program allowed fellows and scientists at the NIH to receive training and a master's degree in clinical research from Duke faculty via a state-of-the-art video classroom at the NIH. It was, indeed, an honor to have Duke be the only degree-granting institution providing clinical research training at the NIH. We also expanded Duke's office of continuing medical education and steadily increased the range of activities offered and the number of participants involved.

In the School of Nursing, we expanded the master's program to include nurse practitioner specialties in primary and acute care for pediatric and adult populations, cardiovascular care, oncology, gerontology, and neonatology, as well as health care leadership, nursing education, and informatics. Dean Mary Champagne also developed an interdisciplinary master's program in clinical leadership. By the time she retired in 2004, near the end of my third term as chancellor, the faculty stood at its highest level, at thirty-eight. Importantly, too, she developed a rigorous standard for teaching and for creative scholarships. In 1993, she led the creation of the Duke Nursing Research Center and by 2004 had laid the groundwork for a new doctorate of nursing practice program and a new facility for the School of Nursing. A turning point for the school came in 2002 with the creation of the accelerated bachelor of science in nursing. In this program, individuals with bachelor's degrees in nonnursing areas could come to Duke and earn a bachelor of science in nursing degree within two years. From 1991 until 2003, student enrollment skyrocketed from 50 to 374. When Mary stepped down as dean in 2004, Duke was among the nation's best schools of nursing. The quality and potential of the school allowed us to build a state-of-the-art nursing education building and to recruit Catherine L. Gillis from Yale to be the new dean. Our decision to go "all in" on nursing turned out to be the right one.

— — —

As noted earlier, Gordon Hammes served as a key leader in overseeing the reorganization of biomedical research. By 1997, Gordon was interested in stepping down within the next year, and his departure prompted me to rethink my own roles and responsibilities. With the development of DUHS on the horizon, I realized there would not be enough time for me to also fulfill my duties as both chancellor for health affairs and dean of the School of Medicine. It made sense that Gordon's successor might serve not only as the head of academic affairs but also as dean of the School of Medicine. After all, a major function of the dean is to oversee academic affairs. Thus, in 1998 we began a search for an individual who could assume the responsibilities of Duke's next medical school dean. We needed someone well recognized as a competent biomedical researcher, educator, and academic leader in clinical medicine.

We found such a rare individual in Edward W. Holmes. I had known Ed since 1972, when he was a fellow in the laboratory of Bill Kelley, then chief of the Division of Rheumatic and Genetic Diseases at Duke. We enjoyed a long history of working together, and he knew Duke's medical center very well, having been a professor of medicine at Duke until 1991, when he left to become chairman of the Department of Medicine at the University of Pennsylvania. In 1997, he left Penn to go to Stanford University's School of Medicine, where his wife, Judith Swain, also a good friend and longtime Duke faculty member, became chair of the Department of Medicine. I considered Ed the right person for this job, and he agreed to come back as Duke's next dean of the School of Medicine. This condemned him to a bicoastal life, with his wife remaining at Stanford.

Ed's appointment in January 1999 coincided with my tenure as chair-elect of the Council of Deans of the AAMC. Fellow deans wanted me to serve in this position, which was an important one in that organization and the leadership of the AAMC, and I could hardly refuse. For me to take that on, however, Nan Keohane had to agree to allow me to assume the role as executive dean of the School of Medicine, thereby enabling me to continue to play a role in the AAMC. My leadership role within the association proved to be an important asset for Duke as its medical enterprise occupied center stage within the nation's largest organization representing all academic medical centers. It also provided me with an important bully pulpit to advocate for new models of health care—personalized health care in particular.

Ed did a superb job as Duke's dean for approximately a year, but his bicoastal balancing act proved unworkable. He decided to return to the West Coast to become vice chancellor at the University of California, San Diego.

Having Ed as dean for only a year and a few months was certainly disruptive, and of course I was sad to lose him. But we were fortunate to find an equally stellar individual to replace him: R. Sanders "Sandy" Williams. Sandy also grew up at Duke, as a fellow in the laboratory of Bob Lefkowitz.

I had known him for many years while he was training and then as a faculty member at Duke. Sandy was a renowned cardiovascular researcher and chief of cardiology at the University of Texas Southwestern Medical Center. He and his wife, Jennifer, a physician's assistant at Duke during his time here, were a highly visible and extremely popular and productive couple. Sandy came back to Duke in July 2001 as dean of the School of Medicine and vice chancellor for academic affairs. We worked very closely and amicably together for the remainder of my third and last term.

As dean, Sandy played a major role in creating a new generation of chairs and in doing so greatly increased their diversity. In 2000, Mike Sheetz resigned as chair of cell biology to go to Columbia. Harold P. Erickson, a member of the department, took over as interim chair and he remained in that position until 2002, when Brigid L. M. Hogan, the first woman chair in the history of the medical school, was recruited. Brigid, a world-renowned developmental biologist at Vanderbilt, was a superb choice for this large and important basic science department.

A department of Biostatistics and Bioinformatics was created in 2000 in recognition of the importance of this area of inquiry for academic medicine. William E. Wilkinson served as interim chair from 2000 until 2009. Bill received his PhD in mathematical statistics from the University of North Carolina and spent his entire postdoctoral career as a member of the Duke faculty.

Jerry Reves, chair of Anesthesiology, left Duke in 2001 to assume the role of dean of the College of Medicine and vice president of the Medical University of South Carolina. After a national search, I realized the best choice for Jerry's successor was Mark F. Newman, chief of the Division of Cardiothoracic Anesthesiology at Duke in 2001. In 2014, Mark was elected president of the Duke PDC.

In 2002, Dale Purves, the first chair I recruited, retired as chair of the Department of Neurobiology. James O. McNamara, a strong internal candidate known for his work on epilepsy, replaced Dale. Dean Williams's next recruitment was again historic in terms of enhancing diversity among our medical school chairs. When Chuck Hammond retired as chair of OB/GYN after twenty-two years, a national search identified Haywood L. Brown, a noted maternal-fetal medicine specialist and professor at Indiana University, as the best candidate. Haywood became the first African American chair in the medical school.

In 2003 Bart Haynes stepped down as chair of the Department of Medicine, and Harvey J. Cohen, a highly regarded leader of our Aging Center, became interim chair. Harvey and I had been classmates at SUNY Downstate Medical Center, and we both came to Duke as interns in 1965. Later in 2003, Pascal J. Goldschmidt became the permanent chair. I had recruited Pascal in 2000 from The Ohio State University College of Medicine to be chief of the Division of Cardiology and director of the Duke Cardiovascular Center for Genomic Sciences. I thought very highly of his creativity and was pleased that he became chair of our largest department. He subsequently left Duke in 2006 to go to the University of Miami, where he served as senior vice president for medical affairs, dean of the School of Medicine, and chief executive officer of that university's health system.

In 2003, Bob Anderson retired as chair of the Department of Surgery and was replaced by Danny O. Jacobs, our second African American chair. Danny was formerly chair of surgery at Creighton University. Danny left Duke in 2013 to become executive vice president, provost, and dean at the University of Texas Medical Branch at Galveston.

Christopher G. Willet arrived in 2004 from the Massachusetts General Hospital as chair of the Department of Radiation Oncology, replacing interim chair, Len Prosnitz, who had replaced Ed Halperin in 2002. Ed had stepped down as chair to become vice dean of the Duke School of Medicine and associate vice chancellor for academic affairs.

Thus, by the time I stepped down, of the chairs that were there in 1989, only Carl Ravin in radiology and Richard F. Kay in biological anthropology and anatomy remained in place.

Another major accomplishment in medical education centered on the creation of the Duke-NUS Graduate Medical School. Beginning in 1999, Duke's School of Medicine became interested in internationalizing its unique approach to medical education and began visits to Singapore, a highly innovative and entrepreneurial society whose leaders were determined to make it a regional resource for all issues related to biomedicine. In April 2002, during my third term, Singapore sent a delegation to Duke led by Tony Tan, the then deputy prime minister who eventually became president. The delegation sought to lay the foundation for an American-style medical school in Singapore, the goal being to train the best leaders in medicine and medical research to enhance that small country's capability to provide leadership in this area throughout Southeast Asia.

Tony Tan and I immediately developed a strong and trusting relationship, and although the delegation had been scheduled to visit a number of other institutions, Tony and I had a handshake agreement to pursue the development of a Duke-led medical school in Singapore. Numerous visits occurred at Duke and in Singapore from April 2002 until June 2003, when I traveled there to sign a memorandum of understanding defining and enabling the creation of the school between Duke and the National University of Singapore. In April 2005, we formalized the partnership and by August 2007 the first class of students took their seats. The Duke-NUS Graduate Medical School is a shining example of collaboration between our School of Medicine and the health system in Singapore. It now occupies the Khoo Tech Puat Building, dedicated in 2009, and is a world leader in the creation of new models of medical education.

— — —

It was clearer than ever by my second term that the field of genetics was critical to forming the foundation for new ways of understanding health and the evolution of disease. In 1990, Duke researchers discovered the role of the APOE-4 gene in the development of susceptibility to Alzheimer's disease. Duke researchers also linked the BRCA1 and BRCA2 gene mutations to breast cancer. In 1996, we created the Duke Center for Human Genetics, headed by the nationally recognized Margaret Pericak-Vance and her husband, Jeff Vance. This center created the DNA bank and tissue repository, one of the largest academic DNA banks in the country. By the mid-1990s, it was evident throughout the United States that the human genome would ultimately be sequenced and that genetics would provide tremendous opportunities to understand and treat human disease. This recognition stimulated the creation of several centers for genetic research. I was determined that Duke would host one of the very best of the lot.

To realize such ambition cost money, of course, so it was no coincidence that in 1998 the university began a major fund-raising campaign. President Keohane challenged her senior leadership team to create an inspiring opportunity for an imaginary philanthropist willing to give the university $200 million to fund an important idea. Hearing Nan describe this theoretical opportunity and knowing it would require a university-wide operation, I began doodling on a napkin. I drew a daisy with a then notional institute for genome science and policy at the center; distributed around the center were petals representing all the schools and components of the university that could be involved in taking a broad approach to understanding the future of genomics. The School of Medicine, the health system, biomedical research, law, ethics, and policy—all would be involved. Hence, the concept of the Institute for Genome Sciences and Policy (IGSP) filled that napkin. The idea generated immediate interest and won the strong support of Nan and the university provost. In 2002, the Duke IGSP opened its doors, with its areas of expertise including ethics, law, and policy; genomic medicine; computational genomic sciences; genomic sciences in society; population genomics; evolutionary genomics; systems biology; and genome sequencing and analysis. The distinguished genomics researcher and leader Huntington F. Willard from Case Western Reserve University in Cleveland became the founding director. By the time I stepped down as chancellor, the IGSP had approximately 100 faculty members representing more than twenty-five departments and more than 125 staff.

I think it is fair to say that, by 2004, each of the medical center's core missions had been transformed from its condition in 1989. Moreover, a new overarching mission to create better models of health care was taking firmer shape. In addition to these changes, several initiatives were particularly novel and, in my view, important in academic medicine: establishing translational and clinical research as an academic priority, bringing the patient and his or her holistic needs front and center in care through integrative approaches, creating the highly successful academic health system, and defining entirely new approaches to health care. Importantly, we developed a coherent focus on enhancing institutional diversity, inclusion, and synergistic relationships with the Durham community. Each of these initiatives is described more fully in the subsequent chapters.

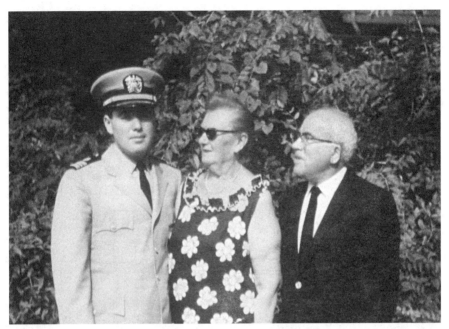

FIG. GALLERY 1.1 Ralph Snyderman with his parents, Ida and Morris Snyderman. Ralph Snyderman was a commissioned officer in the U.S. Public Health Service from 1967 to 1970. Photo from personal archive of author.

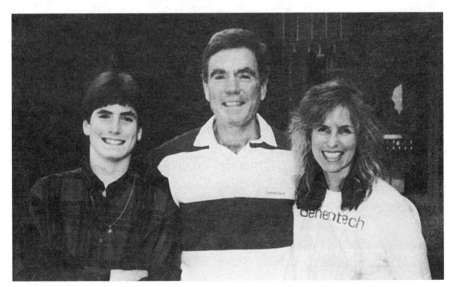

FIG. GALLERY 1.2 Ralph Snyderman with his wife Judith and son, Ted, 1989. Photo courtesy of the Duke Medical Center Archives.

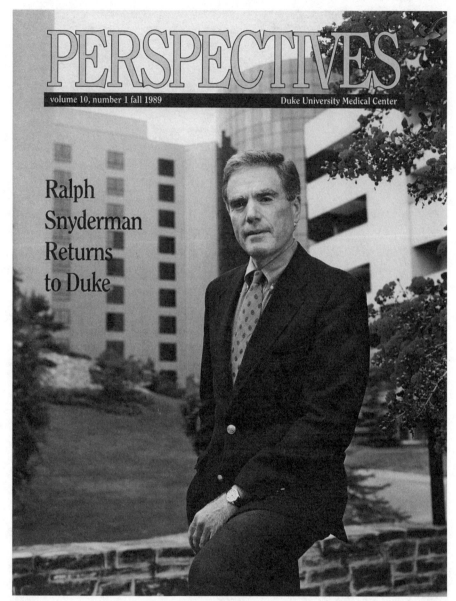

PERSPECTIVES

volume 10, number 1 fall 1989   Duke University Medical Center

Ralph
Snyderman
Returns
to Duke

FIG. GALLERY 1.3 Ralph Snyderman returns to Duke as chancellor for health affairs and dean of the School of Medicine, 1989. Photo by Butch Usery. Courtesy of the Duke Medical Center Archives.

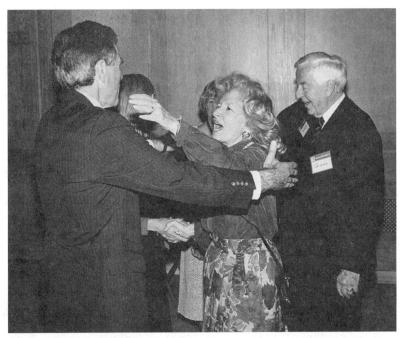

FIG. GALLERY 1.4 Mary Duke Biddle Trent Semans and James H. Semans at a reception welcoming Ralph Snyderman back to Duke in 1989. Photo by Duke Photography. Courtesy of the Duke University Archives.

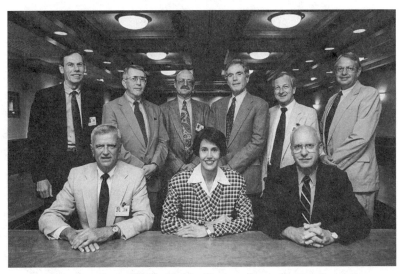

FIG. GALLERY 1.5 Chancellor for health affair's staff in 1989. Standing, left to right: William Donelan, James "Pete" Bennett, Jim Good, Ralph Snyderman, John Robinette, Larry Nelson; seated, left to right: Bernard McGinty, Lynn Proctor, Robert Winfree. Photo from personal archive of author.

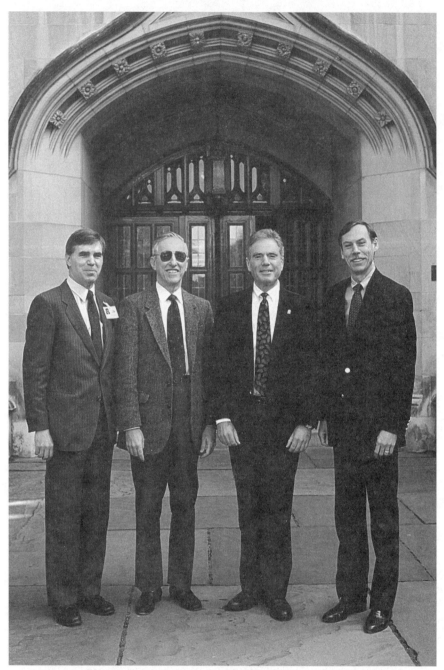

FIG. GALLERY 1.6 Vickery Stoughton (CEO, Duke Hospital), Gordon Hammes (vice chancellor for academic affairs), Ralph Snyderman, and William Donelan (vice chancellor for medical center administration and chief financial officer), 1991. Photo from personal archive of author.

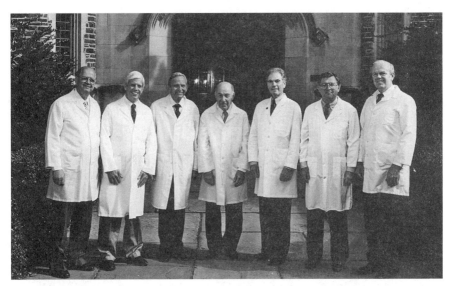

FIG. GALLERY 1.7 Medical School deans, 1993. Left to right: Arthur Christakos, Dan Blazer, Ewald Busse, William Anlyan, Ralph Snyderman, Charles Putman, and Doyle Graham. Photo by Duke Photography. Courtesy of the Duke University Archives.

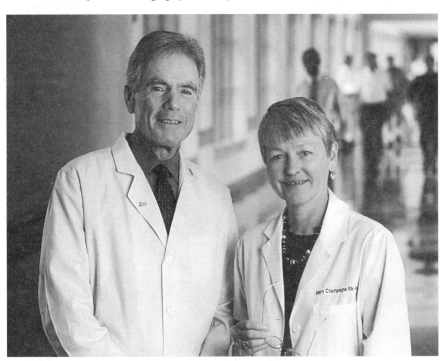

FIG. GALLERY 1.8 Mary Champagne, dean of the School of Nursing, and Ralph Snyderman, 2001. Photo by Duke Photography.

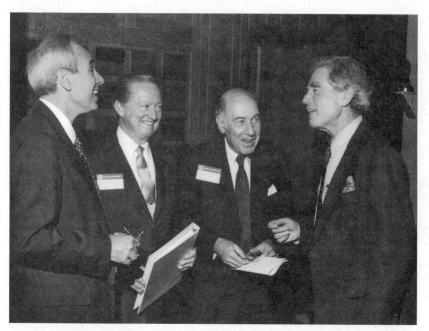

FIG. GALLERY 1.9. Keith Brodie, president, Duke University; Philip "Jack" Baugh, chair, Duke University Board; William Anyan, chancellor emeritus; and Ralph Snyderman, early 1990s. Photo from personal archive of author.

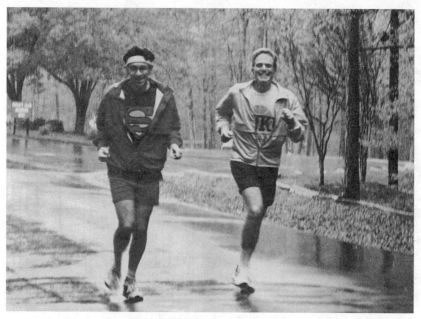

FIG. GALLERY 1.10 Bob Lefkowitz and Ralph Snyderman on one of their runs in the late 1990s. Photo by Gale McCarty.

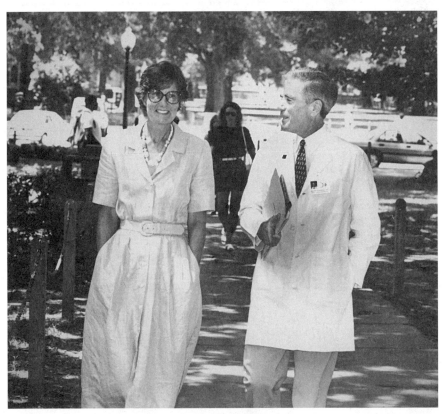

FIG. GALLERY 1.11 President Nan Keohane and Ralph Snyderman on Duke campus, 1993. Photo by Jim Thompson. Courtesy of the Duke Medical Center Archives.

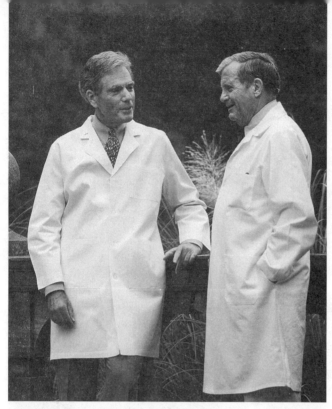

FIG. GALLERY 1.12
Dave Sabiston, chair, Department of Surgery, and Ralph Snyderman, 1994. Photo by Will and Deni McIntyre.

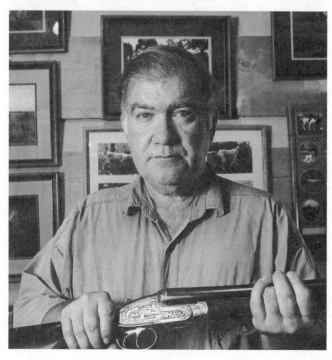

FIG. GALLERY 1.13
Joe Greenfield, chair, Department of Medicine, 1994. Photo by Will and Deni McIntyre.

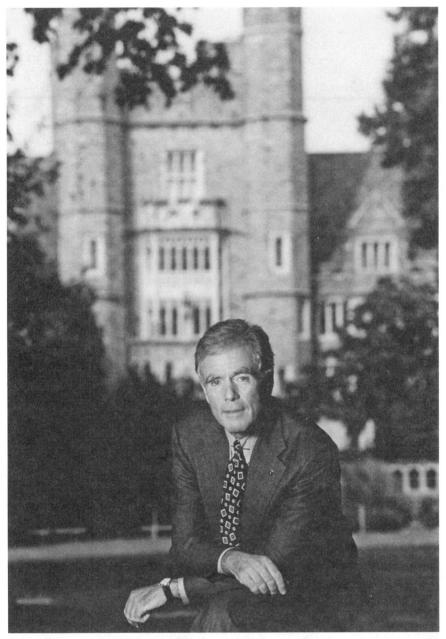

FIG. GALLERY 1.14 Ralph Snyderman in front of Davison Building, 1995. Photo by Will and Deni McIntyre.

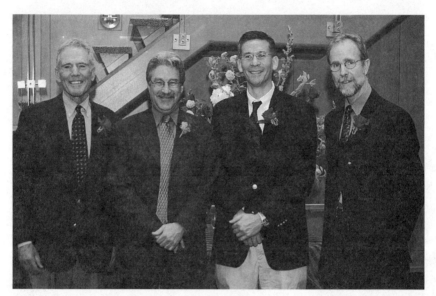

FIG. GALLERY 1.15 Ralph Snyderman, Richard Klausner, Kim Lyerly, and Sandy Williams following the Chancellor's Lecture given by Dr. Klausner, 2003. Photo courtesy of the Duke Medical Center Archives.

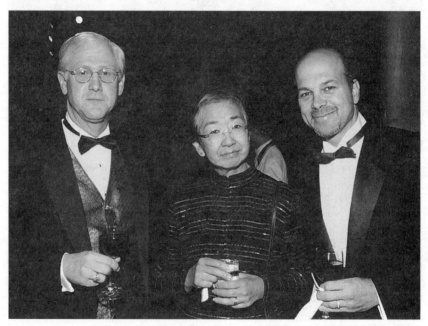

FIG. GALLERY 1.16 Gary Stiles, vice president and chief financial officer, DUHS; Vicki Saito, associate vice chancellor for communications; and Steve Rum, vice chancellor for development and alumni affairs, at the Bravewell Leadership Award Dinner, 2003. Photo courtesy of the Bravewell Collaborative.

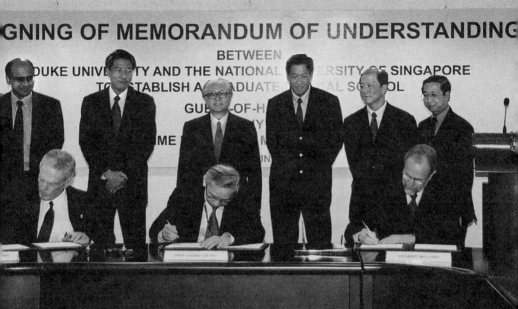

FIG. GALLERY 1.17 Signing the memorandum of understanding between Duke University and the National University of Singapore, 2003. Seated, left to right: Ralph Snyderman, Choong Chi Tat, and Sandy Williams; standing, left to right: Tharman Shanmugaratnam, Teo Chee Hean, Tony Tan, Ng Eng Hen, Moses Lee, and Tan Ser Kiat. Photo courtesy of the National University of Singapore.

II
MAJOR INITIATIVES

9

—

Enhancing Diversity, Inclusion, and Community Relations

Being a southern institution in Durham, North Carolina certainly impacted DUMC as it was in part a reflection of its local environment. While Duke Hospital was formally desegregated in 1963, its de facto segregation and insensitivity to racial issues lasted far longer. When I first came to Duke as an intern in 1965, the medical school had yet to graduate its first African American physician. It was still strikingly a reflection of its segregated past, and I was woefully unaware of the magnitude of this issue. As chancellor, one of my major goals was to address ongoing inequities while making Duke a caring and effective workplace. The stratification of African Americans in the lower paying and service components of the workforce was clear. This helped create the vision of Duke as a "plantation" in the minds of many of its African American workforce.

There were other signs of legacy racism as well. This was brought home to me during a meeting I had with the physician leadership of Durham Regional Hospital in 1997 (see chapter 11). As Duke was seeking to lead the operations of Durham Regional, I had numerous meetings with their constituencies to learn more about them and their needs. At one such evening meeting, an African American physician across the table from me asked if I recalled him. I indicated that while his face looked familiar, I did not remember when we met. He indicated that he had been an applicant to the fellowship program in Duke's Rheumatology Division when I had been its division chief in 1978. I immediately thought to myself, "Oh my God, I hope we didn't turn him down," and I asked him why he had not come to Duke. He indicated that during his interview, I took him around to various outpatient clinics and he saw that Duke continued to be a segregated institution—one not segregated based on race but on economics, thereby accomplishing the same thing; i.e., separating the poorer African Americans in the medical outpatient clinics from the wealthier Caucasians in the private diagnostic clinics. He told me he withdrew his application because he did not want to come to a segregated institution. He was, of course, correct.

While Duke Hospital and the ambulatory services officially desegregated in 1963, the institution's clinical operations remained organized as "public" and "private" services until early 1995. In clinics and in the hospital, patients were sorted by whether they did or did not have medical insurance, thereby creating a two-tiered system. Those with insurance were seen in the private clinics by Duke medical faculty and, if admitted to the hospital, they resided in private wards. Those without insurance went to public clinics and wards and were treated by house staff and fellows who were supervised by faculty. This system generated not only an economic segregation but also a de facto racial separation. Very few private patients at that time were African American, while most public patients, whether in the clinics or the hospital wards, were black. As a clinical trainee and then a medical attending, I understood this economic dichotomy, but frankly I did not appreciate the full significance of the racial segregation at that time.

In retrospect, my lack of a full appreciation of the nature and lasting impact of Duke's segregated past surprises me (I suspect the same is true of most whites). Like many others, I gave little thought to the presence of duplicate bathrooms and drinking fountains in the older sections of the clinical facilities. In segregated times, duplication was necessary to separate blacks and whites. Understanding the impact of the region's segregated and unequal past became an important part of my education as chancellor. As I understood the consequences of our two-class private and public clinical enterprise, I became committed to changing it. My inherent ethics of fairness and compassion for the underserved, as well as a view of the need for improving the work environment, made me intent on addressing the historical inequities. In retrospect however, it surprises me as to how long it took for me to understand (if I do today) the full magnitude and insidious nature of the effect of segregation has had on African Americans and the culture of our institution.

In 1993 we recruited Arthur A. McCombs, an African American who headed human resources at Yale New Haven Hospital, to be associate vice chancellor for human resources of Duke's medical center. We formed a minority task force consisting of approximately a dozen African American hospital employees as an advisory group to help us identify and remedy issues negatively affecting our employees. My focus on social issues was sharpened in 1994, when the hospital announced the need for a workforce reduction of more than a thousand employees (see chapter 8). This news was met with shock and dismay within the Durham community. The understandable concern was that the layoffs would disproportionally affect blacks, who occupied the lowest-paying and most expendable positions. This was not the intended case or eventual outcome, but it was generally believed to be true in the community. I was fortunate to receive a call late one evening from Kenneth Spaulding, the chair of the Durham Committee for the Affairs of Black People. He and his group were intent on ensuring fairness and preventing discrimination by Duke. We had a productive phone conversation during which Ken asked me to appear before the committee and the black community at the White Rock Baptist Church. I asked Ken only that I be treated fairly and be allowed to have a constructive discussion. Ken agreed, and the meeting was mutually respectful and productive. To this day, I value Ken Spaulding's frankness and fairness. Through these difficult and initially adversarial times, I believe I ultimately became far more understanding of the inequities that continue to fracture race relations. Fortunately, the combination of a hiring freeze and early retirement packages allowed all 1,040 jobs to be trimmed with only 24 forced layoffs—all at the management level.

Recruiting and promoting African Americans to senior leadership positions in the medical center became a high priority. During an intensive discussion on this topic with the Board of Trustees in mid-1997, trustee Melinda Gates, a Duke alumna and cofounder of the Bill & Melinda Gates Foundation, said that there had been enough talk; action was needed. Early the next week, I contacted Jean G. Spaulding, Duke medical school's first African American female graduate, who did her residency in psychiatry under Keith Brodie. Jean, a member of the Duke University Board of Trustees at the time, agreed to become vice chancellor for health affairs in January 1998. Jean was recruited to serve as a senior member of the medical center's leadership team. Her role was to enhance both recruiting and mentoring of medical center faculty and students, as well as to serve as a resource to help us better focus on the needs of underrepresented minorities and women. She also helped oversee community health programs that largely provided care to the underserved African American community

To help advise my senior leadership team and me on how we could be more open and effective in dealing with African American students, clinical trainees, and faculty, I appointed newly retired Charles Johnson in 1997 as a consultant. I had gotten to know Charlie, who was among the first African Americans to be appointed to the medical school faculty, when I interned at Duke and was a fellow in endocrinology. At that time, interns were poorly treated as the bottom of the pecking order in the clinical training program. Charlie was different in that he was both a kind and an excellent teacher, and he proved to be very helpful in communicating to the African American community that we were very serious about changing the nature of our organization and embracing diversity.

MaryAnn E. Black joined us in 2002 as director of community affairs for the health system. As described in chapter 11, MaryAnn, an African American who was then chair of the Durham County Commissioners, played a major role in the negotiations resulting in Duke's assuming operations of Durham Regional Hospital. A prominent local leader as well as a clinical social worker, MaryAnn provided valuable insight and expertise to strengthen the delivery of health care to underserved populations in our community. Mark Gordon, also an African American, became chief operating officer of Durham Regional Hospital.

The first African American chair of a department at Duke University arrived in 2002 when Haywood Brown filled the position of chair of the Department of OB/GYN. The second African American chair, Danny Jacobs, was recruited in 2003 to head the Department of Surgery. Haywood and Danny were valued members of the clinical chairs.

When I arrived as chancellor, 8 percent of medical school students were African Americans, a number quite common for all but historically African American medical schools. Wanting to increase diversity in our medical school class, in 1996, I took a chance in appointing as associate dean for medical education, Brenda E. Armstrong, an African American member of the Department of Pediatrics, who was known as a firebrand undergraduate at Duke. She was among those who had occupied the president's office in a 1968 sit-in, an event that ultimately led to the replacement of Doug Knight as president of Duke. Brenda was a passionate advocate for the underserved. When she was being considered for this position, we had a long talk about her goals as the prospective head of admissions for the School of Medicine. We agreed that while Brenda would focus on increasing the percentage of qualified underrepresented minorities in our medical school class, her primary function would be to improve the quality of the entire medical school class. In the time that Brenda served in this role while I was chancellor, she performed her job admirably. The proportion of underrepresented minority students rose from 8 percent in 1989 to 24 percent in 2004, outpacing most U.S. medical schools other than those schools that had been established specifically for minority students.

— — —

As we embraced the need for more equity and diversity, being a caring and productive member of the community became a higher priority for us. With the recruitment of Jean Spaulding and the able leadership of Susan D. Yaggy, who founded the Division of Community Health at Duke and served as its division chief from 1996 to 2008, we created several community initiatives.

One such program, Promising Practices, arose from a study aimed at understanding the high level of nonreimbursed care we experienced at Duke Hospital. The study found that a vast majority of these patients were indigent members of the Durham community. Thus, Promising Practices arose in 1999 to provide free preventative care to patients who frequented the emergency rooms of Durham hospitals. We identified patients with limited resources and inadequate access to ongoing medical care, and endeavored to provide medical care in their homes as well as in clinics. This program was meant not only to provide better care for the underserved but also to save Duke Hospital money by avoiding needless underreimbursed emergency room visits. The program took a holistic approach to health care, assessing, in addition to medical needs, nutrition and education needs, and the environment in which the patient lived. Ongoing follow-up and support for patients' health care needs and development of an overall plan to improve their wellness became a focus of the initiative. This nationally recognized program combined meeting society's needs with innovative health care approaches to meet the needs of the diverse community. Promising Practices fulfilled its mission to provide care particularly for people in Durham suffering from diabetes, asthma, and hypertension. A grant from the Duke Endowment via the Neighborhood Partnership Initiative allowed the program to expand and reach even more areas of Durham. The medical and financial outcomes of Promising Practices revealed significant improvement in the level of diabetic control, as well as substantial savings in overall cost of care, most of which was attributable to a decrease in hospitalization cost.

The Department of Community and Family Medicine and the School of Nursing also collaborated to create programs for the underserved or disadvantaged, including the elderly, the homeless, and underinsured and uninsured children. Services ranged from dental and medical care to mental health services and provided education and teaching of effective health practices.

— — —

Among President Keohane's and my priorities were to broadly enhance diversity and to raise the status of women throughout the university. Nan put this issue on the university-wide agenda in 1994, and the medical center's leadership took it very seriously. At that time, no woman had ever served as chair of any medical school department at Duke, and few women worked at the level of professor. While there were roughly equal numbers of women and men in the School of Medicine, there were far fewer women in post-doctorate training or the MD/PhD program. The distribution of women in the faculty was heavily oriented toward non-tenure tracks and in clinical departments and primary care rather than specialty practices.

To better understand the issues behind these disparities, I conducted numerous focus groups with women from all areas of the medical center. We met at my home on many occasions in what I called, after FDR's example, "fireside chats." Among the most valuable information we learned is that women often chose career paths based on family responsibilities, including childbearing and child raising. These responsibilities often occurred at the precise times that tenure and promotion were in the offing. Women generally had far less flexibility in their working hours than men due to their family obligations. In addition to needing child care arrangements, women needed role models, and mentors. We identified ameliorating these factors as crucial goals for the medical center.

In September 1995, the medical center issued a policy statement reaffirming and strengthening its commitment to diversity, and in October 1996, it issued an affirmative action plan. We undertook specific initiatives to address the needs of medical students, house staff, and faculty, particularly junior faculty. Revisions in maternity leave policy, enhancing the flexibility of tenure-track requirements, mentoring programs to enhance grant writing, and a commitment to hiring and retaining women became major goals of the medical center. We modified recruitment and search processes to ensure that women and underrepresented minorities would be sought out and evaluated fairly.

In 2002, Nan undertook a major project called "The Women's Initiative at Duke University." This comprehensive, university-wide study included medical center representation. This initiative examined each component of the university from employees and students all the way through the Board of Trustees. In response to this report, the medical center appointed Ann J. Brown, an assistant professor in the Departments of Medicine and OB/GYN, to also be associate dean for women in medicine and science. Her role was to spearhead initiatives to study and enhance the environment for female faculty and learners within the medical school and to fulfill the goals of the initiative. Indeed, as noted in chapter 8, Brigid Hogan, a developmental biologist from Vanderbilt, became the first woman chair in the history of the medical school, when she became Chair of Cell Biology in 2002.

Duke understandably needed to move from its segregated, white male–dominated past to an open and inclusive institution valuing our employees, students, faculty, patients and their families, and visitors. The changes we made, I believe, were the result of a genuine commitment to engage and honor our entire Duke family, listen to their views, and do all we could to ensure upward mobility, equity, and diversity throughout the system. While the job is not yet done, I believe the strides we made created a more just and embracing institution. It has been a long time since I've heard the term, "Duke Plantation," and that is a very good thing.

10

—

Duke Clinical Research Institute

My first reappointment as chancellor allowed our team to make progress on a range of initiatives whose impacts played out over subsequent years. As hard as it may be to make decisions, it is often much harder to implement them successfully. One of the long-term efforts we set in motion in the early 1990s deserves special description because it remains one of the medical center's preeminent accomplishments, and one of which I am very proud.

Duke has a long reputation of trendsetting in clinical research. In 1966, under the leadership of Gene Stead, chair of the Department of Medicine, Duke, more than most of its sister institutions, recognized the importance of clinical research. I was a resident when Gene initiated the use of computers in medicine at Duke, beginning what later became known as the Duke Cardiovascular Database. This first-of-its-kind system collected long-term information about how heart patients responded to care. It created a "living medical textbook" that has become the world's oldest and largest cardiac outcomes database. Both Gene and his successor, Jim Wyngaarden, understood the critical importance of high-quality clinical investigation at academic medical centers, recognized the need for the training of clinical investigators and felt that the specialty was underappreciated at other academic institutions. I shared these views.

In the early 1990s, I began discussions with Robert M. Califf, a professor in the Department of Medicine, about further expanding Duke's presence in the field of clinical investigation. Rob, one of the best academic clinical investigators in the world, was also a great proponent of clinical research and of the value of the clinical investigator. He understood clearly that the practice of medicine was about to be transformed by biomedical research, but that clinical research was needed to translate these discoveries into sound, reliable clinical applications. As Rob put it, physicians must have evidence that the medicine they practice really works, or at least some sense of the extent to which it works. A way to accumulate such evidence is through clinical trials. Such trials, however, not only must be designed accurately but also must have transparency. In pharmaceutical drug development, this was not the general rule.

Pharmaceutical companies usually worked with commercial contract research organizations (CROs) to conduct most of the clinical trials needed for regulatory approval. The trials invariably went forward on company terms, and negative outcomes of clinical trials were rarely published. The result, in Rob's opinion and that of many others, was that the companies sponsoring clinical trial research accrued the clinical data and possessed undue influence over the publication of clinical results. Rob and I believed strongly that academic medical centers could add to the creativity of clinical trials and act as honest brokers through the free publication of clinical trial information. Indeed, academic medical centers might objectively provide the evidence to determine what constituted effective clinical therapeutics.

Rob and I started collaborating on clinical research trials while I was at Genentech, and for good reason. Genentech had been preparing to commercialize Activase, a genetically engineered protein known as tissue plasminogen activator (t-PA), which quickly dissolved clots obstructing coronary arteries and thus could save the lives of millions of people who would otherwise die from heart attacks. One of my jobs as head of research and development at Genentech was to finish the clinical development of Activase and get the drug approved by the FDA. Eric J. Topol, who was then at Cleveland Clinic, and Rob led many of the clinical trials that demonstrated the clinical value and safety of t-PA, so I got to know Rob and Eric well. Activase won approval for the treatment of acute myocardial infarction in November 1987 and provided a breakthrough therapy for a leading cause of death in the United States.

A year after its being marketed, however, published findings by European researchers suggested that t-PA was no better at saving lives than the older and far cheaper standard, streptokinase. We greatly doubted these conclusions, since many studies showed that t-PA worked far more quickly than streptokinase and, therefore, should save more heart muscle. Regardless, Genentech needed to prove this contention. To do so, Genentech chose to again work with Rob and Eric. This constituted a gamble for the company because the trials were very expensive and complex, and if t-PA didn't outperform streptokinase, the investigators were free to—and undoubtedly would—publish that information. Nonetheless, Genentech believed that objective data always should be made available, and if t-PA really wasn't better, it should not and would not be commercialized as planned.

In many ways Genentech's early success depended on the quality of the clinical trials conducted by Rob, Eric, and others. I witnessed firsthand the power of outstanding clinical investigation. Rob and his team set up an extensive network of hospitals and doctors across the United States and the world to conduct a trial, called Global Utilization of Streptokinase and t-PA for Occluded Arteries (GUSTO), comparing the survival benefit of t-PA versus streptokinase. Some study sites were academic medical centers, but most were community hospitals located in fifteen countries. A twenty-four-hour center was established to randomize newly enrolled patients from around the globe. Within two years, more than forty-one thousand patients participated in the trial, which found that using t-PA saved the lives of two thousand heart attack victims a year in the United States alone.

Under Rob's leadership at Duke, the Division of Cardiology in the Department of Medicine had developed a remarkable capability to perform large clinical trials such as GUSTO—multiple-center clinical research of the highest caliber. Rob's enterprise was prolific and profitable, and he wanted to expand it. From conversations with Rob, along with the help of numerous individuals including Bill Donelan, the vice chancellor for administration and chief financial officer, and Bob Taber, the newly recruited head of the Office of Science and Technology, we discussed the possibility of moving Rob's clinical investigation operations from the Division of Cardiology to an institution-wide entity. This would be necessary to broaden the scope of the clinical research being performed. In any case, neither the Division of Cardiology nor the Department of Medicine had the resources to expand Rob's program. Thus, the concept of the Duke Clinical Research Institute

(DCRI) took root: an institutional research structure to enable first-class clinical research in any clinical department throughout Duke. Nothing like this had ever existed at Duke or at any other medical center.

The creation of the DCRI was neither straightforward nor without risk. Rob operated administratively within the Division of Cardiology of the Department of Medicine, and the department chair distributed the revenues Rob's research generated. Moving such a highly regarded entity out of its founding department's purview, especially one generating surplus revenue, was bound to meet with resistance. And it did, specifically from Joe Greenfield, the department chair.

Expanding this program from a cardiology focus into an institutional role also required the infusion of considerable resources from the central administration. As chancellor and dean, I presumably had the authority to order this move, but there was little in the way of surplus resources available to me at that point to finance it—and overcoming the resistance of the chair of medicine proved to be a feat in itself. We nevertheless came up with the funds, and the Department of Medicine ultimately acquiesced, but not without prolonged and difficult negotiations.

We spent nearly a year designing the organizational structure and the business model for the DCRI. Based on my experience at Genentech, I knew that success depended on entrepreneurial-minded and focused leadership, as well as tremendous energy and creativity. The ultimate structure we devised can be likened to a corporation established within an academic medical center. It resembled a public corporation in that the DCRI had its own officers, board of directors, and so forth. There was also broad representation from other clinical departments, and we recruited outside experts to help run the operation. Fittingly, the DCRI was not formally incorporated, remaining wholly under the supervision of the medical center. By organizing the project in this way, the DCRI overcame the silo mentality so common in academic medical centers. Rob became its director/CEO, of course, and I assumed the role of chairman of its Board of Directors.

The DCRI initially received faint praise and even a bit of scorn from the academic deans of other leading medical schools. When I started talking about it at a meeting of the AAMC Council of Deans, the audience was highly skeptical. Several of my colleagues—from places like Harvard and Penn—asked me, in essence, why I was wasting my time on this type of endeavor. Top-tier academic institutions championed investigator-initiated laboratory research—that, the argument went, was where major original discoveries were made and where honor and praise were bestowed. Clinical research was dismissed as *applied* research and therefore less creative—or so went the line. Teams, not individuals, were required, and it was less lucrative professionally because the NIH inadequately funded it.

It was true that clinical research findings, while extremely valuable for clinical practice, rarely produced the "eureka" discoveries that came from investigator-led biomedical research. With NIH dollars and research discoveries as coin of the realm, clinical investigation assumed a second-rate status. Understandably, most medical school deans put far greater value on their faculty performing investigator-initiated laboratory research. While we fully valued and supported discovery research at Duke, we still pursued the DCRI track aggressively because it was important, and I could see that new computerized means of manipulating "big data" resources would empower clinical research to do things few at that time imagined were even possible. I believed that clinical investigation would soon become a major pursuit for academic medicine and that our leading institutions needed to step up to their role in recognizing it. As we developed the structure for the DCRI, we engaged many leading academic medical centers to join us in a collaborative effort. Despite herculean efforts, we found no takers. So, we went it alone.

Our desire to encourage and enable academic institutions to play a greater role in leading industry-sponsored clinical research led to the creation of the DCRI in 1996 during my second term. The impact of our actions far exceeded any of our initial ambitions. Indeed, the DCRI generated substantial benefit for Duke, academic medicine, and health care in general. Today, Duke's DCRI is the world's largest academic clinical research organization, with more than 1,100 employees, including 200 faculty. Since its inception, studies have been conducted at 37,500 sites in more than sixty-five countries. Over 1.2 million patients have been enrolled in clinical trials in more than twenty therapeutic areas. Further, the DCRI continues to expand into new fields, such as genomics, and the institution is capable of conducting any clinical research project, from the smallest pilot study to truly global trials, as well as postapproval analyses and health economics studies. Faculty have published more than 8,300 articles in peer-reviewed journals, and in 2008, Duke's sister school in Singapore launched the Singapore Clinical Research Institute—the DCRI's first "franchise."

An initial goal of the DCRI was to facilitate Duke's ability to conduct large national and international clinical trials, particularly for emerging biotherapeutics. The DCRI's success is evidenced by the number of trials, and the amount of revenue, it has produced. It has funded both the spectacular building that houses the DCRI and an expansion in manpower that has already outgrown that building. The DCRI gave Duke the appropriate infrastructure to allow its faculty to successfully pursue large clinical research grants and conduct outstanding research; Duke's dramatic ascent in the rankings of NIH grant recipients to a substantial degree flowed from the creation of the DCRI and the culture it fostered.

Put simply, the creation of the DCRI helped establish Duke as an innovator and leader in academic medicine. The initial reluctance of top-tier academic institutions to support clinical research dissolved quickly as the spectacular successes of the DCRI became evident. Indeed, the creation of the national Clinical Research Forum in 1996 followed close on the creation of the DCRI. Today, the forum is composed of fifty of the nation's most prestigious and acclaimed academic health centers and professional organizations, which are energetically involved in pursing clinical research investigation along the pathway laid by the DCRI.

Perhaps the most singular effect of the DCRI has been in sparking cultural recognition of the intrinsic value of the academic clinical investigator. In a seminal article published in 1979, entitled "The Clinical Investigator as an Endangered Species," Jim Wyngaarden had decried academic medicine's lack of focus on clinical investigation.[1] He pointed out that one of the reasons the clinical investigator had become an endangered species was that little nurturing or recognition existed within the academic institutions that provided its ecosystem.

We decided to do things differently at Duke. To support academic clinical researchers, we created a clinical research tenure track to allow the development of a strong academic research faculty. The DCRI provided a home for such individuals on our faculty and demonstrated to other academic institutions that this was an appropriate recognition of creative clinical investigation.

Moreover, we acknowledged through the DCRI that clinical investigation required training unlike that needed to be successful as a bench scientist. Clinical investigators needed to understand the science of clinical investigation, issues regarding human subjects, clinical trial design, and biostatistics—all critical skills for a well-trained clinical investigator. To train these investigators, we created a Clinical Research Training Program leading to a master's degree in clinical investigation, which quickly became among the strongest in the country. Once the program was established, I collaborated with my colleague John I. Gallin, NIH clinical director, to make Duke the degree-granting institution for clinical investigator trainees at the NIH. Since the creation of the NIH Clinical Center in the fall of 1998, through 2016, the center, in partnership with Duke University, has enrolled 229 individuals from various NIH institutes and centers, and 111 of the graduates have received degrees from Duke University. In 2000, the Department of Biostatistics and Bioinformatics was created to strengthen the academic infrastructure needed to foster clinical and translational research.

Duke established a culture that acknowledged the work of clinical investigators and heightened their status by encouraging clinical trainees to enter this increasingly important field. To provide professional opportunities for top-notch clinical investigators, the medical school created a new tenured clinical investigator track. This allowed clinical research faculty to devote up to 50 percent of their time to clinical research. Promotion depended on the quality of their clinical research as well as excellence in patient care.

Meanwhile, the NIH, under the leadership of its director at the time, Elias Zerhouni, increasingly understood that one of its important functions, in addition to funding investigator-initiated discovery research, was to create processes to translate discoveries into clinical use and adoption. The DCRI allowed Duke to compete successfully for the newly created Clinical Translational Science Awards (CTSA), which were designed to support translational research. Duke was among the first institutions not only to receive such a grant but also to receive the highest score of any competing institution.

More important than Duke's status, the DCRI has had a tremendous impact on the improvement of public health in the United States. Where pharmaceutical research was once strictly controlled by the businesses that funded the trials—they agreed to work with you only if they owned the data and had final say on whether to publish—we changed all that. We decided early on that the DCRI would be co-owner of all clinical research data collected during trials, and that the faculty within the DCRI would have the rights to publish the findings whether or not they supported the goals of the commercial entity that funded the research. In other words, we insisted on research transparency at a time before the concept took on its current importance. In time, even the drug companies themselves admitted this was a prescient decision. Indeed, in some ways it was the foundational forerunner of the decision between the NIH and several major pharmaceutical companies to share data on key basic pharmacological research.

The DCRI will have an increasingly important impact on the quality of health care delivery as we move forward in the genomic age. The development of novel therapeutics requires unbiased and accurate analysis that only professional-quality clinical investigation can provide. Not only are the research findings extremely valuable for evaluating therapeutics, but the policy the DCRI established and has firmly held to ever since also provides a shining national example of an academic medical center's ability to evolve in fulfilling the need for outstanding clinical investigation.

Fittingly, in 2004 I was pleased to author an article in *JAMA* entitled "The Clinical Researcher: An 'Emerging' Species."[2] This was an appropriate bookend to Jim Wyngaarden's "endangered species" article; mine demonstrated the emergence of a new understanding of the vital need for the support of academic clinical investigation to improve health care. I am proud to have contributed to a conversation that Jim Wyngaarden commenced. Perhaps even more fittingly, Rob Califf was appointed as Commissioner of FDA in 2016.

11

—

Duke University Health System

The financial viability of the medical center depended on complex cross-subsidization using margins from those operations that produced a financial surplus to support essential functions that could not fund their own activities. The vast majority of funds to support education and research came from margins created by Duke Hospital or clinical department practices operated by the PDC. By 1991, margins from clinical revenues had declined in all the departments, threatening the viability of the institution as a whole. Evaporating margins from Duke Hospital added to the more austere clinical environment.

Several factors caused the shrinking of clinical margins. Changes in government regulations reduced reimbursement levels for Medicare and Medicaid patients. Private insurers followed suit, and an emphasis on cost reduction ensued. Then came managed care—a new, ultimately insidious movement out of California. Paul M. Ellwood, Jr. and Alain Enthoven of Stanford developed the concept of managed care in the mid-1980s. These leading clinical scholars recognized that the practice of medicine could be greatly improved by making primary care physicians responsible for coordinating all of the patient's care. Such coordination promised to minimize unneeded and expensive specialty care and was motivated by a noble and medically positive intention.

Alas, Ellwood and Enthoven failed to anticipate what would happen when nonmedical managers and insurance companies got hold of the managed care system. Insurers and employers quickly figured out a way to reduce health care costs by restricting an individual's access to expensive clinical interactions and interventions, whether medically indicated or not. Insurance companies began demanding that care be directed by primary care physicians acting as "gatekeepers" for services. Referrals would be heavily restricted by decisions rendered by those who were not medical professionals. More important, referrals would be limited to approved physicians and hospital networks whose rates were held low through competitive bidding.

Managed care competition had drastically cut income from patient care on the West Coast and was moving rapidly across the country. Many prominent academic medical centers felt the pinch, with some selling their teaching hospitals to for-profit corporations. It became increasingly obvious in my second full year as chancellor that for DUMC to survive, we needed to develop a more coherent and synergistic approach to the practice of medicine. We had to figure out how to deliver better care for less money.

The 1991 Long Range Plan helped us find the answer to the challenge. By 1993, as our thinking evolved, we had envisioned the need for a new Duke University health system to be a regional provider of cost-effective care. That meant providing a geographic extension of our services through a broad network of primary care affiliates who would refer patients to the central operation. The idea was that the health system would resemble metaphorical "hub and spokes." The hub would be situated within a strong campus core, and the spokes would radiate out, forming a network of both collaborating primary care physicians, many of whom were our own alumni, and other regional hospitals and clinics. We formed an integrated planning group consisting of representatives from Duke Hospital, the PDC, and clinical departments to engage in strategic planning, the aim of which was to develop a comprehensive program in managed care.

A huge concern for Duke's entire clinical enterprise back in 1991 consisted of the highly specialized Duke Hospital and roughly nine hundred PDC faculty clinicians whose clinical practices were almost entirely specialty-based. Referrals came from physicians with no connection to Duke who wanted their patients to get Duke-quality care. As these physicians became members of networks that were not affiliated with Duke, their referrals to our physicians diminished drastically. Thanks to the sudden proliferation of managed care, referrals now had to stay "in network," and these lower-cost networks often did not include Duke.

By the early 1990s, Duke's clinical practice operations were becoming increasingly problematic financially for a number of reasons. All clinicians practicing in Duke Hospital and its clinics were members of clinical departments and, as faculty, were expected to teach and often do research as part of their responsibilities. For many, clinical work played only a secondary role within their overall professional responsibilities. In addition, the clinical faculty were almost all specialists, so that the composition of their practice rarely met comprehensive clinical needs. These specialists also faced increasing competition from outside providers, many of whom trained at Duke but were actual competitors. Finally, no overall coordination of the various clinical practices existed. The clinicians were members of divisions within their own departments but with few links to other clinicians they might have needed for consultations on complex issues. Clinical consultations among Duke faculty operated within informal professional networks based on who knew whom, and getting things done often required a personal call. There was no central appointment system, let alone strategic oversight of the system, to facilitate efficient coordination. The incentive structure pointed in a different direction; clinical faculty were hired and retained by chairs whose individual needs and goals were generally narrow and parochial. As a result, the ability to coordinate patient care suffered, and further threatened the bottom line.

The nominal operating entity for the faculty practice, the PDC, allowed clinical faculty to have private medical practices, and thus income, outside their university responsibilities. From its inception in 1931, the PDC had been a for-profit entity, but in 1972, its tax status faced an IRS challenge. In response, the PDC reorganized itself as a general partnership and entered into a formal agreement with Duke Hospital and the university dictating a "5(b)" revenue stream to the medical center for use of the facilities in lieu of rent. The reorganization stipulated that only Duke faculty could practice in the PDC. When patients required hospitalization, they were generally admitted to Duke Hospital and cared for by the admitting physician and the hospital house staff. While the PDC performed many of the administrative services necessary to practice medicine (such as billing and collections), it was not designed to coordinate the practices or provide strategic oversight. The PDC was organized into two divisions—the Medical PDC and the Surgical

PDC. The board met annually at a perfunctory session, but the real operations depended on direction from the department chairs and their designees. This arrangement served the functions of the chairs and the hospital until the late 1980s, but pressing needs for greater efficiency and the coherence that could produce it were putting great strains on the entire clinical operations.

Among the greatest challenges of my first term was dealing with the need to coordinate clinical care. This was made difficult by the independent structure of the PDC and the outright resistance of the chair of medicine to any change. The chancellor had no authority to oversee the PDC other than removing clinical chairs—a difficult step I was forced to take. My best option was to cultivate consensus among the clinical chairs regarding the need to coordinate and rationalize care, and then to work with them to modernize the PDC operations in the direction of a comprehensive clinical practice.

Fortunately, as the issues with Joe Greenfield were resolved, medical center administration and the chairs did join together to reform our clinical practice. By 1995, the PDC had created four committees to oversee its operations: clinical affairs, managed care, PDC affairs, and primary care. Together we created an administrative board with Chuck Hammond, chair of OB/GYN, as its first chair. Paul R. Newman, a competent and fair administrator, assumed the task of the executive director of the PDC. Paul was an honest broker who worked effectively to bridge the needs of the PDC with those of the medical center and health system. Thus, by my second term, we were well on the way to transforming Duke's clinical practice from an example of atavistic medical feudalism to a form of shared governance. The independent nature of the PDC as a limited liability company remained unchanged throughout my tenure and continues through 2016. Nonetheless, over the years, increasing trust and collaborations have allowed the health system and PDC to work synergistically.

Meanwhile, there were fewer than fifty primary care physicians among all the Duke clinical departments, and Duke lacked any clinical network of its own to refer patients to its specialists, let alone an ability to manage care according to the new paradigm. Duke's specialty clinical enterprise thus became highly vulnerable in this new managed care culture. Insurers saw Duke's weakness and aggressively pursued contracts with decreased reimbursement for our service. This further undermined the stability and financial underpinning of the entire medical center. It is impossible to overstate the vulnerability this created. The situation grew so dire so quickly that it shocked many veterans of the Duke team into denial.

To help address these issues and to facilitate the creation of a genuine and financially viable health system, we established the Office of Managed Care to analyze the emerging changes in health care and their impact, extant and potential, on our clinical business. To that end we recruited Steve Sloate in 1992 from the University of Florida and named him vice chancellor for medical center planning. Along with the medical center leadership, Steve began developing a detailed understanding of Duke's clinical operations, professional referral patterns, and the demographics of patient referrals. With sufficient information gathered, we developed strategic plans for the creation of a health care network that could provide better and more co-ordinated care and that could, at the same time, sustain the outstanding specialty operations at Duke Hospital and clinics. Bill Donelan, along with Steve Sloate, Mark Rogers, and Al Swinney, played important roles in planning these next steps. Collaboration with the more operationally effective PDC was critical to the coordination and design of the system.

We envisioned the hub-and-spokes model as a clinical distribution system for patients in the geographic regions we served. We would develop primary care networks in areas from which our patients were generally referred and facilitate access to Duke-affiliated specialists and community hospitals located within these areas. When appropriate, the system would refer patients to the medical center at Duke. We also cultivated strategic relations with more distant community hospitals that referred patients to Duke. Duke specialists and clinics would be dispersed geographically to meet the referral needs of local primary care physicians and to provide convenient access to Duke's quality care. Duke Hospital, at the center of the campus hub, would be a major resource for tertiary and quaternary care for the entire region, the nation, and the world.

As time went on, we expanded this concept to include an even more comprehensive health system that provided nursing care, home infusion services, hospice care, and health insurance. This vision represented a major conceptual transformation for the role of the academic medical center, one that would assume a new overarching mission to utilize our skills in education, research, and clinical care to develop new models of health care delivery to benefit the people we serve. In ways we never could have anticipated, the relentless smaller innovations and improvements we set rolling from the outset provided the building blocks we ultimately used to build the larger system that saved the medical center from financial collapse.

To establish primary care physicians in our major referral areas, the medical center created Duke University Affiliated Physicians (DUAP) and purchased the practices of approximately fifty primary care physicians. This move established an important precedent because the medical center, not the clinical departments, hired these physicians as employees. We really had no choice since the clinical departments had neither the resources nor the desire to hire primary care physicians. To assure quality and synergies among the clinical departments, we recruited DUAP physicians jointly with the appropriate departments, and the physicians maintained clinical faculty appointments within them. These physicians were carefully selected for their skill, their location, and the nature of their practice. Unlike other academic medical centers that invested vast amounts of money to purchase the practices of hundreds of primary care physicians, Duke entered this area cautiously, selectively, and prudently. We carefully linked the numbers and natures of hired physicians to the system's needs.

Another part of the plan involved creating a strong contracting network to improve our negotiating strength with insurers. To do this, we formed an independent practice association called PrimaHealth, which created an opportunity for non-Duke primary care physicians in our referral areas to affiliate with DUAP and the PDC for the purpose of negotiating insurance contracts. Such a large and comprehensive physician network made it virtually impossible for insurers to exclude their members from our panels. This amounted to a form of collective bargaining in which we increased our market power. PrimaHealth began operations in 1997 with twelve hundred physicians, four hundred of them private community physicians from Durham, Orange, Franklin, Granville, Person, and Vance Counties. This network proved crucial to Duke's ability to create highly desirable primary care networks. In addition, to foster referrals from an even broader area and to improve regional care, the medical center developed close affiliations with hospitals throughout North Carolina and the Southeast, including Lumberton, North Carolina; Danville, Virginia; Beaufort, South Carolina; and Naples, Florida. By 1995, after the start of my second term, Duke operated a health care delivery and referral network that covered a large part of the Southeast and involved relationships as far away as Buenos Aires, Argentina.

Our operational plan assumed the need for close relationships with community hospitals in Durham and nearby counties—particularly Wake County, where the greatest population growth was occurring. A direct presence in Wake County, moreover, would enable us to expand into Johnston and Franklin Counties to the east. In 1996, the leadership of Rex Hospital in Raleigh also recognized the need to affiliate with a larger, more robust health care network. Two members of Rex Hospital's board began negotiations with Bill Donelan and me to determine if we could arrange a mechanism to bring Rex into the Duke network. As the conversations continued, it became clear that important conceptual differences existed between us. Rex wanted local independence and control; Duke needed the Raleigh hospital to be fully integrated with the Duke health system.

While our difficult negotiations with Rex proceeded, we learned of the pending sale of the 218-bed Raleigh Community Hospital by the Hospital Corporation of America, which was divesting itself of a number of community hospitals. By owning Raleigh Community Hospital, Duke could control its own clinical destiny in Wake County. We hoped initially to purchase Raleigh Community Hospital and still have a strategic relationship with Rex Hospital along the lines previously envisioned. But as our plans to purchase Raleigh Community Hospital became clear, the leadership of Rex shifted their negotiations toward the University of North Carolina. We ultimately purchased Raleigh Community Hospital in 1998, changed its name to Duke Hospital Raleigh, and built what is now a thriving community hospital with primary and specialty care clinics staffed by Duke and other community physicians. Rex Hospital eventually became part of the University of North Carolina Health System.

Duke's interest in Durham Regional Hospital had begun back in 1995 when I received a call from Richard Myers, president of the Durham Hospital Corporation, the parent organization of Durham Regional. He indicated that the hospital was doing poorly—in fact, it was in danger of financial collapse. He asked me whether Duke would help sustain the viability of Durham Regional Hospital. We could hardly have been more pleased to be the recipient of that question. By that point, we considered a strong relationship with Durham Regional Hospital as an absolutely essential piece of the Duke health system strategy. Over the next six months, the Duke and Durham Regional leadership teams met on numerous occasions and worked out mechanisms whereby Duke would take over responsibilities for managing Durham Regional Hospital and assure its financial viability. Just as we were about to reach an agreement with the Durham Regional board, however, the Durham County Commissioners suddenly made it clear that they would play the leading role in deciding the fate of Durham Regional Hospital. The hospital, after all, was a county-owned entity responsible for the health care of the citizens of Durham. The commissioners' intervention delayed matters for well over a year.

Regrettably, the relationship between the Durham County Commissioners and Duke University had been and remained rocky at times. Duke, particularly its medical center, was by far the largest employer in Durham, so it was not particularly surprising that the relationship between a major employer and county government would not always run smoothly, especially when it came to matters concerning money. The commissioners thought that Duke, as a tax-exempt organization, was not paying its fair share of taxes. They thought this despite the obvious fact that Duke employees who lived in Durham paid county taxes, and that many of them either would not have decent jobs or would not stay in the area without Duke.

Other issues besides money intruded as well. Many county residents, including a large portion of the African American population, worked at Duke and viewed the institution as racist, referring to it as a "plantation" that excluded African Americans from upper-level positions. To my knowledge, this had not been by design; those upper-level positions required the professional education and training that few African Americans in the area had access to at that time. Ironically, in an attempt to ease unemployment in Durham and to provide meaningful jobs at Duke, then president Terry Sanford and chancellor Bill Anlyan hired thousands of African Americans at Duke to operate the newly installed data terminals in the clinical facilities. The data terminal operators were entry-level positions and were occupied largely by African Americans, thereby further increasing their preponderance in lower-paid positions. We soon began to understand, however, that we needed to and could do more to mitigate the inequities of the past, and this became a focus of our attention as was discussed in chapter 9.

Tax revenue and racial legacies aside, the issue of health care delivery in Durham County was plenty complex. Prior to the early 1960s, Durham County had three hospitals. Watts Hospital served the white population and admitted no African Americans; Lincoln Hospital served the African American population; Duke, meanwhile, accepted both whites and African Americans but was strictly segregated. The segregation at Duke Hospital lasted until 1963 and generated strong negative and painful memories among the local black population. While racial segregation at Duke ended in 1963, de facto segregation continued far longer as a consequence of the economic stratification of clinics.

One story that resurfaced during the time we were seeking to oversee Durham Regional Hospital was that of Dr. Charles Drew, a noted black scientist and surgeon who pioneered research on the use of plasma transfusions. On April 1, 1950, Dr. Drew died of injuries suffered in an automobile accident not far from Durham. It was rumored that he died because a white hospital refused to treat him and, ironically, that he bled to death for lack of a transfusion from a segregated hospital. Some falsely believed that Duke Hospital was involved. In truth, Dr. Drew was treated by two white surgeons in the emergency room of the segregated Alamance General Hospital but died of his wounds.

Even more ironic, eight months later, Maltheus Avery, a student at A&T College in Greensboro, was in a serious car collision and was brought to the same Alamance General Hospital emergency room. The physician on call judged that Mr. Avery's head injuries were so severe that he needed to be sent to a neurosurgeon at Duke Hospital. By the time Mr. Avery got there, the Duke surgeon concluded that he would not benefit from brain surgery and instructed that he be taken to Lincoln Hospital because there were no beds for blacks available at Duke. Maltheus Avery died shortly after arriving at Lincoln. The full truth of the role of segregation in Mr. Avery's death cannot be known, but this story, along with that of Dr. Drew, understandably made a deep and lasting impression that segregation had hurt the health care of blacks in Durham. It also created a lingering animosity in some for the role that Duke had played in it.[1]

In 1976, when Watts Hospital and Lincoln Hospital merged to form the new county-owned Durham Regional Hospital, many in the African American community remained concerned about the ability of Durham Regional to provide them with the same quality and access to health care as Lincoln Hospital had done. Thus, as Duke sought to acquire Durham Regional Hospital, many old issues and past inequities surfaced. Would Duke be sensitive to the needs of all the citizens of Durham County, or would it treat all but white people as second-class patients?

After exhaustive and exhausting discussions, the county commissioners determined that rather than allow Duke to assume control of the four-hundred-bed Durham Regional Hospital, there would be a competitive bidding process for a long-term operating lease. The bidding began in late 1996; Duke, the University of North Carolina, Health Management Associates, and Tenet Health Care all submitted bids. Over the next six months, my number one priority was to ensure that Duke obtained this lease. I knew it would not be easy; several of the county commissioners seemed determined that Duke would not win the right to lease Durham Regional Hospital.

To better understand the concerns of the African American community and how Duke could address them, we scheduled question-and-answer sessions with any group in the community that was interested in speaking with us. On April 30, 1997, more than a hundred people filled the pews of the Union Baptist Church, a historically important institution in the civil rights movement in Durham in the early 1960s, to attend a two-hour program hosted by the Durham Committee on the Affairs of Black People. Richard Meyers, Evelyn Schmidt of Lincoln Community Hospital, and I were there to discuss the merger of the two hospitals. After our introductory remarks, I asked for questions from the audience. The first person to take the microphone was Howard Clement, an outspoken African American member of the Durham City Council. As Howard moved to the aisle to address us, a large banner hanging behind us from the ceiling commemorating the hundredth anniversary at the church came crashing to the ground. As the startled audience tried to regain its composure, Howard, being an excellent and theatrical speaker, did not skip a beat. He proclaimed: "That sign fell down, and whether that's symbolic or something we need to be concerned about. . . . We're in God's house. I want things done right. When I look up there, I'm not too positive whether or not things will be done right."

Despite this shaky and sometimes contentious start, the open and honest conversations between the Duke leadership and the community proved useful in enabling those of us at Duke to better understand the concerns of the community. Early on some of the commissioners leaned heavily toward choosing Tenent, a for-profit hospital chain, to lease Durham Regional. Through numerous meetings with many constituents in the community, the commissioners ultimately believed in the sincerity of Duke's commitment to provide all of Durham's citizens the best health care possible. With the leadership of MaryAnn Black (then chair of the Durham County Commissioners), the Durham County Commissioners and Duke ultimately agreed on a long-term lease for Durham Regional Hospital that has provided an outstanding solution for all.

During the tough selection process for Durham Regional and the hard negotiations that followed, I came to know and respect MaryAnn Black. MaryAnn, a social worker with a master's degree from the University of North Carolina, had worked in the Community Child Guidance Clinic at Duke between 1973 and 1982. In 2002, when she decided to leave politics, I offered her the position of director of community affairs—a key part of my leadership team. When we discussed her position, she asked how she could work for me as her boss when we had previously been equals in a hard bargaining situation. I said that if she joined us, we would work together as partners. MaryAnn often cited that conversation, noting happily that the arrangement worked out beautifully. I highly valued our partnership, and she continues to lead the DUMC's community health programs.

During our discussions with the leadership of Rex Hospital, Raleigh Community Hospital, Durham Regional Hospital, and the county commissioners, it became clear that we needed an organizational structure that could effectively operate a complex health system and also provide representation for entities within it. We needed the Durham community, Durham Regional Hospital, and Duke Hospital Raleigh all to be represented on the governing bodies of Duke's health system. The organizational structure of our health system at that time was in no way designed to allow community or regional representation on a governing board. Indeed, no specific governing body existed within the university or the medical center to oversee a broadly distributed health system with complex clinical operations and financial underpinnings. As structure follows from function in the human body, so it must do so in collective human endeavors.

Until 1998, the governance of Duke University, including the medical center, lay solely with the university's Board of Trustees. The chancellor for health affairs was responsible for the School of Medicine, the Graduate School of Nursing, and Duke Hospital and reported to the university president, who reported to the board. Oversight of the medical center by the university board included an annual presentation on the part of the chancellor for health affairs to the full board of the university. In addition, a subcommittee of the Executive Committee of the Board of Trustees oversaw the medical center, but it could in no way deal with the complexity and intricacies of an expanding clinical enterprise.

What we needed became obvious from our immersion in the new world of health care as it collided with business. Our vision emerged not from any stroke of genius but from a pragmatic and analytical recognition of reality. To survive this uncharted new world of health care, we needed to abandon the upside-down pyramid at Duke: high-margin specialty care delivered in a costly specialty hospital with no primary care base to refer patients to Duke or to lower-cost community hospitals when appropriate. Our medical practice and hospital were totally dependent on others referring high-margin patients to us, but all the incentives for them to do so were quickly disappearing. We needed to develop our own feeder network, that hub-and-spokes architecture for patients to receive an appropriate level of care. That meant, in turn, that we would have to invest money and energy to build a network and do things differently.

To keep the Board of Trustees better apprised of and involved in these changes as they were occurring, I created an informal group including key members of the trustee committees, the board chairman, the president, and me. We would gather for breakfast in my office before each meeting of the board, thus engendering the name "Breakfast Club." While this group became far more informed and involved with the medical center's clinical strategy, its purpose was not to oversee the health system we were building. There was simply no way that part-time laypeople could do that.

To help envision the organizational structure best suited to govern Duke's new clinical enterprise, we brought in David Anderson, principal with Health Care Futures, LP. David suggested several potential governing structures, and by late 1996, we in the medical center favored the concept of an entity called the Duke University Health System (DUHS), an independent, not-for-profit corporation wholly owned by Duke University. The DUHS concept rationalized the operations and governance of an increasingly complex and far-flung medical operation within a university and also allowed regional constituencies to serve on its governing board. In addition, it made the creation of a true DUHS Board of Directors possible. The board would include key university representation along with national health leaders and community representation to help guide us along our path. This would be a profound departure from the existing model of an academic medical center. No American medical center, anywhere else in the country, had put itself so far over its skis.

As we refined the checks and balances of what we considered appropriate within the university, I presented the concept of a corporate health system to a group of the university's leadership, including the chairman of the board, Randall L. Tobias. Suffice it to say, Randy's first response to our proposed creation of an "independent" health system owned by Duke University but not reporting directly to its president or board was not positive. He asked, "Why in the world would we want to do this?" The conversation abruptly ceased.

Over the succeeding months, however, the rationale for our proposal became clear to the board and to President Keohane. Nan appreciated the overarching importance of the medical center's success to that of the university itself, and it was obvious to her that Duke needed to create a new model of health care delivery to adapt to a changing environment. Roughly two-thirds of the university's budget related to the medical center, and the medical center's financial failure would crush Duke University's financials as well. So Nan supported the creation of DUHS, and through her we developed a general understanding and acceptance among the board members. Indeed, Randy Tobias became one of our greatest champions. On February 27, 1998, the board approved a resolution authorizing the incorporation of DUHS.

We paid careful attention to balancing a health system so that it would be sufficiently independent to succeed but not separate from the university. There needed to be university oversight of the emerging health system, but the medical complex had to be able to differentiate, take appropriate risks, including financial ones, and have the specialized leadership needed to run a complex integrated health operation. We determined that all members of the DUHS board would be appointed and retained by the university board. The university president and seven members of the university board would sit on the board of directors of the health system. The DUHS board would contain five independent members. The chancellor for health affairs would also be the president and CEO of the health system and a member of its board and would report to the health system board for his health system responsibilities. The new corporation included Duke Hospital and the affiliated business and clinical operations of the hospital, but it did not include the medical school and faculty or the PDC. We began operation of the health system in July 1998 with an absolutely outstanding Board of Directors consisting of twenty-one members. We soon developed one of the best regional health delivery systems in the country. The complete slate of the first DUHS Board of Directors is listed below:

MEMBERS OF THE BOARD OF TRUSTEES OF DUKE UNIVERSITY:

1. Ernest Mario, Chairman of the Board
   CEO, Aliza Corporation
2. Roscoe R. Robinson, Vice Chairman of the Board
   Vice chancellor emeritus, Vanderbilt University Medical Center
3. Roy J. Bostock
   Chairman and CEO, McManus Group
4. Edwin N. Sidman
   President, the Beacon Companies
5. Randall L. Tobias
   Chairman of the board and CEO, Eli Lilly Corporation
6. Harold L. Yoh, Jr.
   Chairman of the board and CEO, Day and Zimmerman, Inc.
7. Daniel T. Blue, Jr.
   North Carolina representative, partner, Thigpen Blue Stephens & Fellers Attorneys at Law

INDEPENDENT MEMBERS:

8. Frank A. Sloan
   McMahon Professor of Health Policy and Management and professor of economics, Duke University
9. John B. Anderson, Jr.
   Medical director and physician, Duke University Affiliated Physicians
10. Carl E. Ravin
    Professor and chair, radiology, Duke University Medical Center
11. Charles B. Hammond
    Professor and chair, OB/GYN, Duke University Medical Center
12. Jean G. Spaulding
    Vice chancellor for health affairs, Duke University Medical Center

13. Nannerl O. Keohane
   President, Duke University
14. Ralph Snyderman
   Chancellor for health affairs and dean of the School of Medicine,
   president and CEO of DUHS
15. William J. Donelan
   Vice chancellor for administration and chief financial officer of
   DUMC
16. Michael D. Israel
   Vice chancellor and CEO, Duke Hospital
17. Tallman Trask III
   Executive vice president, Duke University

INDIVIDUALS CHOSEN FOR THEIR ABILITY TO
CONTRIBUTE TO GOVERNANCE:

18. Mitchell T. Rabin
   Distinguished institute scholar, Institute for Education and Research, Beth Israel Deaconess Medical Center
19. Uwe E. Reinhardt
   Professor of political economy, Princeton University
20. Joe W. Bowser
   Durham county commissioner
21. Gary S. Wilson
   Hoskin Davis and Wilson

Following the incorporation of DUHS, its operational components included Duke Hospital and clinics; Durham Regional Hospital; Raleigh Community Hospital (now Duke Hospital Raleigh); DUAP; and NYL Care (later Well Path), a managed care company. The health system had numerous other strategic relationships with regional as well as distant hospitals and also collaborated with Galloway Ridge, a senior living facility, in Chatham County. It also created a joint venture with St. Josephs of the Pines, Triangle Hospice, and Chartwell Southeast, with the acquisition of United Methodist Retirement Home in the pipeline.

The university's health system was designed to integrate the best features of the corporate world with the uniqueness of its academic missions.

Most would agree that DUHS has been tremendously successful in this. By having an outstanding Board of Directors, with the DUHS CEO and president reporting to them yet remaining fully responsible to the president of the university as chancellor for health affairs, we managed to create that elusive, delicate balance between the corporate and academic worlds.

— — —

While serving as DUHS's first CEO and president, I was also fortunate to serve on the Board of Directors of Procter & Gamble (P&G), the world's leading consumer-product company. Procter & Gamble, similar to DUHS, also exhibits a hub-and-spokes model, with Cincinnati, Ohio at the center of the hub and marketing organizations throughout the world. Products and major corporate services flowed from Cincinnati, but the market development organization governed the businesses selling products in unique geographies.

There are obviously major differences between a consumer-product company and an academic health care delivery institution, but my experience on the P&G board and my contacts with major leaders of industry proved helpful in the development of DUHS. Indeed, as the concept of the distributed health system developed, I assembled an ad hoc group of advisers consisting of John Pepper (CEO of P&G), Roy Bostock, Ernie Mario, and Karl Von der Hayden (chief financial officer of PepsiCo). This group, along with my key senior leadership team, spent many hours with me discussing the concept and potential elements of an academic health network. Among the concepts we ultimately enacted were the clinical service units (CSUs), which organized major clinical areas such as cardiovascular disease, oncology, women's health, and musculoskeletal services as "product lines," with all their operating units integrated to deliver patient services across the entire system.

For example, in cardiovascular disease, the CSU was an ensemble of medical cardiology, cardiac imaging, cardiothoracic surgery, and cardiac anesthesiology in one organizational structure. This allowed services to be better organized, even created if necessary, and delivered to all patients who needed them. This concept is not altogether different from what occurs in industry, where, for example, P&G's Crest brand and its multiplicity of products are organized as a product line run out of Cincinnati but are sold in broad geographic areas such as the United States, Western Europe, Asia, and elsewhere. The creation of DUHS, in synergy with the academic components of the medical center and the university, allowed a degree of creativity and capability to create an entirely new model for academic medicine. As a consequence of Duke's novel and comprehensive approach to care, *Time* magazine devoted a full issue to the health system initiatives in October 1998 (see chapter 15).

— — —

In 1998, as DUHS began and my second five-year term as chancellor ended, I thought perhaps 1999 would be a good time for me to leave Duke and move on to other things. I also believed that the medical center might benefit from new leadership as it began its new enterprise. I raised this possibility with the leadership of the university and the board, but its members strongly expressed their desire for me to continue for another term. I took this request into account, but at that point I was genuinely undecided.

Then, once again, ten years after I left Genentech, another *beshert* (fated) evening in California bound me to Duke for another five years. I sat at dinner with Ernie Mario. He and I were discussing the fate of the new health system and sharing a bottle of wine in one of my favorite restaurants, 231 Ellsworth, in San Mateo. By the end of the evening, each of us had extracted a promise from the other. I would stay on for another term as chancellor and the first president and CEO of DUHS so long as Ernie agreed to be its first chairman of the board. This agreement turned out to be crucial to the new health system's eventual success.

In retrospect, it is clear that our health system design enabled Duke not only to succeed in an increasingly competitive and risky health care market but also to innovate and vastly improve the quality of care. We gave citizens throughout a large portion of North Carolina the opportunity to receive a full continuum of care from Duke, ranging from prevention and wellness through specialty care and ultimately hospice care. The success of DUHS played a major role in positioning the entire medical center as an engine of creativity and identifying it as among the best of the best in the country and the world.

The financial impact of DUHS has been huge, as well. When I arrived at Duke in 1989, medical revenues totaled $400 million; when I stepped down as chancellor, they exceeded $2.2 billion. During my final year as CEO, DUHS produced more than $100 million in cash flow from operations. By 2008, approximately $350 million had already been transferred to our medical school from the margins the health system had generated. To be sure, DUHS secured the finances of the School of Medicine, made possible new cross-disciplinary institutes, provided a source of superb health care throughout North Carolina and beyond, and helped found the field of personalized health care. Duke had made the future its friend; the alternative was too dire to contemplate, so I never did.

12

—

Integrative Medicine

One of my great joys as chancellor was starting most days by walking through the grand front doors of the Davison Building on the Duke campus. Before entering, I would frequently gaze up and admire the building's beautiful Gothic architecture, then open the heavy wooden doors, ascend the few stairs, and, before turning left to enter my office, look at the colorful posters in the corridor announcing visiting speakers.

One morning in 1995, I couldn't help but notice a large poster with a picture of hands above a human abdomen with the title "Healing Hands: The Power of Touch." A closer look revealed that the Duke Faculty group on integrative medicine was sponsoring the talk. I knew of no such program or group at Duke. Given that the term had a connotation of alternative and complementary therapies, I was surprised that we had an organization interested in and evidently promoting this approach. Primarily out of curiosity, I asked my assistant to invite the leaders of this group—Drs. Martin J. Sullivan and Larry Burk—to my office so that I could learn about it.

The concept of integrative medicine was not entirely new to me at the time. I had recently read a manuscript by Harvard physician David M. Eisenberg calling attention to the vast use and recent growth of complementary and alternative therapies in the United States. Dr. Herbert Benson, also of Harvard, had recently published several fascinating articles concerning the power of the placebo effect and the relaxation response, both features of mind-body interactions. Additionally, I had been exploring the ideas of billionaire Sir John Templeton, founder of The John Templeton Foundation, who was funding projects focusing on the importance of spirituality in medicine. John Templeton was introduced to me by my good friends, John and Joy Safer, loyal Duke supporters. Even more important perhaps was my recent visit to Atlantic Beach, North Carolina, where I had participated in a brief program demonstrating the power of guided mental imagery in relieving stress. So I looked forward with anticipation to my meeting with Marty and Larry.

When they entered my office, the two doctors, knowing nothing about my budding interest in the subject, appeared anxious about having been summoned to see me. I later learned that they feared they were being taken to the woodshed for engaging in unscientific, "flippy" activities unbecoming of a serious institution. That was not the case at all, as they soon found out to their great relief. During the meeting, they explained their interest in exploring alternative approaches combined with traditional care; they also described a program in anodyne imagery they hoped to bring to Duke. Anodyne imagery provides patients with techniques to reduce their perception of pain while undergoing potentially painful procedures. I found this approach interesting given my recent experience with guided imagery. Based on my conversations with Marty and Larry, I agreed to provide a small amount of central support to bring in an anodyne imagery instructional team to see what impact it might have at Duke.

Not surprisingly, when I discussed this idea with our clinical chairs, skepticism filled the air. One chair in particular, Allen Frances of the Department of Psychiatry, sent me an e-mail stating (tongue in cheek, I hope) that for some time he had wondered if I was losing it; now he knew I was. He was clearly suggesting that anodyne imagery was comparable to Shirley MacLaine–style pyramid power and other "new age" hallucinations. He was mistaken, and once Marty and Larry demonstrated the technique to physicians in the Department of Anesthesiology, they were impressed enough to begin evaluating its effectiveness. Several months later this approach found its way onto a national TV news feature that highlighted a patient at Duke receiving anodyne imagery prior to a coronary artery procedure. The patient indicated that among multiple such procedures he had previously endured, this one was the least traumatic and was, indeed, pleasant.

Perhaps encouraged by the lack of obstruction, and with guarded support from the medical center administration, Marty, Larry, and their colleague, Jeffrey Brantley, cautiously began to lead efforts to bring integrative medicine to Duke. I was supportive, though not effusive beyond what the science allowed us to suppose.

Privately, however, I was more optimistic than I let on. In the fall of 1996, I had attended a major mind-body conference at the Hotel Europa in Chapel Hill where the keynote speaker was Jon Kabat-Zinn, who developed the Mindfulness Based Stress Reduction program at the University of Massachusetts Medical Center. Jon was well known for his work in clinical applications of mindfulness meditation and had published several popular books, one of which, *Wherever You Go, There You Are*, became a best-selling primer on the subject. I went to hear Jon speak and sat in the front row. His presentation was spectacular, exciting, and invigorating. His talk opened my eyes to the potential power of mindfulness meditation. Jon was able to engage those around him to be "in the moment" and thereby have a finer appreciation of ordinary experiences that are almost invariably missed in the hurried flow of everyday life.

Jon demonstrated how simple techniques can focus attention to create vivid experiences. He illustrated this by leading the audience through the process of eating a raisin mindfully. After passing one raisin to each attendee, he asked us to envision grapes growing in the warm sun over the summer as they slowly dry and increase their sugar content. We were led to explore the sight and feel of the raisin as we rolled it between our fingers, to inhale the raisin's intense aroma, then to feel it as we put it on our lips and tongue. When we finally bit the raisin, its taste virtually exploded in our mouths—a far cry from the usual experience of gobbling down a handful of raisins at once.

Jon also described a way to condition the mind to be present in the moment and more aware of the importance of time and place. The richness and power of mindfulness were astounding. In my view, the benefits of mindfulness required mental conditioning, similar to the physical conditioning I had developed by being a committed runner since the age of thirty-seven. Running had become a major factor in improving my health, well-being, physical conditioning, and ability to handle stressful situations. It seemed as though mindfulness training could have similar and perhaps even more powerful effects on the brain.

At the end of Jon's talk, I rose and embraced him and asked if we could talk at greater length. He and I went to his hotel room, where we spoke for at least two hours. I plied him with questions, and he tried to formulate answers that would satisfy my ingrained scientific skepticism. I didn't doubt that the methods worked; what I wanted to know was how and why they worked. Jon kindly and generously shared his thoughts. I had the sense of having wandered through a desert, hot and parched, and having suddenly come upon an oasis.

My exposure to Jon Kabat-Zinn and mindfulness meditation opened my curiosity to concepts and techniques that were not a part of conventional Western medicine. Until late 1996, I based my thinking about medicine, and even life, on my training and experience as a physician-scientist. I truly believed, although I never gave it a great deal of conscious thought, that science and technology would eventually solve all medical problems. I paid little attention to fields outside of science. I was a normal, Skinnerian-age reductionist, a typical late-twentieth-century positivist who did not have enough philosophical knowledge to realize it. This soon changed.

In my annual presentations to the Duke University Board of Trustees, I typically described important research discoveries made at Duke during the prior year and then extrapolated on their potential benefits for the future treatment of disease. There was something exciting to say every year—such were the continuous power and creativity of the Duke research operation. That said, in preparing for my board presentation in 1996, and after assembling the most important research discoveries made at Duke and elsewhere, I concluded it would take two decades or longer for most of the recent discoveries to make a difference in medical care. Still more troublesome, even in their aggregate the discoveries would likely not address more than 20 percent of the complex problems our patients faced day in and day out. I was beginning to appreciate that science and technology alone were but partial solutions to our medical challenges.

As a practicing physician, I had treated many patients suffering from rheumatoid arthritis, a chronic, destructive disease of the joints. I recall one particular patient with whom I had developed a close physician-patient relationship. She suffered from severe rheumatoid arthritis, and at that time, there were no effective therapies to blunt the progress of the disease. The best I could do was to jiggle her aspirin dosage to provide better relief. At the end of her appointments, I frequently thought to myself, "You fraud;

you haven't helped her at all. Her disease will continue as though you weren't even here." Only many years later did I understand how foolish I had been. This woman kept coming back because she valued a caring relationship with her physician. I had been oblivious at the time to the critically important distinction between curing and caring. While I couldn't always cure, I could always care, and the latter could be as powerful as the former in helping patients manage their heath challenges.

Over time I came to understand that those two concepts, curing and caring, needed to be brought together in practice. As I became more appreciative of integrative approaches, it finally dawned on me that for us to provide better care for the patients we served, we needed to explore therapeutic opportunities beyond those derived from strict laboratory-based research. Though I had given lip service to this notion before as a form of medical-professional diplomacy, I had failed to really see the practical potential of integrative medicine. Its central feature is awareness of the patient's whole set of relationships—to his or her self, loved ones, physician, and environment—and making these interactions more humane and effective in addressing the patient's health needs.

By 1997, I wished to explore more fully the field of integrative medicine to learn what it had to offer in practical terms—terms that could perhaps be institutionalized in some useful programmatic ways. In no way did I then, or since, leave my scientific roots and my firm belief in the power of science to improve medicine. The conviction, after all, is borne out each day. However, I now entertained the view that medical science needed to embrace a more compassionate and thoughtful analysis of how to fully respond to the needs of our patients. I was intrigued with the potential of mindfulness meditation.

In February 1997, Marty Sullivan; William E. Kraus, a Duke cardiologist focused on cardiovascular prevention; and I visited with Jon Kabat-Zinn at his Center for Mindfulness at the University of Massachusetts School of Medicine. Jon's program was fully integrated with the medical services at the University of Massachusetts Medical Center. He had clinics with perhaps three dozen patients undergoing mindfulness meditation in addition to their usual therapies. Jon and his colleague, Saki F. Santorelli, had accumulated substantial data indicating that for many people, mindfulness meditation greatly improved their ability to deal with their clinical problems. From that time onward, I embraced the need to better understand the integration of curing and caring.

This was not a radical alteration of my attitudes but rather an indication of what I considered a mature growth in them. There were plenty of undocumented and outlandish claims for alternative and complementary therapies. I had not become more susceptible to them; rather I was opening my mind to the possibility that not all alternative approaches were futile. I appreciated the power of perception in creating feelings of well-being and enhancing responses to therapy. I began to accept nontraditional therapies if they worked, but not the unscientific mechanisms often ascribed to them. I became increasingly aware of the importance of caring and compassion on the part of physicians to more fully meet the needs of patients—that is, going beyond the traditional offerings consisting of drugs and procedures.

This change in my thinking was perhaps most evident when it came to the needs of patients with cancer. A cancer diagnosis may be the worst news an individual can receive; it is a wrenching emotional experience. The patient requires the best in medical, surgical, and radiation therapies, but this is clearly far from sufficient. He or she also needs to deal with the anxiety, pain, and potential depression and with the grueling consequences of long-term chemotherapy. I hoped that a more organized approach to holistic care would provide patients with services ranging from access to support groups and wigs for hiding hair loss, to instruction in mindfulness meditation, nutrition, and therapeutic massage. To focus only on medicine, surgery, and radiation oncology, and to ignore the power of compassion, overlooked the needs of patients as human beings. Medicine, I now believed, should get past the image of patients as essentially broken bodies. It should see them instead as whole human beings—not to satisfy any philosophical urge but because this would produce more effective clinical outcomes.

The need for such comprehensive services became vividly clear to me one day when I received a call from a woman, a CEO in Philadelphia whom I had met several weeks earlier at a conference. During the call, she indicated that she had just learned she had breast cancer. Despite leading a successful company and having excellent health insurance, she was anxious, fearful, and lost. She needed help in navigating her medical, surgical, and radiation oncology care, but she also needed hope, a plan for success, and a greater level of support to achieve that success.

I was beginning to understand more completely that the predominant approach to health care nationally and at Duke was reactive. It focused on identifying and treating disease. Starting with medical education through medical practice to therapy, the role of the physician in this paradigm was to define the cause of the patient's present illness and to expunge its specific cause and thereby mitigate the problem. This "find-it and fix-it" mentality based on a century of the application of reductionist science to the practice of medicine had yielded great breakthroughs in the treatment of many diseases, but it was proving increasingly inadequate in dealing with more complex, chronic diseases with multifocal causes. Importantly, the care of patients with chronic disease was focused largely on addressing the specific disease pathology rather than appreciating the more multifactorial and holistic needs of the individual in dealing with his or her condition.

As I continued to learn about and embrace the thoughts of leaders in the field of integrative medicine, I realized there were important disciplines focusing heavily on how to best engage individuals in their own health and well-being that lay outside the parochial areas of medicine in which I had spent my entire professional life. Given that most physicians and medical scientists considered alternative and complementary strategies to have no place in conventional medicine, I found myself increasingly at odds with the orthodox professional consensus. But I nevertheless felt confident in embracing a concept of integrative medicine that elevated the status and utility of adjunctive strategies such as mindfulness meditation, nutrition, therapeutic massage, and perhaps acupuncture to more fully address our patients' needs. Medicine as a kind of guild can be very conservative, and not always in a way that benefits patients. Change sometimes takes a little bravery. I realized that if a hard-nosed scientist in the field of medicine, like me, could understand that improving care might require at least entertaining, and perhaps embracing, selected strategies not yet proven effective through rigorous research, then others might follow.

With all this in mind, in 1998 I encouraged and supported the creation of the Duke Center for Integrative Medicine (DCIM) and appointed Marty Sullivan as its first director. With a grant from the Duke Endowment and the leadership of Drs. Sullivan, Burk, and Brantley, Duke's first mindfulness-based stress reduction program came into being. The Integrative Medicine Steering Committee, led by Dan Blazer, the associate dean for medical education and a faculty member in the Department of Psychiatry, developed the center's first business plan, which began with the following mission statement: To improve health care by combining traditional mind-body-spirit, and complementary approaches to medicine through academic leadership, rigorous research, compassionate care, and innovative education.

The DCIM was located on the beautiful campus of the Center for Living, a twenty-six-acre wooded lot about a half mile from Duke Hospital. Here, patients could be seen in excellent clinical facilities outside the main hubbub of the medical center campus. The location also included the Duke University Preventive Approach to Cardiology (DUPAC) and the Executive Health Program. I wanted all three programs to interact so that individuals coming to Duke for executive health physicals or for cardiac rehabilitation could avail themselves of the therapeutic modalities provided by integrative medicine. Similarly, patients coming for clinical programs in integrative medicine could participate in the programs of DUPAC or Executive Health.

An important step forward in the development of integrative medicine at Duke followed a July 1999 meeting organized by Jon Kabat-Zinn. The meeting took place at the Fetzer Institute outside of Kalamazoo, Michigan. The Fetzer Institute is known for engaging people around the world to foster awareness of the power of love and forgiveness in our global community. I had heard of the Fetzer Institute but had never been there or ever thought I would be there. Whatever my expectations, I arrived at this beautiful, warm, contemporary retreat surrounded by dense woods and beautiful nature trails adjacent to meandering streams. Participants included many leaders of integrative medicine from eight universities. I can't recall a more powerful or important conference, with the place, setting, people, and purpose creating a feeling of coming together in a way that I had never before experienced. Each session started with the ringing of Buddhist temple chimes, followed by a period of mindfulness meditation. In a most comfortable way, Jon worked his magic in focusing everyone's attention on the development of a powerful movement in American medicine.

By the end of the meeting, I had made many strong friends and, given my position at Duke and within academic medicine, felt I had an important role to play in planning and fostering the development of more humanistic and holistic approaches to patient care. We would adopt no such approach if we thought it might do any harm; in no way did I believe that experimenting with yet scientifically unproven methods should be unbounded. That determination, too, had to remain within the limits of what we knew from conventional academic medicine.

An important related concept arising from the Fetzer meeting was the recognition that academic medical institutions provided an important resource to foster the development of integrative care. The Academic Consortium on Integrative Medicine, an association of academic health centers dedicated to the adoption of integrative medicine, took root at that meeting. The consortium initially included participants from Duke, Harvard, Stanford, the University of California San Francisco, the University of Arizona, the University of Maryland, the University of Massachusetts, and the University of Minnesota. All agreed that the consortium's role was to support chancellors in advocating integrative medicine at their own institutions. Given my friendship with and admiration for Jon, as well as my role as chancellor for health affairs at Duke, I became actively engaged in and committed to establishing a base of scientific knowledge and appropriate clinical expertise regarding how integrative medicine and mind-body perspectives could positively influence health care.

After the historic meeting at Fetzer came a retreat in September 2000 at the Miraval Retreat Center outside of Tucson, Arizona. Miraval is an elegant, yet rustic, resort in the desert adjacent to a nearby mountain ridge that lends the place an aura of beauty and drama. A gorgeous outdoor amphitheater faces the ridge, and from it one can observe spectacular sunrises over the Sonora Desert. At this meeting, representatives from the Albert Einstein College of Medicine at Yeshiva University, Georgetown University, and Thomas Jefferson University joined the original eight academic institutions. Jon Kabat-Zinn again created an almost magical environment for discussions on how academic medicine could embrace the emerging concepts of integrative medicine. The sessions started as they had at Fetzer with a period of mindfulness meditation, with most individuals sitting in yoga positions on pillows or on the ground. The group officially changed its name at that meeting from the Academic Consortium on Integrative Medicine to the Consortium of Academic Health Centers for Integrative Medicine.

As a consequence of my involvement with integrative medicine, I developed a friendship with Andrew Weil, a highly visible spokesperson for the field, best-selling author, and frequent guest of television host Larry King. Prior to meeting Andy, I had questions about his standing as a physician, since some of his views seemed far beyond mainstream medicine. As I got to know him and his thinking, however, I became fascinated by his deep knowledge of medicine and botany, as well as his sincere commitment to improving care. I was also impressed with the training programs that he had established at the University of Arizona. Likewise, Tracy W. Gaudet, the leader of Andy's fellowship training program, was a Duke graduate whom I had met when she was a medical student. I was impressed by Tracy's contributions to Andy's program as well as by her creativity in bridging the best in conventional medicine with her deep commitment to providing patients with all the resources needed to meet their health needs.

As I became increasingly interested in a paradigm of health care embracing a more holistic view of patients' needs, my day job continued to focus on Duke's medical center, its health system, and my role within the AAMC. In 2000, I became chair of the AAMC Council of Deans with responsibility for creating the program for the council's annual meeting. I seized the chance to introduce my fellow deans to Andy's thinking; indeed, I invited him to be the meeting's keynote speaker. This was, of course, a bit controversial and more than a little risky, to say the least. I suspected that most medical school deans were not yet ready to embrace alternative and complementary approaches, and probably held at least as skeptical a view of Andy as I had before I got to know him. Nevertheless, Andy came to the meeting and presented what I considered an eye-opening plenary talk entitled "From Genomics to Ginkgo Biloba." The response was mixed; he was treated politely, of course, but some deans were clearly wary. Most were not yet ready to open their minds to the emerging field. Regardless, with integrative medicine as the main agenda item for this national meeting, it was clear that a movement was beginning.

In May 2000, I invited Tracy Gaudet and Richard S. Liebowitz (Tracy's spouse at that time) to visit Duke to determine whether Tracy would be suitable to lead our new center. Tracy was an OB-GYN and Rich was a primary care physician who practiced integrative medicine. By the end of 2000, we were able to recruit both of them to Duke. The DCIM now had legs. The effort then gained financial support in the form of a $5 million pledge from Christy and John Mack. The purpose of the DCIM was to develop educational and research programs dedicated to introducing integrative medicine approaches into conventional medicine. The center was also designed to have a clinical focus delivering "full immersion" into integrative care consultations and services such as mindfulness meditation, yoga, and acupuncture. Tracy and I spelled out our definition of what integrative medicine was meant to be at Duke in an article for the journal *Academic Medicine*. In the article, we delineated the mission of Consortium of Academic Health Centers for Integrative Medicine as follows: "to help facilitate the transformation of health care through rigorous scientific studies, new models of clinical care, and innovative educational programs that integrate biomedicine with the complexity of human beings, the intrinsic nature of healing, and the rich diversity of therapeutic systems."[1]

A critical step in making integrative medicine more mainstream took place at Miraval in 2001. Organized by the George Foundation and led by Penny and Bill George of Minneapolis, that meeting went by the humble name of "Conversation at Miraval." It fit the sponsors. Bill George was then CEO of Medtronic and a strong supporter of his wife, Penny, who was firmly committed to the concepts of integrative medicine. The meeting brought together academic leaders, well-known practitioners in the field of integrative medicine, and a group of philanthropists sympathetic to the approach. With some similarities to the Fetzer meeting, Miraval 2001 produced a spectacular outcome.

The meeting started in an unusual way. We were all asked to assemble at the outdoor amphitheater late the afternoon of the first day. We did so, said our hellos, and introduced ourselves to individuals we did not know. As we wondered what this first event was all about, a tall, fiftyish, handsome, sun-worn man wearing authentic black cowboy gear appeared before us. He said his name was Wyatt. In a warm, Western accent, he asked, "Why are you here?" I looked around for hidden cameras and microphones; I detected none. After a few moments of hesitation, some attendees started offering answers: "I'm here because I'm interested in integrative medicine and want to have my institution involved." Wyatt would look that person in the eye and say, "Fine. But why are you *really* here?" Other people in the semicircle raised their hands and answered in a similar fashion: "I want to help humankind through better models of health care." "Yes, but why are you *really* here?" This went on for about five minutes, with invariably rational answers given to the question of "Why are you here?" Finally, Jon Kabat-Zinn raised his hand and said, "I don't know why I'm *really* here." Wyatt agreed, and an important point shone forth.

What was that point? Questioning a person's motivation for doing something can produce honest responses that are nevertheless tactical and superficial. It can produce what some social scientists call performance rituals that are heavily conditioned by social expectations grounded in a given culture. We are so habituated to providing such performance rituals that most people come to believe that the answer offered is the real answer, or even the only answer to a given question. But underlying these kinds of responses are deeper reasons that almost invariably are based on emotional, not fully rational or consciously understood, quests. People do things all the time without knowing exactly why. We often ascribe motives to our actions, believing them to be correct whereas the true reason remains unappreciated, and requires deeper contemplation to be identified. This understanding certainly has relevance to health care, as I learned later when I became involved in personalized medicine.

This session got the meeting off to an outstanding start by making us all think more deeply about what it is we do when we engage with patients— and with each other as doctors. The entire meeting would have been worthwhile for this lesson alone. But there was more. Indeed, Miraval 2001 turned out to be a marvelous coming together of all involved, including warm and rich interactions with many leading philanthropists. When it ended, it seemed that we were on the verge of something really important: the creation of the field of integrative medicine.

As a leader of one of the nation's more prestigious academic medical centers, I was asked frequently during the meeting what I thought we needed to move this initiative forward. At one of the final sessions, calls for action mounted. People wanted to actually do something. John Mack, CEO of Morgan Stanley, a nationally known leader in banking and a highly influential member of Duke's Board of Trustees, locked his gaze on me and, out of the blue, asked, "Ralph, how much money would it take to get an academic consortium for integrative medicine started?"

It is a dream of all academic leaders to be asked such a question by a potential donor. It's the sort of experience that can temporarily annul the law of gravity. In my entire career I had never before been asked such a question. My mind raced through a budget that had to be practical but not unimaginative. "About $5 million would get such a consortium up and running," I said, matter-of-factly. John did not blink an eye. He turned to his fellow philanthropists and said, "OK, hands up; let's get the contributions right here and now." He did not pull a gun. He didn't have to. John is a strong, decisive figure, and although he did not elicit pledges for $5 million on the spot, he did well enough to get the effort off the ground. He created the Philanthropic Collaborative for Integrative Medicine to fund the Consortium of Academic

Health Centers for Integrative Medicine. Thus the Bravewell Collaborative, as it is now known, got its start.

John's wife, Christy Mack, who was an expert in reiki therapy and whose father was a physician, had a long-standing interest in approaches to enhance wellness and healing. As I came to know Christy better, we increasingly shared interests in determining how Duke's medical center could be positioned to develop programs that could improve health and serve as a launching pad for national initiatives in integrative medicine. Her support and commitment meant a great deal to me personally. Through her philanthropy, she also spurred the development of integrative medicine at Duke. The George Foundation also supported the center with a grant of $500,000 for the DCIM Holistic Mentoring Program in 2001.

By January 2002, thirteen major academic medical centers had joined the consortium. The group included Duke, Harvard, Columbia, the University of Michigan, the Albert Einstein College of Medicine at Yeshiva University, Georgetown University, Thomas Jefferson University, Stanford University, the University of Arizona, the University of California San Francisco, the University of Maryland, the University of Massachusetts, and the University of Minnesota. The consortium currently has fifty-two members.

Under Tracy's leadership, the DCIM heightened its visibility through a health system–wide physician and consumer survey initiated in 2002 to determine views about integrative medicine. For physicians, integrative medicine was defined as the appropriate, safe, and effective use of conventional medicine blended with evidenced-based complementary and alternative therapies and modalities. This included lifestyle and wellness, diet and nutrition, exercise, movement, and mind-body domains. For consumers, integrative medicine and complementary and alternative medicine (CAM) meant an approach that seeks to improve medical care by combining the best of conventional medicine with mind-body-spirit approaches shown to be effective in complementary techniques. The survey demonstrated a high degree of agreement among physicians that their patients would consider CAM therapies. Indeed, a large percentage of Duke physicians turned out to be surprisingly open to the development of this field at the university. For example, 96 percent indicated that they would refer patients to high-quality programs utilizing integrative medicine approaches. Similarly, patients indicated a high degree of potential utilization of CAM resources and an interest in having such programs available at Duke.

On the other side of the stethoscope, Tracy believed that medical school training should reflect the understanding of the stresses imposed by the rigorous curriculum. She developed excellent programs in which medical students received training in mindfulness mediation and concepts of integrative medicine early in their medical school career. Research led by the DCIM also benefited from a Center for Medicare and Medicaid Services grant to study the role of patient-centered personalized and integrated approaches to the treatment of chronic disease, in this case, cardiac disease and diabetes.

The DCIM's collaboration with Christy Mack continued to grow, and her support and enthusiasm played a significant role in its success at Duke and nationally. In 2002, before I stepped down as chancellor, Christy and John Mack demonstrated their extraordinary commitment to integrative medicine by providing a $12 million grant from the C. J. Mack Foundation to build an integrative medicine facility on the Duke Center for Living campus.

In January 2007, Duke Integrative Medicine opened the doors to its new home, a 27,000-plus-square-foot building. This first-of-its-kind medical building was specifically designed by Duda/Paine Architects in Durham to be dedicated solely to the practice of integrative medicine. The new facility was described as a "living laboratory" for the exploration and demonstration of innovative models of care, treating the whole person, not just the disease or injury. The building features a variety of rooms—some of them sun-filled and grand and others intimate and sheltering. It includes a sitting room/library and indoor and outdoor meditation spaces, therapeutic treatment rooms, conference and workshop spaces, fitness facilities, and a state-of-the-art kitchen for healthy cooking demonstrations and meals. The building and grounds are integrated to create a sense of connectedness between the indoor spaces and the surrounding woodlands and streams of the Duke Forest.

— — —

In November 2003, the Bravewell Collaborative hosted a major event—a black-tie gala held at the Regent Wall Street in New York City—to highlight progress in the field of integrative medicine and choose the recipient of the inaugural Bravewell Leadership Award. One of six finalists would be honored with this important achievement award and also would be presented with a check for $100,000 to enable the individual to pursue his or her interest in the field. I was one of the finalists, but I attended this glorious affair without seriously believing I had much chance of winning. I had strongly supported integrative medicine, but I was hardly one of its foundational developers.

None other than Walter Cronkite, anchor of the CBS Evening News, hosted the evening's proceedings. I had the honor of sitting at the same table with him and his wife, Betsy. Even better, my close cousin Edith, my childhood role model as a research physician at the University of Pennsylvania, sat with us as well. Cronkite was as impressive in person as he was as a national newscaster, but he was also a warm, genuinely interesting, and humble person. When he walked to the stage to announce the winner, his presence gave the event the pageantry of the Academy Awards.

Only a small number of people knew the winner's identity. I watched attentively as Cronkite accepted the envelope from Christy Mack and proceeded to open it. By this point, I believe my breath had stopped as I waited for him to call out the winner, totally prepared for it to be anybody other than me among the deserving finalists—all of whom I knew and respected. When I heard him read "Ralph Snyderman," it was among the most magical moments of my life. I was truly surprised—no, shocked. Honored and humbled by this unexpected recognition, I initially thought that receiving the award was extremely generous because integrative medicine had done more for me, had made me a better person and doctor, than I had ever done for it.

As these thoughts blurred my mind, I looked out to find myself standing at the podium with Walter Cronkite on one side and Christy on the other. I don't remember how I got up there. Looking out into this spectacular room full of well-dressed people, I spoke for perhaps ten minutes being totally mindful of the moment but without being fully aware of what I was saying. I spoke from the heart, totally connected with everybody in the room.

— — —

Although my role as chancellor at Duke occupied the preponderance of my time, I found myself often being asked to be a spokesperson for integrative medicine. I did so mainly through interviews in health journals and lectureships at academic institutions. I did this gladly when time permitted because I was becoming increasingly convinced that current models of care were minimizing our true responsibilities to our patients, actually preventing us from providing them with what they needed for optimal outcomes. When I stepped down as chancellor in June 2004, my role in directly affecting the practice of integrative medicine diminished. However, in 2005, an extremely important opportunity came my way, largely through Jon Kabat-Zinn. Jon was organizing a scientific dialogue with His Holiness the 14th Dalai Lama on the healing power of meditation, and he asked me to participate. So, in DAR Constitution Hall in Washington, DC, leading Buddhist scholars, researchers, and philosophers convened for three days to discuss the healing power of meditation from the perspective of knowledge acquired using Buddhist approaches as opposed to Western medicine. The Dalai Lama himself participated in every one of the five sessions. My role in the last session, entitled "Integration and Final Reflections," was to summarize for the Dalai Lama and the audience all that had been learned in the previous sessions. For approximately an hour I sat center stage at DAR Constitution Hall with the Dalai Lama and his interpreter, Dr. Thupten Jinpa. I can't think of a more challenging assignment than this one, yet the nature of the meeting, the warmth, sincerity, and commitment of all who attended, and the gracious comfort provided by His Holiness made the task exciting and fulfilling.

Following the meeting, the speakers and a small select group met with the Dalai Lama, who as is customary, presented each of us with a Tibetan Buddhist prayer shawl. Immediately after the meeting, I flew to New York for the second annual Bravewell Leadership Award banquet to honor the Collaborative's newest awardee. While making introductory remarks at the podium, and again looking out at a magnificent black-tie audience, I unfolded the prayer shawl from my suit pocket, placed it around my neck, and described the powerful feelings I had just shared with His Holiness the Dalai Lama.

I continue to be asked to speak about integrative medicine, and as I do so, my understanding and commitment to its principles deepen. One profound experience occurred during my visit to the Dana-Farber Cancer Institute as the Leonard B. Zakim Visiting Professor in November 2005. In addition to delivering a major lecture, I made rounds on the integrative medicine services at the hospital. The team prepared me to meet a patient being treated for recurrent breast cancer and indicated that her chemotherapy was being withheld because her platelet count was too low, and the doctors were try-ing other ways to get the count back up. As the door to her room opened, I was met with scents of aromatherapy and notes of gentle new age music. A woman was lying on a massage table in a dimly lit room. She had a pad over her eyes, and acupuncture needles lined her from head to toe. A physician who appeared Asian was manipulating the needles on her legs. I looked at him and asked what he was doing. "Stimulating the thrombocyte (plate-let) meridian," he replied. My immediate private thought as a scientist and physician was "bullshit." But then I looked at the patient, who removed the cover from her eyes and looked at me. I asked, "How are you feeling about this therapy?" She stared deeply into my eyes and said softly but forcefully, "Empowered!" The impact on me was immediate and profound. She believed that acupuncture would bring her platelets back up. Perhaps it did. But even if in this case it did not, what physician wouldn't want their pa-tient to approach a medical challenge with such hope and positivity?

— — —

In conversations with Christy Mack and a team at the Bravewell Collabora-tive, I had been asked how they might best leverage their resources to call national attention to the values of integrative medicine. I suggested that they form an association with the highly regarded Institute of Medicine. Through the initiative of Christy and Dianne Neiman, representing the Bravewell Collaborative, the Institute of Medicine agreed to host an event dealing with integrative medicine. My suggestion became my job, which seemed only fair. So I organized and chaired a summit whose purpose was to examine the scientific basis of integrative medicine and to discuss its potential for improving the health of the nation.

After two years of planning, the February 2009 Summit on Integrative Medicine and the Health of the Public attracted one of the most diverse au-diences ever to examine the practice of integrative medicine, its scientific basis, and workable solutions for improving the health of the nation.[2] More than six hundred people attended the three-day discussion, which focused on integrated approaches to health care—approaches that engage the pa-tient as an informed and empowered participant while personalizing the care to best address the individual's unique needs and circumstances. The diverse approaches emphasized prevention, health maintenance, and early intervention. The meeting was among the largest ever held by the Institute of Medicine, and its president, Harvey V. Fineberg, attended every session and addressed the group twice.

Setting the stage for the meeting, I began by sharing my vision and passion for personalized health care, focusing on prevention through healthier behaviors and my belief in the power of emerging technologies to quantify susceptibilities to disease, to detect disease early, and to intervene successfully using integrative approaches to care. The plenary sessions covered the vision for integrative medicine, models of care, the underlying science, workforce and education needs, and economic and policy implications. Speakers included Donald M. Berwick (Institute for Healthcare Improvement), George C. Halvorson (Kaiser Foundation Health Plan, Inc., and Kaiser Foundation Hospitals), Michael Johns (Emory University), Mehmet C. Oz (Columbia University), William Novelli (AARP), Sean Tunis (Center for Medical Technology Policy), Dean M. Ornish (Preventive Medicine Research Institute and University of California San Francisco), and Dame Carol Black (Academy of Medical Royal Colleges), with the closing keynote delivered by Senator Thomas R. Harkin. In addition to these distinguished speakers, the Prince of Wales provided a prerecorded statement highlighting the groundbreaking nature of the summit.

The press widely covered the summit and helped us establish a successful starting point for developing more coherent and effective approaches to health care reform. The timing of the summit couldn't have been better: it occurred as the Patient Protection and Affordable Care legislation was being drafted. Certain concepts emphasized at the summit—preventative care, patient-centered care, and shared decision making—found their way into the legislation, which was signed into law in March 2010.

Being involved in integrative medicine became a professional passion for me. I realized the critical importance of humanizing our approach to patient care and accepting responsibility for more than treating the pathophysiology of patients' diseases. Integrative medicine also changed me as a person, opening my eyes to the importance of caring, tolerance, and the consideration of things I had not formerly put stock in. The practice of mindfulness meditation also helped me cope better with stresses I experienced personally and professionally. It is perhaps interesting in this regard that President Nan Keohane wrote the following in my performance review in July 2001: "On a more personal level, I noted that you have become a more mellow person in the past year; you shared some of the reasons why this is so, including a focus on mindfulness. . . . This development on your part has surely eased working relations around the senior officers table, as well as with me personally, and I commend you for taking the initiative to deepen this aspect of your life."

I've always considered my engagement in integrative medicine as that of an interloper in a field where others had done the heavy lifting. Given my position at Duke, however, and my background as a research-based physician-scientist with a deep commitment to the scientific approach to medical care, my voice as a proponent of integrative medicine gave the approach a great deal of weight within academic circles. Thus, being chancellor for health affairs at Duke allowed me to bring attention and a degree of credibility to the concepts of integrative medicine. I am humble about, yet still proud of, these contributions.

My professional goals also changed as integrative medicine enriched my view of the clinical calling. I learned that what was ethically sound was also pragmatically more effective. It taught me that rationality and emotion are complements, not opposites, in every human personality. As a result, I developed the concept of personalized health care, an approach that combines the best scientific knowledge of genomics with the holistic approach of integrative medicine. It has become the primary focus of my current work.

13
—

Personalizing Health Care

By 2003, Duke had won national recognition for envisioning personalized health care, an entirely new approach to care with the potential to transform the practice of medicine vastly for the better. Rather than treating disease events long after the underlying problem becomes chronic, personalized health care (initially called prospective health care) focuses on enhancing health, minimizing disease, and personalizing therapy. This proactive approach is built on the concept that diseases and health evolve dynamically as a consequence of one's genetic inheritance modified by environment over time. Thus, rather than reacting to diseases that have already developed, health care can be personalized, predictive, and preventative. Personalized health care synthesizes the power of predictive and precision technologies with the concepts of integrative medicine. In practice, personalized health care carefully quantifies a patient's health status and risks for disease, then devises a plan to mitigate that risk and improve health, and when available, uses personalized therapies to meet the individual's needs. The approach tracks progress and encourages patients to be fully engaged in their own care. This proactive and personalized approach focuses on prevention and minimization of disease. Prevention of chronic disease is essential because nearly three-quarters of health care spending today goes to treat chronic diseases that are preventable. Personalized health care improves the effectiveness of emerging concepts of patient-centered care and uses precision medicine whenever applicable.[1]

But the development of new models of health care, now clearly in sight, took time to coalesce. What looks clear today appeared anything but as events were unfolding. Back in 1989, Duke's highly fractured and uncoordinated clinical enterprise was growing increasingly incompatible with pressures to reduce costs via so-called managed care and other means. Changes in the clinical delivery system, which commenced in 1994, not only allowed Duke to deliver excellent contemporary care more effectively but also allowed the evolution of novel ways of thinking about new models of health care delivery. As the components of Duke's clinical services became better integrated, broader perspectives emerged for improving health care delivery.

As my team and I grew in experience, we began to understand how Duke could develop vastly better ways to deliver care—how it could translate emerging perspectives into actionable programmatic changes. From my position within the institution and nationally, it was painfully apparent that the nation's overall approach to care was deeply flawed. Health care, as well as the education of physicians, focused on identifying the root cause of a patient's disease or disease events. The underlying concept—for every complicated clinical problem there is a single causative factor, and the function of health care is to "find it and fix it"—worked well with certain diseases (such as infections), but it did not align with the reality of more common complex chronic diseases whose causes, often predictable and preventable, are multifaceted. Indeed, I myself had been trained in the "find-it, fix-it" tradition from medical school through clinical training and as an internist and rheumatologist. The emphasis on treating the manifestation of disease left little time for attention to long-term treatment of chronic disease or caring for the holistic needs of patients facing complex clinical problems. Even further from consideration was any serious attention to how chronic diseases could be prevented.

Throughout the 1990s, I came to appreciate that the way we delivered care did not comport with what we knew about how disease develops or what our patients really needed. The evolution of DUHS helped me see what we were lacking because it put all the necessary "dots" into a single visual-cognitive field. By the late 1990s, Duke's health system ran three hospitals, connected thousands of physicians and clinics in the networks throughout the Research Triangle area, and had strategic relationships with hospitals throughout the Southeast. These connections added almost two million patient visits per year and involved perhaps a hundred thousand hospital admissions. We delivered excellent conventional care within a fully integrated health care delivery system capable, at least in theory, of providing cradle-to-grave care. But it was excellent only if measured by the "find-it, fix-it" model. As good as we were by contemporary standards, I appreciated that Duke and American medicine could do much better even with the same technical and therapeutic resources, which would surely continue to grow as technology and know-how advanced.

The first stage of my enlightenment came from my interest in integrative medicine. As I became more involved in integrative medicine, I began to understand the benefits of intensive patient engagement and the continuum of care, as opposed to the current treatment of brief episodes of disease. I also understood the broader needs patients have when faced with the challenges of navigating serious illnesses and the vast array of uncoordinated resources, some of which are considered alternative or complementary therapies.

I had become increasingly dismayed, for example, by the prevailing national approach to the treatment of cancer patients. Conventional oncology dealt with a patient's tumor through a combination of surgery, chemotherapy, and radiation therapy. With their lives turned upside down by a life-threatening diagnosis and dangerous, unpleasant therapies, patients would clearly benefit from a compassionate environment, support systems, and a plan to help them get through their cancer therapy. This thinking led to the development of the Duke Cancer Survivorship Program. Individuals with newly diagnosed cancer received the opportunity to see a "navigator"—a trained individual who would create a survivorship plan to guide them through long periods of cancer therapy. Each patient, in collaboration with their navigator, developed a personal health plan that, in addition to their cancer therapies, included additional therapies, such as mindfulness meditation, yoga, nutrition, stress reduction, and acupuncture along with mentoring by the patient's navigator. This program was the right thing for our patients because it emphasized the concept of coordinated, integrated care over a period of time and because patients loved it.

Unfortunately, the health care reimbursement system did not love what we were doing. It still does not support many of these activities. The old legacy system still creates by far the greatest obstacle to the implementation of more rational models of care. Nevertheless, over time, the concept of patient-centered, coordinated care has become increasingly accepted by health care professionals across the country. This is the direction in which health care needs to go, and all but the most hidebound in the medical community know it. Health care expenditures by the late 1990s already accounted for 15 percent of GDP, and health care was rapidly becoming unaffordable. We knew even then that almost seventy-five cents of every health care dollar was being spent on the treatment of preventable chronic diseases. This, in my view, made the need to develop new models of care an obligation on the part of those who had the power to change the system.

So at a meeting of the senior executive team in 1997, I challenged the group to think of a way that we could maximize our potential to develop new and effective models of health care delivery. Together we came up with a challenge grant of $250,000 to any clinical group at Duke that could design a pilot program to deliver care that would improve quality and reduce costs measurably over two years. We advertised this challenge grant broadly. Before long, a cardiology group in the Department of Medicine, led by Christopher M. O'Connor, proposed to study patients who had been discharged from Duke Hospital with congestive health failure—a serious and expensive medical condition.[2] Patients in one group would be treated as they always had: given appropriate medications and instructed to see their physicians on what was thought to be an appropriate schedule. Those in the other group would be given intensive education about their clinical condition, a plan for how and when their medication should be taken, and careful dietary instructions. They would report their weight weekly to a health care coach, who would provide support and monitor their condition as weight is extremely important in congestive heart failure because excess fluid retention indicates that the condition is worsening.

The results of this clinical trial could not have been more dramatic. Over the course of the year, those individuals who were given intensive instruction, encouraged to take responsibility for their own care, and provided with a plan that could be tracked by the patient and his or her coach experienced a dramatic reduction in the severity of their disease and in the number of hospital admissions. This approach reduced costs by a median of $8,571 per patient per year from $16,025 per patient per year prior to enrolling in the study. This favorable outcome reflected a major decrease in hospitalizations, which more than offset a slight increase in outpatient costs due to more frequent clinic visits for patient monitoring.

But here is the punch line: because reimbursement is structured to compensate at a higher level for inpatient versus outpatient services, by decreasing admissions, the health system lost revenues, making the innovation economically unsustainable. The better we did medically, the worse we did financially. This feature of the reimbursement system, rewarding high-cost interventions at the cost of lower-tech services, made the more effective clinical model economically unsustainable. I thought long and hard about this "outcome of the outcome." We had dramatically improved clinical care and significantly decreased real costs, but the perverse incentives in the health care reimbursement system made such an approach untenable. This was maddening. Fortunately, Thomas A. Scully, administrator of the Centers for Medicare and Medicaid Services (CMS), learned about the results of this study while he was at a Health Sector Conference at Duke and disseminated them widely. He also initiated a CMS-funded program to support these trial approaches. Duke's approach to congestive heart failure and the reimbursement system that prevented its adoption became a cause célèbre for health care reform. The Duke Heart Failure Program was the subject of a case review by the Harvard Business School and was also cited by representatives of the White House as an illustration of the need for health care reform.[3]

— — —

By 1999, embracing both integrative medicine and what we had learned through the more personalized and coordinated approaches to congestive heart failure, I became heavily focused on envisioning new and transformative models of health care delivery. At the time, very serendipitously, dramatic biomedical research breakthroughs emerged as well. In the late 1990s, the NIH created the Human Genome Project to sequence the entire human genome through a Manhattan Project–like initiative.[4] J. Craig Venter, an aggressive entrepreneurial and iconoclastic researcher, decided to race against the government genome effort using a much less expensive "shotgun" approach. By 2000, both groups reached the finish line virtually simultaneously and with great fanfare: the entire sequencing of the human genome had been achieved.

This was a truly revolutionary accomplishment. For clinical matters, it meant that technology was now available, or would be soon, to decode individual human blueprints, making predictive, personalized care possible for the first time ever. While the initial sequencing took years and incurred great expense, it was clear that rapid advances and decreasing costs would follow. Other major biomedical research breakthroughs bore additional clinical implications. Proteomics (identifying hundreds of different proteins in biological samples), metabolomics (the ability to identify thousands of metabolites in biological samples), advances in biostatistics, and the development and analysis of databases, along with nanotechnology and related qualitative improvements in medical instrumentation—all heralded great progress in the treatment of human diseases.

One day it dawned on me that even as this biomedical research revolution provided far greater understanding of diseases, it might also provide an entirely new capability that could turn the practice of medicine on its head. In the aggregate, genomics, proteomics, metabolomics, and the ability to collect and analyze vast amounts of clinical data, would for the first time provide increasingly accurate ways to predict an individual's risks for specific diseases, to track whether those risks were increasing or decreasing, and to predict specific disease events, such as development of a heart attack or a stroke. By understanding an individual's specific risk, we could develop revolutionary personalized, predictive, and preventative approaches to care. We could take a fine-tuned strategic approach that would make the disease-reactive and essentially one-size-fits-all approach of the past a historic relic.

I became convinced that contemporary health care, as good as it had become, was essentially backward-looking. It started at the point of disease and tried to reverse its cause. Care was reactive and directed toward fixing an unwanted event that had already occurred. But health and disease are dynamic; they are a consequence of one's genetic inheritance as it is affected over time by what one does or is exposed to. The interplay of genes and environment determines one's health over time (figure 13.1). Contemporary care lacked any sense of this dynamic understanding and also lacked a strategic vision in identifying health risks at the earliest possible time and developing strategies to mitigate them while improving health. Thus, the concept of personalized health planning as a new approach to care evolved.

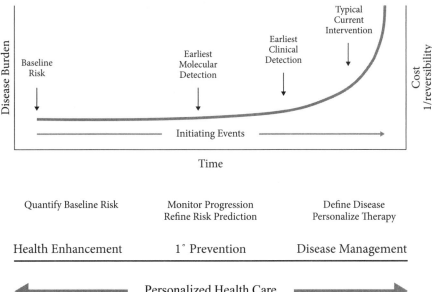

FIG. 13.1 *Inflection curve of disease development.* The concept underlying personalized health care is that disease develops over time and pathology accumulates subclinically until an initial clinical event signals its presence. Available and emerging technologies enable early quantification of risk, measurement of disease progression, and early targeted intervention, thereby enabling a new personalized, proactive model of care.

Personalized health care mandated major changes both in medical education and in the relationship between patients and their physicians. Rather than seeing their doctor only during illnesses, patients would interact with their physician to develop a personalized health plan to meet their longer-term needs, whether to enhance health and well-being, prevent disease, or manage disease most effectively. The plan would define the individual patient's current health, identify his or her impending health risks, develop jointly agreed upon goals and plans to meet them, and define exactly how to measure progress toward achieving goals. The basic structure of this approach is adaptable to virtually all health-related needs and cohorts—from pediatrics to geriatrics and everything in between.

While this concept seemed glaringly obvious to most of us within the health system at Duke, many others thought it grandiose and unlikely to be implemented. When I presented this approach at a meeting of the DUHS board in 2000, the chair of the Duke University Board of Trustees, gruffly stated, "It'll never happen." He claimed it would be too expensive and that people would never buy into it. He made the case that most people, and particularly insurers, engage in short-term thinking and would not embrace such dramatic changes to how health care is delivered. My Duke colleagues and I, however, did not succumb to such pessimism. We continued to refine our thinking about what personalized health care might look like in practice, and I began speaking about it nationally.

The more I thought about the concepts of personalized health care and the more I discussed it with forward-thinking colleagues, the more obvious it became that we were at the early stages of envisioning an entirely new approach to health care. The approach tracked not only with our understanding of the development of disease but also with common sense. We did not underestimate the vast reorientation of health care delivery that would have to occur to put personalized health care into practice. But it was too logical and beneficial to abandon just because of the intellectual inertia and vested interests in the status quo that stood in the way. I had encountered such inertia and abject resistance to change before, after all, and my experience was that both could be overcome by patience, persistence, and logic. So I proceeded to think, discuss, plan, and advocate on that basis.

Personalized health care, I explained at every available opportunity, was future-oriented and planned, not reactive and incremental like the then-current practice. As part of that effort I presented this radical new approach at national meetings of the AAMC in 2002 and the Association of American Physicians (AAP) in 2003.[5] As chair and president, respectively, of these organizations, I had a ready bully pulpit for the task; I was addressing several thousand people when I presented my paper to the AAMC. *Science* subsequently published an article entitled "Personalized Health Planning," coauthored by Hunt Willard, Sandy Williams, and me.[6]

The concept of personalized medicine gained immediate traction because of its association with the great expectations arising from the sequencing of the human genome. Many initiatives, funded by both government and industry, were raising hopes of rapidly explaining susceptibility to inherited disease as well as the causal mechanisms of complex diseases. Many anticipated that genomics and related technologies would transform care themselves by personalizing disease prediction, identifying the mechanisms of disease, and developing therapies targeted to the individual's needs.

I was initially attracted by these views, but I had too much experience in what, for lack of a better phrase, were the politics and social psychology of large institutions to think that these changes would come about automatically, ineluctably, simply as a result of scientific and technological progress. I knew that personalized health care was more than genomics applied to medicine. To advance, medical professionals would need to be willing to change the way they thought and practiced—not an easy task. More important, and perhaps the most difficult, would be the necessity for a dramatic change in medical reimbursement. The still prevalent fee-for-service model which rewards intervention for disease events would need to be changed to one of rewarding prevention and effective outcomes. Since the health care industry which accounts for one-seventh of the GNP is based on fee-for-service payments, changes in reimbursement would need to be carefully introduced and, as of 2016, progress has been very slow. Finally, the seemingly straightforward concept that good health is among the greatest resources any nation possesses had to take root in the minds of medical professionals, the public, and the country's business and political elite. The latter, after all, would have to push the medical establishment as well as be pulled by it.

I did some tugging of my own in addressing a prestigious roundtable of the nation's leading CEOs in 2003. I enjoyed asking them, why, if they had strategic plans for their businesses, they had no such plans for their most valuable asset—their own health and the health of their employees. Why, I continued, should health not be managed strategically, just as one would manage any valuable asset? The CEOs were nonplussed; they had no choice but to see the simple but compelling logic of prospective, personalized care.

I was pleasantly surprised in 2003 when Gary Stiles, the chief medical officer of DUHS, came to me and said, "Boss, we're ready to roll out personalized health care to the employees of Duke University." Unbeknownst to me, Gary took the concept of personalized health care and ran with it, all the way to the point of coming up with an initial model that could be offered to Duke employees. The major components included a health risk assessment and personal health plan, the involvement of primary care physicians and health care coaches, and, when appropriate, disease management.[7]

Unfortunately, this approach could not be implemented for the broader population of patients seen at Duke because, again, health care reimbursement did not pay for preventative measures, let alone the innovative approaches conceived in Duke personalized health care. However, because

Duke University was self-insured for its employees, delivering more cost-effective care would benefit both the employees who chose to participate and the university. During the first two years, medical costs for high-risk individuals decreased by 3.5 percent; emergency room visits and hospital stays also decreased. At the end of two years, Duke's health care costs averaged $5,298 per employee, well below the national average of $7,498. Duke more than recovered its initial investment to launch the program. This new model of care was among the nation's first to be directed toward personalized, predictive, preventative care with intensive participation on the part of the individual. I was very proud to have been chancellor when this major demonstration of the concept occurred.

Since stepping down as chancellor in 2004, my commitment to the advancement of personalized health care has become even more focused. Under my direction, the Duke Center for Research for Personalized Health Care was created to provide a platform for encouraging and participating in research directed toward developing better models of care. The center serves as a creator of clinical models and a think-tank to facilitate the development of personalized health care.[8]

As practical models of personalized health care continued to be refined, it became obvious that what we learned from our initiatives in integrative medicine were necessary components of the personalized care model. Personalization of care brings the needs of the individual front and center. Understanding patients' health needs as an integrated whole and building on their readiness to engage and change their lifestyle to embrace healthier behaviors are key components of developing and implementing successful care. Since the inception of personalized health care in 2002, the perceived value of patient engagement and readiness to change has increased tremendously. It is simply beyond question, in my opinion, that the development of personal health goals and plans to achieve them and the availability of appropriate patient support are the best way to prevent and manage chronic diseases.

— — —

I think it is fair to claim that the concept of personalized health care was first developed and saw service at Duke. Duke drew from its approaches to integrative medicine to create the basic conceptual underpinning of real health care reform in the United States. Indeed, as noted earlier, the Patient

Protection and Affordable Care Act of 2010 (a.k.a. Obamacare) embraced many of these approaches, at least in theory. Personalized health care, patient-centered care, patient engagement, predictive medicine, targeted therapy, predictive diagnostics, and most recently precision medicine, are all part of the evolution of health care reform. Unfortunately, getting from theory to practice is not easy. As long as the insurance reimbursement system operates at cross-purposes to personalized health care, its promise will remain unrealized. Alas, Obamacare does not sufficiently address health care reimbursement, which is one of the impediments to real health care reform. Still, changes in reimbursement protocols encouraged by Obamacare are beginning to reward better outcomes rather than volumes of interventions. This is helping to turn things around and is a major step to support personalized health care.

This, plus increasing evidence for the value of patient-centered care, has stimulated a burgeoning movement toward personalized health care. In 2012, the Veterans Health Administration (VHA), the nation's largest health delivery system, asked me to serve as an adviser in designing basic strategies to improve care for our veterans. The VHA has fully embraced these concepts and in its 2014 *Blueprint for Excellence*, personalized, proactive, patient-driven care, and personalized health planning are incorporated as strategic goals.[9]

What began as a concept at Duke in the late 1990s became a concrete proposal in 2002 for a new personalized approach to health care. Currently, there are virtually no academic health centers without personalized medicine programs, and the field, in 2015, is estimated to be a $500 billion industry. Certainly, as a nation, we are now moving to fully embrace the tenets of personalized health care, and as a result the entire country will benefit. When we do get there, my pride and sense of fulfillment, knowing that so much of this movement arose out of initiatives developed at Duke, will be complete. As long as I can, I will continue to support these efforts. I hope to live long enough to see them adopted and result in the better health and economic viability of our nation.

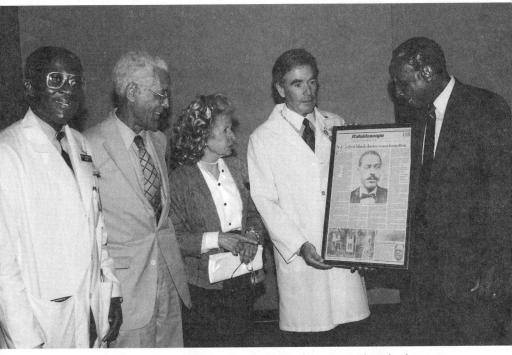

FIG. GALLERY 2.1 Charles Johnson, incoming president of the National Medical Association, being honored, 1990. Left to right: Onye Akwari, associate professor of surgery and physiology; Hubert Eaton, Wilmington physician; Mary Semans; Ralph Snyderman; and Charles Johnson. Photo by Duke Photography. Courtesy of the Duke University Archives.

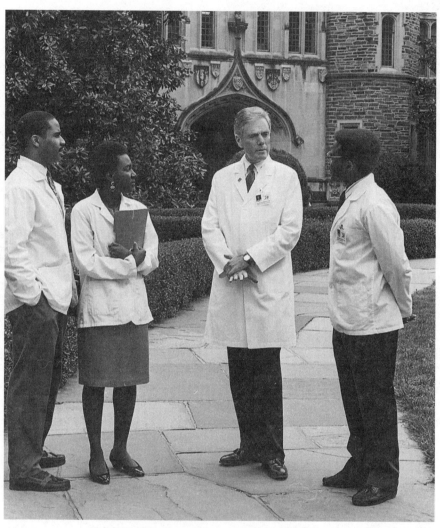

FIG. GALLERY 2.2 Ralph Snyderman meeting with medical school students, 1993. Photo by Duke Photography. Courtesy of the Duke University Archives.

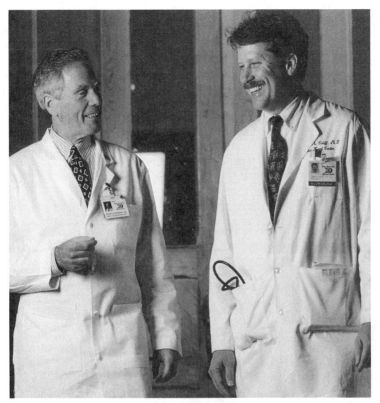

FIG. GALLERY 2.3 Rob Califf, vice chancellor for clinical research and founding director of the DCRI, and Ralph Snyderman, 1996. Photo by Will and Deni McIntyre.

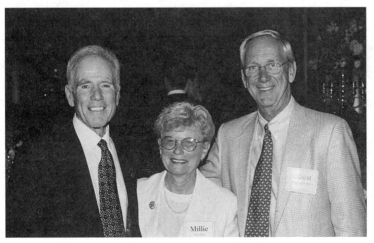

FIG. GALLERY 2.4 Ernie Mario, the first chairman of the Duke University Board of Trustees, and his wife, Millie, with Ralph Snyderman at Davison Club, 2004. Photo by Duke Photography.

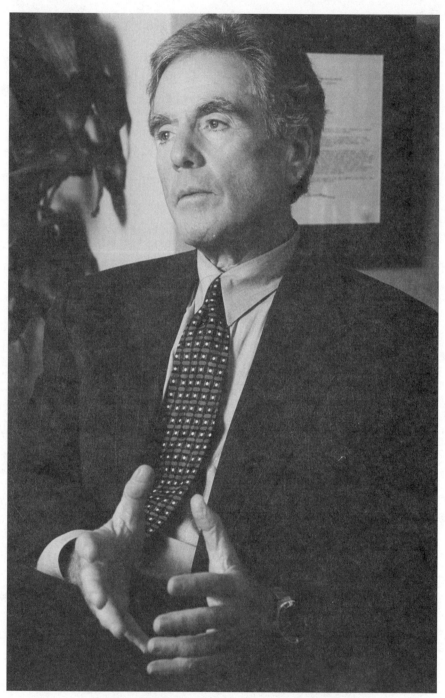

FIG. GALLERY 2.5 Ralph Snyderman, 1998. Photo by Duke Photography.

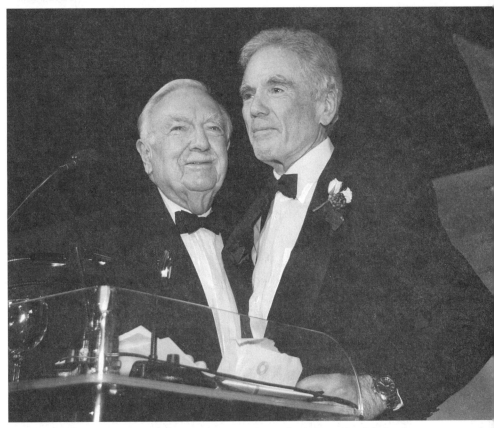

FIG. GALLERY 2.6 Walter Cronkite, CBS Evening News anchorman, and Ralph Snyderman at the Bravewell Leadership Award Dinner, 2003. Photo courtesy of the Bravewell
Collaborative.

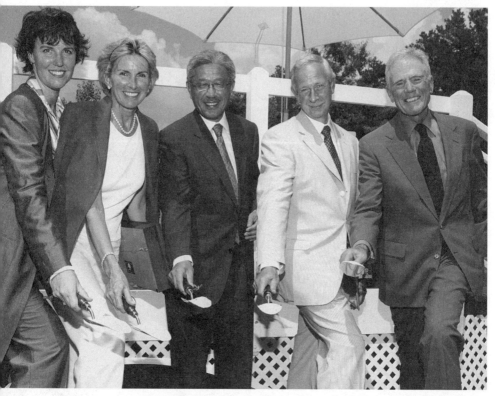

FIG. GALLERY 2.7 Groundbreaking for the Duke Center for Integrative Medicine, 2005. Left to right: Tracy Gaudet, DCIM director; Christy Mack, philanthropist; Victor Dzau, chancellor for health affairs; Richard Brodhead, Duke University president; and Ralph Snyderman. Photo by Duke Photography. Courtesy of the Duke University Archives.

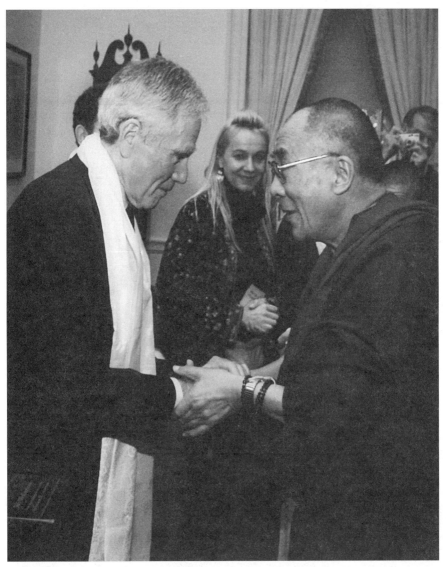

FIG. GALLERY 2.8 His Holiness the 14th Dalai Lama and Ralph Snyderman at the Mind and Life Conference, 2005. Photo by Sonam Zoksang, proprietor of Vision of Tibet.

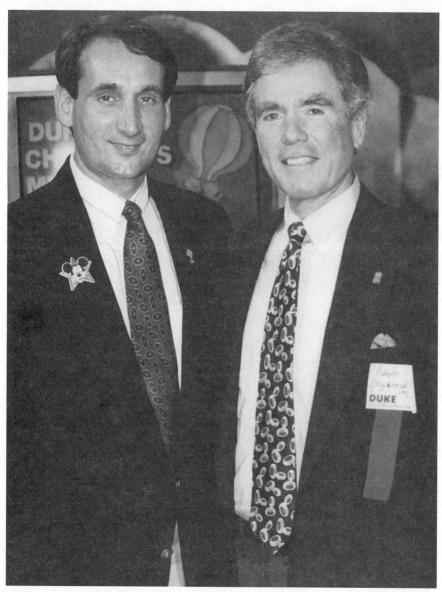

FIG. GALLERY 2.9 Mike Krzyzewski, Duke men's basketball coach and Ralph Snyderman at the Duke Children's Hospital Telethon, 1990. Photo by Duke Photography. Courtesy of the Duke University Archives.

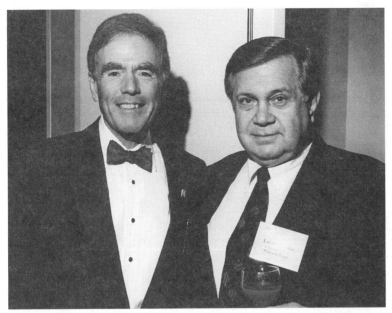

FIG. GALLERY 2.10 Leon Levine, founder of Family Dollar, and Ralph Snyderman at the medical center's Spirit of Caring Weekend, 1993. Photo by Duke Photography. Courtesy of the Duke Medical Center Development Office.

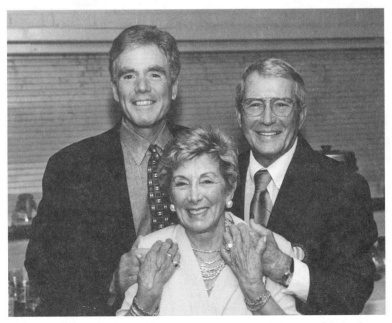

FIG. GALLERY 2.11 Roselle and Perry Como, honorary chairman of the Duke Children's Classic, and Ralph Snyderman, 1995. Photo courtesy of the Duke Children's Hospital Development Office.

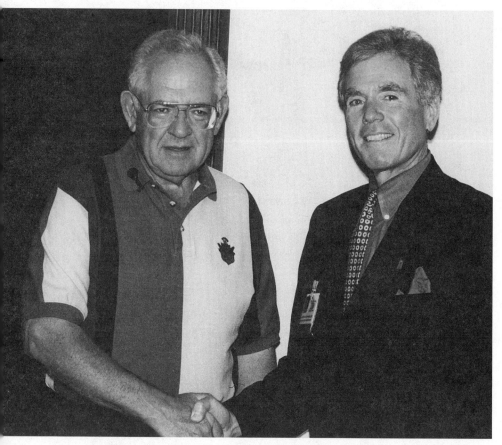

FIG. GALLERY 2.12 Dave Thomas, founder of Wendy's Hamburgers and honorary cochair of the Duke Children's Classic, and Ralph Snyderman, 1995. Photo courtesy of the Duke Children's Hospital Development Office.

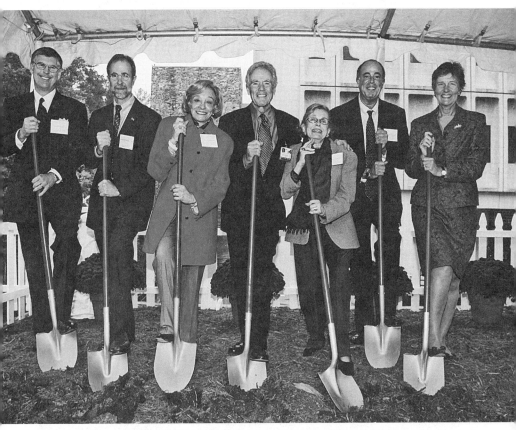

FIG. GALLERY 2.13 Groundbreaking for the Ruth and Herman Albert Eye Research Institute, 2002. Left to right: Harold Shaw, Jr., Eye Center Alumni Campaign chair; Sandy Williams, School of Medicine dean; Roslyn Lachman, Eye Center Advisory Board chair; Ralph Snyderman; Ruth Albert, benefactor; David Epstein, Department of Ophthalmology chair; and Nan Keohane, Duke University president. Photo by Duke Photography.

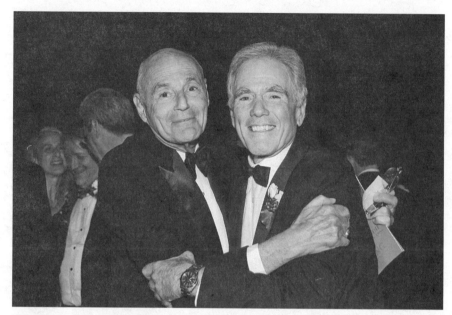

FIG. GALLERY 2.14 Sheppard Zinovoy and Ralph Snyderman at the Bravewell Leadership Award Dinner, 2003. Photo courtesy of the Bravewell Collaborative.

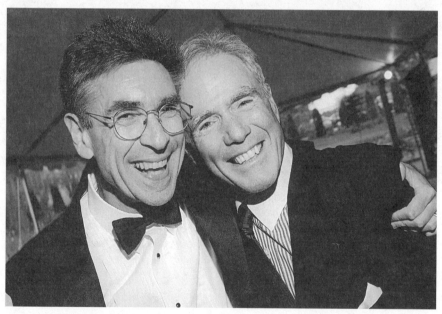

FIG. GALLERY 2.15 Bob Lefkowitz and Ralph Snyderman at Bob's sixtieth birthday celebration, 2003. Photo by Duke Photography.

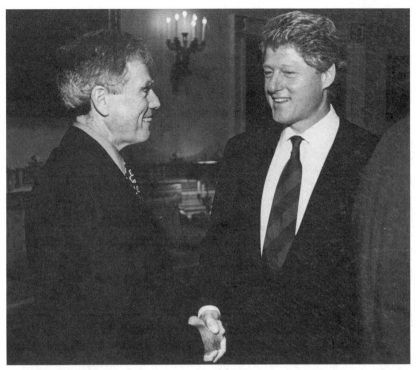

FIG. GALLERY 2.16 President William J. Clinton and Ralph Snyderman at a reception at the White House, 1993. Signed photo given to author by President Clinton.

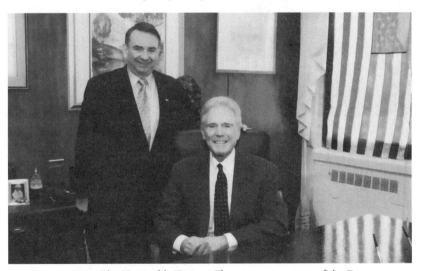

FIG. GALLERY 2.17 The Honorable Tommy Thompson, secretary of the Department of Health and Human Services, and Ralph Snyderman in 2003. Photo given to author by the Honorable Tommy Thompson.

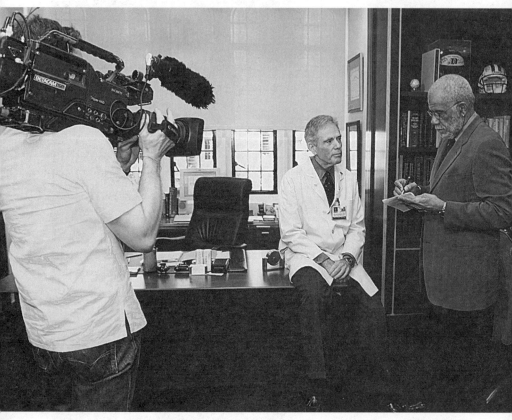

FIG. GALLERY 2.18 Ed Bradley, *60 Minutes* correspondent, and Ralph Snyderman filming "Anatomy of a Mistake," which aired on CBS on March 16, 2003. Photo courtesy of the Duke Medical Center Archives.

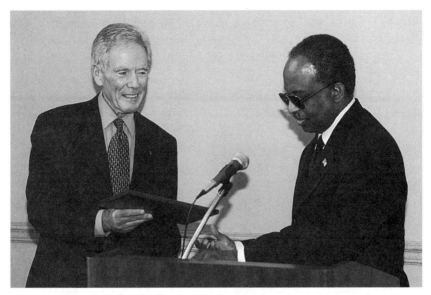

FIG. GALLERY 2.19 William Bell, mayor of the City of Durham, North Carolina, proclaiming May 17, 2004, "Dr. Ralph Snyderman Day" in recognition of Dr. Snyderman's contributions to the Durham and Duke communities. Photo courtesy of the Duke Medical Center Archives.

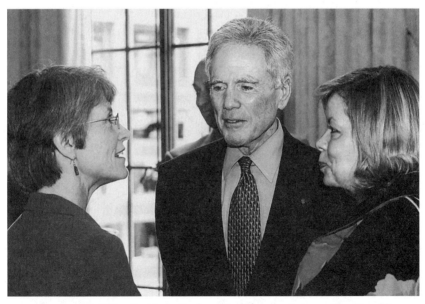

FIG. GALLERY 2.20 Ellen Reckhow, Durham County commissioner; Jean Spaulding, Duke Endowment trustee; and Ralph Snyderman at "Dr. Ralph Snyderman Day," 2004. Photo courtesy of the Duke Medical Center Archives.

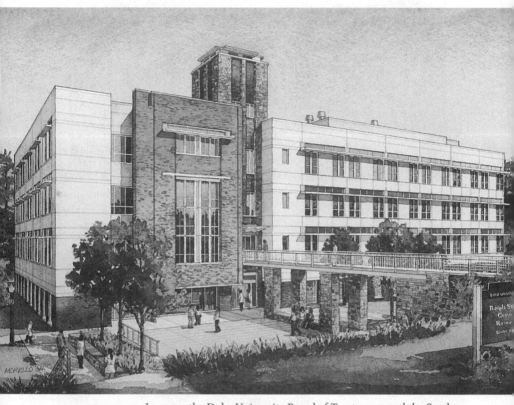

FIG. GALLERY 2.21 In 2004, the Duke University Board of Trustees named the Snyder-man Genome Sciences Research Building in honor of Ralph Snyderman. Photo by Duke Photography.

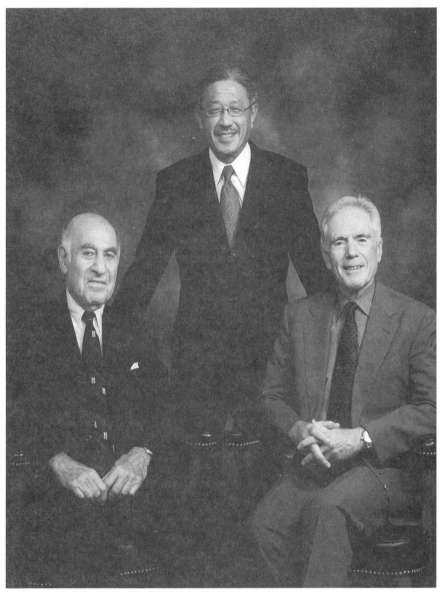

FIG. GALLERY 2.22 Chancellors for health affairs: William G. Anlyan (1964–1989), Victor J. Dzau (2004–2014), and Ralph Snyderman (1989–2004), photographed in 2004. Photo courtesy of the Duke Medical Center Archives.

III

RELATIONSHIPS, LEADERSHIP, AND LESSONS

14

—

Philanthropy and Relationships

Philanthropy is vital and often the only source of funds for creating certain new initiatives, building new facilities, and sustaining important activities not supported by clinical reserves, tuition, or external research grants. The responsibility that I initially had the least experience in or inclination toward was fostering philanthropic giving to the medical center. I've always hated asking people for things, especially money, and have felt this way for as long as I can remember. Maybe it's cultural, or perhaps it's something I learned from my father, but needing to ask people for money has always seemed demeaning to me, and being turned down very painful. But someone had to do it, and I was that *someone* for the Duke University Medical Center—it's in the job description, plain and simple.

When I began my tenure as chancellor, "development" was the overarching, innocuous term for ginning up philanthropic support. Not only did I not relish the task, I really did not understand it. In my simplistic conception, "development" was a euphemism for a transaction in which one who is needy asks one who has excess capacity to give up something out of the goodness of his or her heart. This wasn't a development of anything; the word for this was "charity." This view, of course, is misleading, if not downright mistaken. I ultimately learned that the term "development" means more than enhancement of the institution; it signifies the actual development of a strategic relationship between an individual capable of contributing and an institution capable of creating the donor's vision. Philanthropy, when it occurs on an institutional scale, is a true transaction, akin to a business deal. Like most good business deals, philanthropy is based on mutual need and relationships. The donor benefits from making the contribution as much as the institution benefits from receiving it; developing meaningful relationships is key. It took me a while to learn this, but once I did, the process of creating philanthropic giving to Duke proved to be one of my most rewarding responsibilities. It not only benefited the medical center and created testaments to the wishes of the donors but also enriched me through the lasting friendships I made.

Development officers—which is to say professional fund-raisers—are usually people who are fun to be with. If they weren't, they most likely would not be successful. Bucky Waters, head of medical center development when I arrived as chancellor, was such an individual. Bucky was a tall, handsome, affable former basketball player for North Carolina State University and a former men's basketball coach at Duke. But Bucky had star status even beyond Duke because he was also a television announcer for Division I men's basketball games. Bucky was very easy to talk to, always interesting, and had a comfortable charisma. By 1992, he indicated that, rather than lead the department, he was better suited for raising funds for high-priority projects and as an adviser to me in development. When he stepped down, we appointed him as vice chancellor for special projects. His understudy, Jeff Clark, also an enthusiastic and engaging individual, took the leadership role, but in 1994 he decided to leave Duke to become an entrepreneur.

So, during early 1994, we launched a national search for the next vice chancellor for development and alumni affairs. After seven months, we identified Joseph S. Beyel who was director of medical center development at the University of Michigan. Joe brought talent and experience at a critical time. We knew that creating a margin of excellence depended on philanthropy. Joe's primary mission was to position the development department to increase the level of support for medical center programs by seeking more alumni involvement and generating additional support for such major projects as the Levine Science Research Center, the Medical Science Research Building, a new children's facility, and a planned ambulatory care facility.

In 1996, during Joe's tenure, the university launched the most ambitious fund-raising campaign in its history. The "Campaign for Duke" initially sought to raise $1.5 billion (then increased to $2.0 billion), of which the medical center would raise $550 million. This also was by far the most comprehensive fund-raising effort in the history of the medical center. Joe left Duke in 2000 to become vice president for university advancement at the University of Louisville. After a national search Steven A. Rum replaced Joe. Steve, a former professional baseball player, had directed fund-raising efforts for the Children's National Medical Center Foundation and Special Olympics International prior to coming to Duke in 1995 as executive director of development for Duke's Children's Hospital. Much of his initial effort went into the philanthropic funding of the new Children's Health Center, which provided an attractive, family-friendly setting for a variety of specialized, state-of-the-art pediatric services. These also included the Jim Valvano Day Hospital and linked these to inpatient children services in Duke Hospital. More than $28 million had been raised of the $32.5 million needed to build the children's center.

Steve and I had a special relationship based on the tremendous similarities, yet distinct differences, in our roots and upbringing. I grew up as a Jew in Bensonhurst, whereas Steve was raised as an Italian in Queens. In Bensonhurst, there were only two kinds of people—Jews and Italians. We thought that the entire world was like this because that's all we ever saw growing up. Our groups had an intense love-hate relationship. We lived side by side and went to the same schools, yet we fought with each other all the time. In general, nobody ever got hurt—or at least not too badly. By and large, we had a substantial respect for each other. I liked Steve from the moment I met him when he was head of development for the children's health programs. I was impressed that he combined a savvy fund-raising instinct with the organizational skills necessary in large development programs. When we did a national search for his position, Steve was my first choice. His candidacy was not hurt by the call I received from Mike Krzyzewski, Duke's men's basketball coach, who told me that my ringside seats at Cameron Indoor Stadium would be in jeopardy if I didn't hire Steve.

Each time Steve walked through the door of my office, he would manage to say something that would crack me up and engender a response unlike anything I had used since leaving Brooklyn. Nonetheless, one particular trip with Steve comes to mind and will always be part of the memories of my time as chancellor. In 1999, Steve and I, both avid Duke basketball fans, traveled to St. Petersburg, Florida, for the men's NCAA Final Four, where Duke unfortunately came in second to the University of Connecticut. The morning after Duke lost the big game, a somber occasion, we flew home on a small jet leased by a Duke medical center supporter. At about thirty-five thousand feet, we heard a loud pop, the cabin immediately decompressed, oxygen masks dropped, and the plane dove to about twelve thousand feet in what seemed like seconds. We all looked around, wondering if we were going to survive what seemed to be an impending catastrophic event in this small plane. What had happened was that the copilot's window blew partially out. Thank God, we managed to land safely in Savannah, Georgia.

Steve left Duke in 2005 to become vice president for development and alumni relations at Johns Hopkins. He and I remain close friends, and regardless of how infrequently we see each other, we renew our relationship where we left off because we have a sense of family. I believe this springs from our working together closely and from the similar ways we were brought up. One of the greatest values of having Steve in this position for five and a half years is that I really liked the guy and enjoyed working with him. What really matters, though, is that he left our medical center a far stronger institution as a result of his efforts. Under Steve's leadership, we erected a world-class development organization. The launch of the medical center's campaign, "Keeping the Promise of Medicine," coincided with Duke's comprehensive campaign. We exceeded our goal of $550 million by more than $150 million, raising $706.4 million for the medical center, including the Duke Children's Health Center, Comprehensive Cancer Center, Eye Center, School of Medicine, and School of Nursing. The total included sponsored research, as well as $47.7 million in capital support (mainly for the McGovern-Davison Children's Health Center). These resources provided support for professorships, fellowships, research endowments, and many other areas.

— — —

One of my earliest personal experiences in development in 1989 was traveling with the aforementioned Joel Fleishman, a renowned Duke professor of law and public policy and at that time head of the university's development campaign. Joel, a former close adviser to then Duke president Terry Sanford, and a student of philanthropy who has written the most informative books on the field, asked me to travel with him to Miami to meet Shepard Broad, his children, and several members of his foundation's board.

Shepard Broad was a very wealthy individual who was a major developer of Biscayne Island off the coast of Miami. His wife, Ruth, had recently died of Alzheimer's disease. Joel knew Shepard and his children, Morris and Ann Bussel, very well. I truly enjoyed the opportunity to spend the day with Joel and to get to know Shepard Broad, a magnificent man who not only amassed a fortune but also was an important player along with David Ben-Gurion in providing initial funds and armaments to the Haganah—the pre-state defense force of the Jewish Yishuv in Palestine. As a result of our meeting, the Ruth and Shepard Broad Foundation transferred all its money to Duke to support programs in Alzheimer's research and the neurosciences. This transfer began with $2.2 million in the early 1990s and in 2016 has a market value of assets of nearly $14 million. Since its inception, the foundation has granted more than $7 million to enrich science, the scientific community, and the early careers of brilliant young researchers.

My inspiring engagement with the Broad family and the strength of our long friendship reflect what development is really about. The family created a foundation with a purpose, and they wanted to leverage its resources by supporting an institution they loved and trusted and that could help guide their investments effectively to support their areas of interest. Duke, concomitantly, had strong capabilities in neurosciences as well as a need for additional funding. Duke also had an investment arm, Duke University Management Company, in which foundation money placed within Duke could grow at a far greater rate than if it had been invested almost anywhere else. Thus, everybody was a winner; the Ruth K. Broad Foundation at Duke just celebrated its twenty-fourth anniversary and is still going strong.

Another early personal major philanthropic endeavor related to the gift made by Jack Whitehead to create the Whitehead Scholars Program. As discussed in chapter 5, this $13.7 million gift not only launched a key initiative to recruit star basic science faculty but also greatly pleased Jack Whitehead and his children. Moreover, Jack and I remained close friends until his death, and I remain friends with many notables I met on the ski trips he hosted.

Other noteworthy development experiences for me included obtaining a grant from the Lucille P. Markey Charitable Trust for $7.5 million to help support the recruitment of faculty for the Department of Cell Biology.

Robert Glaser, formerly a dean at New York University, ran the Markey Charitable Trust. He was perhaps two generations before me in internal medicine and, in my view, one of the giants whom I deeply admired. The Markey Charitable Trust was a spend-down trust; its entire $150 million value had to be spent over a period of fifteen years. By the time I got to Duke, about seven years remained. Despite overseeing a vast amount of money, Bob occupied a humble office in a modest business park in Menlo Park, California. Deans like me from far and near visited Bob hoping to obtain his favor in securing funds for their institutions. Like the others, I came to visit Bob in search of money, but I truly did admire and like him, money or no money. I enjoyed talking with him about the great men of internal medicine and sharing the experiences we had in our training. One day I mentioned to Bob that I wanted him to know I would continue to show up whether or not he had any money to give Duke. True to my word, even after a generous gift to Duke from the trust, I continued to visit Bob whenever I was in the Bay Area.

One of the largest gifts I was involved in soliciting and receiving was $10 million from Leon Levine for the naming of the Leon Levine Science Research Center. Prior to my coming back to Duke, Bill Anlyan, along with the university leadership, developed a concept of a large multidisciplinary research facility that would serve as the home for groundbreaking research and also allow collaborations with industry to foster academic-industrial relations. Leon Levine was the founder and CEO of Family Dollar stores, a highly successful enterprise that at that time had well over a thousand individual stores throughout the United States. Bill Anlyan, John Thomas (a major gift officer), and I drove to the Family Dollar headquarters in Charlotte to visit Leon and ask him for a gift. We had lunch together in a pleasant dining room next to his office; during the meal, Leon said something along the lines of "OK, let's get on with it; I know you're here to ask me for something."

At that point, John Thomas started explaining why we were there: Duke University had a major naming opportunity for a new building and enterprise that would foster creative new opportunities for research discoveries and medical contributions. This was probably a good place to start, but John then ventured that such a gift would be propitious at this particular moment because appreciated Family Dollar stock could be the source of the donation. Leon thought for a moment, then looked John in the eye and said, "Are you saying that I should put in appreciated Family Dollar stock because you are aware of something that will cause the price of the stock to go down? Are you telling me that my business is about to take a negative turn?" Leon cut John off, and I don't recall John saying another word. A bit later in the lunch, during which I sat bemused and a bit stunned, Leon looked to me and said, "Why don't you and I go have a little talk." I said sure. So we left the dining room and went to a back room in his office suite.

Having spent my youth working part-time in my father's department store, I was familiar with Jewish-owned retail stores. It was my experience that all such owners had back rooms where the "real" business was conducted. Leon asked me frankly, in a spirit of mutual trust: "Ralph, am I getting a good deal?" I said quickly and honestly, "Leon, this is not only a good deal you're getting, it's an absolute steal. You'd be spending $10 million for naming a building that cost over $60 million. The general rule of thumb is that contributions for naming ought to be 50 percent; you'd be paying less than 20 percent—a bargain by any standards." Then I told him, "I can't believe that they will approve this naming for only $10 million out of $60 million; it's never been done before." He then said, "OK, that's what I'm going to do." Indeed, that's what he did. Bill Anlyan deserves most of the credit for this gift, but I take some pride and comfort in knowing that the trust that Leon had in me might have helped. I am also grateful for the warm friendship I continue to enjoy with him and his wife, Sandra.

A second development luncheon with Bill Anlyan did not have the same outcome. He asked me to join him on a request to the CEO of Burroughs Wellcome for $10 million. The CEO at that time was Philip R. Tracy, a bright, charming, and approachable man who hosted a beautiful luncheon for us in his large, impressive office at the Burroughs Wellcome headquarters in the Research Triangle Park. Over lunch, we eventually got to the topic of why we were there, and Bill Anlyan asked him for $10 million. Phil didn't do a double take but he said nothing for a few moments. Then he said, in a most charming way: "Gee, this is the first time I ever invited someone to lunch and had them ask me for $10 million." We finished a pleasant lunch without a commitment from Phil, and the gift never came from Burroughs Wellcome. It did, however, create a friendship between Phil, his wife, Travis, and me that continues today. Not only did we become good friends, but he agreed to serve on the medical center's Board of Visitors.

Building a children's medical center had been an established goal for decades before my tenure. Because pediatric and children's services in general are among the most poorly reimbursed, such an initiative required philanthropic support. In 1973, Jay Arena, a Duke pediatrics professor, Sam Katz, and Bill Anlyan played key roles in launching the Duke Children's Classic to raise funds for children's programs. Sam Katz describes the history of the Children's Classic as follows:

In the early years of my chairmanship, Pediatrics (as with most University Pediatric Departments then) was in poor financial straits. A faculty member, John Griffith, who had accompanied me to Duke from Harvard, had a brother who was an executive with one of the big oil companies. His brother told us of the celebrity golf tournaments in which many corporate executives played and said because Duke had such a fine golf course, why didn't we initiate something of that sort as a fundraiser. Our good fortune was that one of the older Duke pediatric faculty, Dr. Jay Arena, was a good friend of Perry Como's, at that time a nationally recognized singer. Perry agreed to join us as the leader and to invite many of his colleagues who owed him favors. We talked with Bill Anlyan, the Dean, and he assigned Bucky Waters (former basketball coach who was Bill's Development person) to assist us. We talked with Terry Sanford, then Duke's President, who was most supportive and agreed to attract some of his colleagues to play. The format was that people paid several thousand dollars for the weekend in which they played golf on Saturday and Sunday in a foursome with a celebrity, had a dinner and show Saturday night organized by Perry. It started modestly in 1974 but very quickly became a great success. Many of those who came and paid for the weekend initially included individuals on their own, but with heightened recognition many corporations sent their officers as a "reward" for performance. Celebrities who participated included Dinah Shore, Frank Sinatra, Jay Leno, Buddy Hackett, etc.; sports figures such as golfers Sam Snead, Chi Chi Rodriguez, Arnold Palmer; football, baseball, and basketball stars including Mickey Mantle, Michael Jordan, etc. The celebrities were given a free ride (room and transportation) but no other financial item. With increasing success, we added tennis for those who preferred that to golf and Stan Smith became the leader of that component.[1]

When I joined as chancellor, Perry and his loving wife, Roselle, still were actively involved in the Children's Classic, and we soon became close friends. I was a bit starstruck by this event but found that folks like Perry and Roselle were dear, caring people. When it came time for Perry to step down, we recruited R. David Thomas (founder of Wendy's), Mike and Mickey Krzyzewski, and later on comedian Jeff Foxworthy and his wife, Gregg, to play lead roles. Through these efforts, we helped support much-needed children's programs. The Duke Children's Classic raised $14 million for Duke Children's Hospital over a remarkable thirty-five-year run, and I came to know many remarkable leaders, talents, and dear compassionate people who remain friends today.

Despite the success of the Children's Classic, we still needed a major gift to launch the actual building of the Duke Children's Health. John P. McGovern was a 1945 graduate of the Duke University School of Medicine, a noted philanthropist, and someone I hoped would make a major contribution to his alma mater. A highly successful allergist and an even more successful developer and investor, John had amassed considerable wealth. I first met him in Florida through an introduction from Bill Anlyan and came to like and respect him and to understand a bit of what it must have been like for him to be pursued so energetically by so many asking for donations. In getting to know John, I often got caught up in his stories of being a medical student during the early years at Duke when Dean Wilburt Davison was so intimately involved with the selection and subsequent mentoring of each medical school class. In John's case, he wanted to go to medical school and was waiting in the dean's office for an interview. During the wait, which was longer than John expected, he began looking at the pictures on Dean Davison's walls. There he saw one of Sir William Osler and was gazing at it intensely when the dean entered the office. Dean Davison asked John about William Osler and, since John was an admirer of Osler, "the father of medicine," a rich conversation ensued. John was admitted to Duke medical school. Dean Davison had a profound and lasting impact on John and was one of his heroes.

Many years later, when I was raising money to build Duke's Children's Health Center, I visited John at his apartment in Houston. In speaking with John about philanthropy, I didn't appear to be getting anywhere, but we again started talking about Dean Davison. The idea hit me out of the blue that it might be totally appropriate and quite attractive to link John

McGovern's name with Dean Davison in perpetuity, so I looked at John and said, "Wouldn't it be a wonderful thing to name our new children's facility the McGovern-Davison Children's Health Center? That, I said, "would intertwine your names together at the institution you both dearly loved." John looked me and immediately said, "Yes, I will do that." He contributed $6.5 million to the building that will always carry his and Dean Davison's names. The $32.5 million facility, which opened in 2000, was financed completely through philanthropy.

Dave Thomas was a member of Duke University's Board of Trustees from 1988 to 1997, a patient at Duke University Medical Center, and a major contributor to the Fuqua School of Business through the funding of the R. David Thomas Executive Conference Center. As already mentioned, Dave was affiliated with the medical center through the Duke Children's Hospital and the annual Children's Classic. Dave was also, of course, one of the most recognizable faces in the United States thanks to his ubiquitous presence in all advertisements for Wendy's hamburgers. Dave, who did not complete high school, was an orphan from Dublin, Ohio, who worked his way up from running several Kentucky Fried Chicken franchises. In 1963, he opened his first Wendy's Old Fashioned Hamburgers restaurant in Columbus, Ohio. At the time of Dave's death in 2002, at the age of sixty-nine, the chain had six thousand restaurants in more than thirty countries.

Dave and I met in Fort Lauderdale after one of Duke's many Palm Beach forums. Dave was very proud of his sixty-six-foot motor yacht, *Sunray*, which was one of the fastest motor yachts running. Dave loved to race to Ocean Reef in the Florida Keys with friends who had motor yachts in Fort Lauderdale. Dave and I immediately became friends. He was a warm, humble, and sincere person who evinced a boy's joy in having fun either yachting or playing cards or just sitting around and talking with his friends, many of whom were notable celebrities. My wife, Judith, and I, along with Dave and his wife, Lorraine, spent many fun times together either at their home in Florida or visiting with them at Buckeye Lake, a blue-collar resort not far from Columbus, Ohio. One day while cruising the lake on Dave's boat, I described to him the concept of the emerging Duke University Health System. Dave looked at me in his usual understated and humble way and said, "Doctor, sounds to me like you're developing a franchise system." Because I was sitting with the franchise king of the United States, we had a wonderful and useful conversation dealing with issues I needed to consider as we spread the Duke "franchise" throughout the Southeast. Dave never gave a substantial financial gift to Duke University Medical Center, but he provided a tremendous amount to the institution through his involvement in the Children's Classic and especially through his wise counsel and friendship with me.

One of Bucky Waters's big prospects for a major gift for our Center for Living was Jeno F. Paulucci, who founded Jeno's Pizza and made a lot of money with this and other food-related businesses. Jeno received his medical care at Duke, as well as from his primary physician, Robert "Crusty" Rosemond, a Duke medical school graduate and an excellent and dedicated internist. Jeno lived in Duluth, Minnesota, and had a three-acre fishing camp about a hundred miles farther north, deep in the wilds of Ontario's Lake Country. As a gift to Crusty, Jeno would allow him to invite five other individuals to fly up to the fishing camp in Jeno's two amphibious planes and spend four evenings and five days at some of the best fishing spots in the world. Crusty, being a strong Duke loyalist, indicated that Jeno might be a major contributor to Duke, so for about five years Bucky and I would fly to Duluth during the summer, spend an evening there, and then park ourselves for the next four nights at Jeno's fishing lodge with the hope of meeting with Jeno to solicit a gift in the range of $10 million. Being in this remote fishing camp dozens of miles from the nearest small Indian village, with no way in or out other than by seaplane, sleeping in modest cabins, and eating food prepared by what seemed to be a short-order cook was a unique experience for this kid from Brooklyn. Along with Crusty and Bucky, there were generally three or four other individuals present, virtually all of whom were highly regarded heroes who fought in World War II, many of them naval aviators. We would fish all day, begin drinking at dinnertime, have dinner, and then smoke cigars until the mosquitoes drove us to our cabins. After five years, it became clear that despite getting the opportunity to enjoy these unique surroundings, we would never receive a monetary gift from Jeno Paulucci, and we never did.

Creating the Board of Visitors for the medical center was an important step in assembling a group of individuals with influence, means, and some affinity for Duke who as a group could help advise medical center leadership in their areas of expertise and provide a source of potential philanthropy through their own giving or access to others. Milton and Roslyn Lachman became members of the Board of Visitors. The Lachmans were good friends and supporters of Bill Anlyan, and when Bill introduced them to me, I immediately understood why. Roz was a graduate of Duke University, and Milt was a successful real estate developer. We quickly became friends, and our friendship continues today. Milt and Roz not only contributed generously to the medical center but also organized annual forums in Palm Beach where I met other individuals of wealth and influence who ultimately engaged either with the Board of Visitors or directly with me.

At a Duke fund-raising forum at the Breakers Hotel in Palm Beach, the Lachmans introduced me to Brandt and Belinda Louie. By the time we met, their business, London Drugs, was a flourishing enterprise across much of western Canada. The pharmacy business was one part of a comprehensive retail operation, somewhat like Target. Brandt and Belinda had two sons at Duke, Stuart in law school and Gregory in medical school. The Louies became strong backers of the medical center, as well as dear friends. For many years, they sponsored a Duke forum in Vancouver that featured the medical center's innovative programs. During Gregory's time as a medical student, I found him to be very bright and engaging, and I enjoyed mentoring him. After postgraduate training at Stanford, he joined his brother, Stuart, to work with their father in growing their business throughout Canada.

It was through Milt and Roz that I also got to know Ruth and Herman (Hy) Albert. The Alberts were good friends of the Lachmans, and Milt and Hy were often in business together in development deals. Like the Lachmans, the Alberts had accumulated substantial wealth. Hy was a careful and excellent businessman who loved Ruth greatly. When Ruth developed vision loss and was treated at Duke, Hy wanted much to do whatever he could to please her. Over several years, Ruth, Hy, and I became good friends, and in discussing Hy's wishes to honor his wife, I suggested they consider making a gift to the Duke Eye Institute for a proposed building to enhance the excellent work of our Department of Ophthalmology researchers. Over the period of a year or so, we refined the nature of the gift. Despite one occasion when our head of development offended Hy to the point he was ready to walk away, Hy committed $8 million for the Ruth and Herman Albert Eye Research Institute and $3.5 million to support the Herman and Ruth Albert Lung Cancer Genomics Fund.

An illustration of the nature of the bond between major donors, the institution they give to, and the individuals who consummate such gifts is borne out by my personal interactions with the Alberts. During the course of discussions and negotiations about the gift, Hy developed lung cancer and needed a lobectomy. One of our skilled thoracic surgeons, Tommy D'Amico, performed the surgery and took wonderful care of Hy. For years after the surgery, Tommy and his wife, Ruth, Hy, Judith, and I often met and dined together, becoming good friends. Several years after his surgery, with his lung function already compromised by the lobectomy, Hy suffered a recurrence of his disease, and his clinical course went downhill, leading to his admission to Duke Hospital.

I vividly recall one Friday afternoon in June 2002, when, in my office, I saw Hy Albert's name on a card I received every day indicating "special constituents" who were in Duke Hospital. I made it a practice to visit the hospital and see patients while wearing my physician's white coat. I sought ongoing continuity with patient care, the clinical faculty and staff, and individuals who had a special connection to Duke. That day was the end of a very busy week, and while I was getting ready to leave at about six thirty, hoping to go home for a quiet evening for the first time that week, I recalled that Hy was in the hospital. My immediate feeling was that I could always come back to see him on Saturday, or more likely stop by and see him first thing Monday morning. Then I asked myself, "Would you be doing the right thing not to see Hy Albert tonight?" I often ask myself this sort of question when I'm in a situation where it would be easy to do the comfortable thing, but I know that it would not be the right thing.

So I trekked from my office in the Davison Building to Duke Hospital, up the elevator, to visit with Hy. He was lying in bed, his head on two pillows, looking wan; Ruth and their two children were in the room. He looked at me kindly, our eyes locked, and I took his hand in both of my hands and proceeded to tell him how much I respected him and valued his life and his life's work, as well as what he was doing to honor his dear wife, Ruth. I visited for perhaps twenty minutes, all the while holding Hy's hand and, I hope, comforting him and signifying what I truly believed was the value of a life well lived. We all had tears in our eyes by the time I left. Hy died the next day. I continued to see Ruth, called her frequently, and reminded her how much Hy loved her. The Ruth and Herman Albert Eye Research Institute is visible from my office window, and I spontaneously call her on occasion—an elderly homebound woman in Palm Beach now—to tell her things that I hope will be uplifting. This, too, is what "development" is about.

So it was that the development responsibilities that made me so uncomfortable at first turned out to be a highly rewarding and lasting benefit of my tenure as chancellor for health affairs. The experience taught me that philanthropy is based on friendship, trust, and shared interests in creating a common good. Through my development efforts I met and became associated with good, caring people who are among my closest friends, many years after my fund-raising involvement with them ended. I count Sheppard and Clara Zinovoy, whom I met through my colleague and former Duke cardiologist Judith Swain, who had met them when she was at the University of Pennsylvania, as such friends. Through Judith's high regard for the couple, I invited Shep to become a member of the Board of Visitors, and from the moment we met, we became close friends, with that friendship continuing through today.

It was Shep who told me, as I was stepping down as chancellor, to prepare for the shock that once I left office, hundreds of people I thought of as friends would effectively vanish and I would then understand who my few true friends are. He couldn't have been more correct. It is an illusion to think that one's relationships while in a position of high authority reflect only genuine selfless concerns. Many people, and this is not altogether inappropriate, have a relationship with a *position* rather than with the *person* occupying it. After leaving as Duke medical center's leader, I was fortunate to retain dozens of true friends, many of whom I initially met in my role of a development diplomat for the university.

15

—

Reputation and Crisis

I wanted to do more than enhance the institution's impact in all its core missions and through its innovative programs; I wanted Duke to be recognized as a leading academic health enterprise nationally. Communications, as a corporate service, is among the most important elements required for a complex and expanding medical center bent on being a leader and also being recognized as such. Communicating the excellence of the institution internally and externally is essential. The communications department must create effective capabilities in news services, marketing, and public relations. It must also respond to crises.

When I arrived in 1989, we did not have the kind of communications office suitable for the environment we were in or for the future we were determined to create. The communication function under the leadership of Bill Anlyan excelled in crafting excellent printed material, largely for internal constituents. Realizing that the head of our communications department needed a far broader vision and much wider skills, we conducted a national search for a new leader. As a result, we identified Vicki Saito, assistant vice president for external affairs at the University of Texas Medical Branch at Galveston (UTMB), as our choice for the post.

Vicki had extensive and successful experience at UTMB and before that at the University of California Davis, where she was intimately involved in a highly charged national case involving the issue of affirmative action in admission to the University of California medical schools. Vicki impressed me as someone who combined the needed depth and breadth of experience with a calm and confidential demeanor. I appointed her as assistant vice chancellor/director of medical center communications, and it proved to be a wise choice. Vicki organized and ran a comprehensive and successful office of communications, and most important to me, she became a highly respected adviser in all my duties as chancellor for health affairs. She routinely judged and weighed in on how I was being perceived and how the medical center projected its image internally, regionally, nationally, and internationally. She was candid, totally trustworthy, and she set high standards and developed into a valued colleague.

Under Vicki's leadership, the communications office moved from a focus on publications for internal consumption to news and information, public relations, publications, and marketing communications. Put simply, communications, public relations, and making national news became high priorities as part of the overall operations of the medical center. Over the years, DUMC drew increasing recognition as a center of innovation. It stood out for its establishment of new models of clinical research and health care delivery, as well as the creation of its health system. With notable exceptions, some described in this chapter, Duke's image grew from that of an excellent but not highest top-tier medical center in the early 1990s to one that was increasingly recognized as being among the key centers of medical innovation in the United States.

I needed someone like Vicki more than most chancellors might have. When I was growing up in a blue-collar ethnic neighborhood in Brooklyn, politeness, sensitivity, thoughtfulness, and withholding action while contemplating consequences were not high on my list of virtues. As a teenager in a rough neighborhood, one often acted first, saying whatever was on one's mind and, sometimes, what one did not even know was on one's mind until it got said. These Brooklyn characteristics, which one might call brashness, stayed with me during my early years as chancellor. Slowly, I learned to listen carefully and to contemplate how others might perceive my actions. Vicki and her communications staff helped me anticipate the likely public perception of actions we took, for better or otherwise.

My need to exchange and communicate information grew both as the stature of the Duke medical center expanded and as my role in national medical leadership grew. The latter occurred in part through my participation on the Council of Deans within the AAMC and also as a health system leader in the Association of Academic Health Centers. In 1993, as President Bill Clinton and First Lady Hillary Clinton began to formulate an initiative to create universal health care, I joined approximately twenty leaders of academic medicine to advise the president in formulating what turned out to be the Clinton Health Security Act of 1993. The development of this legislation, led by Ira C. Magaziner and Harold L. Ickes, occurred largely outside the purview of the academic deans, but we convened at the White House from time to time to exchange ideas on issues affecting academic medicine.

As the legislation rolled out, we attended by special invitation several events in the Rose Garden behind the White House, where I was able to speak with the president and First Lady, both of whom were very impressive. Hillary's extensive knowledge of health care was particularly welcome, and I found her extremely cordial and well-informed. But one day, Hillary surprised me when she said that, to pass any legislation, one had to identify a villain to run against. I thought about this remark a lot. I didn't want it to be true, and in the end I concluded that it was true only when people thought and acted as though it was. Unfortunately, this approach is standard fare in American politics today.

Giving me additional exposure on the national scene was my leadership within the AAMC, as councilor in the Institute of Medicine, as president of the AAP, and through appearances at several congressional committees that were evaluating issues related to health care. In addition, I wrote op-ed pieces for national publications—the *New York Times* and the *Wall Street Journal*—and occasionally appeared on national television. Vicki encouraged me to frequent Washington, DC, during which time I developed close relationships with all the North Carolina senators, many representatives, and virtually all congressional health care leaders.

Vicki and the communications department likewise kept a keen eye on opportunities for me to engage broadly on the national scene and to make it easy for local and national press to have access to Duke. It was good for the medical center, good for the faculty, and good for the university. Clearly, Duke's emergence as a model for the academic health system of the twenty-first century was gaining broader attention. I recall at Vicki's behest, a meeting with about forty people from the press. As a result, a member of the group got the bright idea of coming down to Duke to do a feature based on a week in the life of a hospital. *Time* magazine, thought it would be an interesting thing to do and brought an entire crew to Durham. The lead journalists stayed at my house until 11:00 PM one evening discussing various topics. In his book, *Foundations for Excellence: 75 Years of Duke Medicine*, Walter Campbell describes the October 12, 1998 *Time* story as follows:

> . . . *Time* magazine published a 40-page cover story on the medical center at Duke, calling DUMC "one of the crown jewels of American medicine." A masked surgeon looks out intensely from the magazine's cover, his blue surgical uniform acting as a background for the title "A Week in the Life of a Hospital: On the Front Lines of the War between Money and Medicine." The story uses Duke as an example of how America's academic medical centers were dealing with the challenges and opportunities presented by managed care, skyrocketing costs, dwindling federal funding, and widening inequities in care. In one of the story's many brief features, "An M.D. as CEO Redraws the Big Picture," *Time* noted "what Snyderman is doing is not unique, but it is much talked about in medical circles. If it works, he's a genius. If it doesn't Duke could go the same route as the University of Minnesota, which sold its hospital, or the University of Pennsylvania, which reported a $40 million deficit this year. [1]

Duke's medical center continued to create a positive buzz. In September 2000, almost two years after the article appeared in *Time*, the Discovery Channel devoted a thirteen-episode, patient-focused, real-time documentary showcasing a day in the life of a hospital, which was filmed at Duke University Medical Center.

One highly successful initiative in raising national recognition of Duke University Medical Center was the launch in 1994 of what originally was called the Duke Private Sector Conference. My predecessor, Bill Anlyan, and J. Alexander McMahon, a health policy leader at Duke, had initiated this conference years earlier as a way to bring together approximately three dozen health care leaders to discuss important issues facing medicine and particularly academic medicine. After a hiatus of five years, I chose to initiate a modernized version of the Private Sector Conference, and together with a prestigious selection committee, we chose a major topic for discussion and invited some of the most influential individuals from various scientific, business, and government sectors that affected health care.

I had in mind a very specific program format: leaders of academic health centers, health care insurers, commercial health care providers, government officials, representatives of the health insurance industry, and large purchasers of health care—all would attend. The meeting would begin on a Sunday evening in the plush surroundings of the Washington Duke Inn and continue for a full day and a half at the Searle Center at the medical center. Speakers introduced various topics but did not lecture at length in an effort to foster vigorous and intense audience participation. As everyone in attendance knew, the entire proceedings would be recorded, transcribed, and published. A frequent attendee at these conferences was Uwe E. Reinhardt, the noted Princeton health economist. Uwe was often the first evening's keynote speaker, and his description of the foibles of health care would educate and amuse us. Through these meetings, Uwe, his equally prominent wife, Tsung-Mei (May) Cheng, and I became good friends. When the Duke University Health System Board of Directors was created in 1998, Uwe agreed to be a founding member.

At our first Private Sector Conference, we invited John K. Iglehart, the founding editor of *Health Affairs* and the national correspondent for the *New England Journal of Medicine*. John wrote a comprehensive piece covering the Private Sector Conference that appeared in *Health Affairs* and an executive summary in the *New England Journal of Medicine*.[2] The conference (renamed the Duke Health Sector Conference in 2002) convened annually through 2004 and proved to be a highly visible and influential platform for high-level, action-oriented health care policy discussions.

It was at one of these meetings in 1998 that a "personalized health care" program dealing with congestive heart failure at Duke made its debut. The program not only improved care but also saved vast sums of money. DUHS, however, *lost* money on the program because of the perversities of the health care reimbursement structure; although costs were reduced, the benefits accrued to the insurer, not to Duke (more on such perversities is discussed in chapter 13). One advantage of this program was having Tom Scully present; as the head of the CMS, he could create policy to address the revenue discrepancies. In all, the Duke Health Sector Conference placed DUMC at the center of policy discussions regarding a rapidly evolving health care environment. Vicki Saito coordinated the proceedings, and each year we published the edited transcript with the support of the Duke Endowment.

These annual publications captured the excellence and ferment of health care innovation.

— — —

The increasing visibility of DUMC in the news was, of course, a positive factor in enhancing the national reputation of our institution. It was rare for a day to go by without some mention of Duke or one of its faculty in the national media. We wanted everyone working at DUMC to know they were being both watched and praised; it was good for morale and for maintaining a level of vigilance. In an entity as big and complex as DUMC and its emerging health system, it is predictable and ought to be understandable that things will occasionally go wrong. Prior to Duke's high visibility and momentum as a national leader, occurrences such as the hospital workforce reduction in 1995 had generated negative coverage in the local press (see chapters 9 and 11). But the stronger Duke's national reputation became, the greater the risk that anything that went wrong would also gain national attention. So it was that, in 1999, the first of what turned out to be two major setbacks generated unwanted coverage at Duke not only in the local press but also on a national scale.

Monday, May 10, 1999, started like any typical busy week for me. The meeting of the DUHS Board of Directors marked my calendar for Thursday evening, and I had to prepare for it. On Friday, there was a meeting of the Medical Center Affairs Committee of the Board of Trustees, and later that same afternoon, there was a meeting of the Board of Trustees where I was slated to present the status of the medical center. That Friday evening, I was scheduled to present the Hippocratic oath in Duke Chapel to our graduating class of the School of Medicine, followed the next day by a meeting of our Board of Trustees. That evening, I was to give remarks at the Maimonides ceremony at the Center for Jewish Life for the Jewish members of the medical school's graduating class of 1999.

Monday morning began with a meeting of our Executive Management Committee, the senior group of individuals working most closely with me to oversee all medical center operations. What got added unexpectedly to my schedule that day was a 1:30 PM conference call with Michael Carome, chief of the U.S. Department of Health and Human Services' Office for Protection from Research Risks (OPRR). Joining me on this call, among others, were

Ed Holmes, our new dean of the School of Medicine, and John M. Falletta, the head of our institutional review board (IRB). I had been told the call was related to an ongoing investigation of Duke's clinical research programs by OPRR, which began in December 1998. I knew that OPRR had "randomly" selected Duke to review its institutional oversight for protecting research subjects. This fell under the purview of the IRB, which was required to follow all federal guidelines to protect research subjects.

Late in December 1998, OPRR had notified Duke of several shortcomings in its IRB process, all of which seemed technical in nature but nonetheless important to correct. I was informed about the ongoing issue and assumed, incorrectly as it turned out, that these matters were being dealt with effectively. They came under the responsibility of the dean and the head of the IRB and were not a matter that a chancellor would deal with directly on a daily or weekly basis. In February 1999, John, along with medical center officials under the leadership of Ed, proposed a corrective action plan. But that plan was rejected by OPRR several days later, and it was not until late March that the IRB submitted an updated corrective action plan. When I asked Ed about how this issue was going, he indicated to me, in essence, "Don't worry, it's under control," which he and others assumed to be the case.

Thus, the conference call scheduled by OPRR on that Monday, May 10, at 1:30 PM materialized a bit unexpectedly. I assumed there would be a conversation regarding our proposal and perhaps suggested alterations. Gathered around the conference phone, after introductions were made, we heard Mike Carome calmly indicate that I would be receiving a letter later that day indicating that all federally funded clinical research at Duke must be suspended. He indicated that the specific reasons for this action would be stated in the letter and, to reverse this freeze of our clinical research programs, we would need OPRR approval of our remediation.

This news was initially unfathomable. It came just seven months after the laudatory cover story in *Time* about our medical center, which the magazine had offered as an example of American's best hope for the future of health care. Our medical center had championed academically directed clinical research and, at the time, was shepherding approximately two thousand ongoing clinical trials with supporting revenues of approximately $228 million, with a lot of that money coming from the federal government.

I was shocked to hear this news. I had assumed that the IRB situation was under control, since I had been told as much in so many words. Naturally, some of my initial thoughts were: How did this get screwed up so badly? Why had I not been more personally engaged in this? How devastating will this be to Duke's image?

I already knew the answer to that last question. Although no human subjects had been harmed, or even put at risk, the news would tarnish Duke's reputation as a leading health care system. I also understood the devastating effect this would have on our clinical research programs, the faculty members who led them, and the finances underpinning them, as well as on the economic health of the health system and the progress of research being driven by these studies. It also quickly dawned on me that this announcement, which gained international attention the next day, was coming only days before I would address the Duke University Board of Trustees on the progress of our medical center and health system.

This is the sort of episode that momentarily confounds and disorients a person. The shock, embarrassment, and private self-criticism can be debilitating. I was particularly in a quandary over my leadership style. When I first became chancellor, I was criticized, somewhat justifiably, for micromanaging too much from the green zone. I knew that overreliance on my subordinates was not appropriate because, as Harry Truman used to say, come what may, the buck stops at the desk of the leader. Over time, though, I had grown more comfortable with delegating—and now look at the mess we all faced as a result of my relying too much on the judgment of others.

The shutdown of Duke's clinical research programs slapped me back into action. This was a big problem requiring a very complex solution, and I needed to take the lead. Summoning all my strength, I went into crisis action mode, assuming complete responsibility for a rapid solution. I appointed a high-level team led by Ed Holmes, Russel E. Kaufman (vice dean for education in the School of Medicine), Barbara E. Echols (assistant vice chancellor for academic affairs), and John Falletta to review in detail the communication from OPRR and develop a remediation plan. We all committed to work 24/7 if necessary. Russ and I would meet with Mike Carome and the leadership of OPRR to present corrective measures we hoped would lift the ban. Taking a positive, action-oriented approach was empowering. This was an unexpected blow to the medical center and its operations to be sure, but I intended to use it not only to fulfill OPRR's requirements but also to make us a national model for implementing mechanisms to protect human research subjects.

Over the next two days, our team worked ceaselessly to find solutions to meet OPRR's demands, and on Thursday, May 13, we chartered a plane to fly the team to Bethesda, Maryland, for a morning meeting with OPRR. We needed a private plane because I had to be back at the medical center early that afternoon for the Duke Chapel service in memory of my dear friend and colleague Charles E. Putman, senior vice president for research administration and policy at Duke, who had died unexpectedly that week of a heart attack at the age of fifty-seven. What was more, that evening the DUHS board would meet, and as its CEO, of course I had to be there. I could only shake my head at having this horrible event in the news directly before my presentations to the boards of both the health system and the university.

The meeting with OPRR went well. Although offended that OPRR had taken such visible and, I thought, unnecessarily stringent actions, I did not say so. Rather, I explained that Duke wanted to become the national model for human subject protection and that OPRR could benefit from working with us to set a national example. These words seemed to have a powerful effect. We left the meeting with our remediation plan and worked diligently on the way back on the plane to answer the remaining questions that OPRR had posed during the meeting. By the time we arrived back in Durham, we had revised our plan and, blessedly, by the next day we received notice that "the regulatory requirements for the protection of human subjects were satisfactory overall."

My presentation to the Duke University Board of Trustees on Friday afternoon, May 14, 1999, is one I will never forget. I had planned a positive update about all the good things we were doing and the progress we were making, and I had plenty of evidence to support my optimism. Then the OPRR bombshell had hit, spreading reputational shrapnel everywhere. Now I needed to discuss in detail the cause of the clinical research shutdown and the steps we had taken to get it rescinded.

My presentation was open, honest, and comprehensive. I followed the dictum of former House Speaker Sam Rayburn: "Always tell the truth; that way you don't have to remember what you said." After I finished presenting, one of the trustees, John Mack, the CEO of Morgan Stanley and a man known to be a strict leader (some called him "Mack the Knife"), leaned over the table, looked me in the eye, and asked: "Whose fault was this?"

This question surprised me. My first inclination was to blame the dean, who had assured me that everything was under control. But then I pictured

Harry Truman sitting in the Oval Office with his "The buck stops here" sign. I looked back at John Mack and said, "I'm responsible. I'm the one who screwed up and I'm going to see that it is fixed." That seemed to satisfy John and the rest of the board, but had OPRR failed to rescind its shutdown of our clinical research programs that very day, my answer might not have set as well.

We all were certainly glad that the rescindment came so quickly, but it left us with a lot of work to do. While we could resume enlisting patients in clinical research and our clinical research studies, about 250 research projects that had enrolled patients with insufficient IRB oversight needed to be reviewed. That would take months. Additionally, it became clear that we had to focus far more resources on our IRB and also create a second IRB to accommodate our high volume of clinical research.

The issues raised by OPRR, which we addressed in our response, were largely administrative failings in documenting appropriate IRB procedures for research protection. As I have already indicated, no one was harmed or came close to being harmed by Duke's clinical research programs. The administrative failures involved how minutes were to be collected at meetings; taking quorums at each vote; documenting guidelines for pediatric clinical research; and discrepancies in the recorded minutes, such as the actual number of individuals in the room at times of voting. To address these failures, we created an administrative oversight position for all human subject protection; we recruited national experts in clinical research subject protection to advise us; and we reflected on what it would take and what it would mean to be a national leader in protecting those individuals who so generously and selflessly engaged in clinical research.

The press attention to the clinical research shutdown at Duke was extensive, as we had expected. Articles appeared in newspapers throughout the country, as well as in the major scientific journals, including *Science* and *Nature*.[3] Many indicated that Duke had gotten tagged as a scapegoat because it had the largest clinical research program in the country; OPRR wanted to send a strong message to others by bringing the largest clinical research operation to its knees.

We at Duke did not become involved in this speculative debate. We kept our heads up and did all we could to make this a learning experience. We hoped to turn adversity into advantage by leading in the development of improved national standards for human subject research protection. Indeed, the January 28, 2000, issue of *Science*, published an article by Ed Holmes and me entitled "Oversight Mechanisms for Clinical Research."[4] In addition to describing the history of regulating human clinical subject research protection, we described Duke's experience in the growth of clinical research and proposed recommendations whereby IRBs and academic medical centers could create state-of-the-art means to protect human subjects.

This episode, which lasted well over half of the year from the time of the shutdown to the publication in *Science*, once again taught me that in addition to all the responsibilities of institutional leadership, all the planning and oversight mechanisms one can devise, there would still be times when an unexpected event could shake the leader and the institution to its marrow and deflect it from almost everything it was doing until the problem was solved. While such events are inevitable, it is the reaction to them that matters. The reaction can make or break a leadership cadre and affect the strength of an institution. The old intern adage, "If it doesn't kill you, it's a learning experience," again served me as a guideline. Alas, this was not the last such event I would face as the head of Duke's medical enterprise.

— — —

February 2003 proved to be among the most difficult and tumultuous times for the medical center, the university, for me, and, most tragically, for Jesica Santillan and her family. It all started back in 1999, when seventeen-year old Jesica Santillan and her mother, Magdelena, entered the United States illegally from Tamazula, Mexico. They had come looking for a better life and for the medical attention Jesica needed for her worsening health issues. She suffered from a cardiomyopathy that eventually resulted in cardiac failure and secondarily compromised her lungs.

On February 7, 2003, in a hospital surgical suite at Duke, the pediatric cardiac surgeon James Jaggers and his surgery team transplanted a newly arrived heart and set of lungs into Jesica. They used skills and technologies at least the equivalent of sending a man to the moon and returning him safely. Out of this heroic attempt, however, a tragic mistake not only led to Jesica's death but ultimately threatened to bring our medical center to its knees.

Once the heart and lungs were in place in Jesica's chest and her blood was reinfused, it became apparent to Jim that something was wrong. The color of the organs did not look right upon this reperfusion. Jagger's concern turned to alarm when he learned from the transplantation laboratory that the transplanted organs were incompatible with Jesica's blood type. In other words, Jim and his team had transplanted mismatched organs into Jesica's body, and the organs would likely be rejected by her immune system. The transplant team immediately initiated high-dose immunosuppressive agents, as well as plasmapheresis to prevent immediate organ rejection. Duke instantly notified UNOS (United Network for Organ Sharing) that a new heart and lungs were needed to save Jesica's life. Jesica was transferred to the intensive care unit and maintained on mechanical ventilation and all means of appropriate support. Jim also informed the family and their supporters about the mistake in blood-type matching.

I first learned about this horrible incident on Monday, February 10, three days after it occurred. At that point, Jesica continued on mechanical ventilation and received a procedure called ECMO (extracorporeal membrane oxygenation) to support her life. We used every state-of-the-art medical therapy to keep her alive while new organs were sought.

While they were in the United States awaiting her transplant, Jesica and her mother had come to the attention of Mack Mahoney, a builder in Louisburg, North Carolina. He helped support the family and was committed to Jesica's well-being. Mr. Mahoney was a contentious individual, however. He suspected that Duke was not doing enough to procure a new set of organs for Jesica and felt that generating negative publicity might improve the likelihood of her obtaining a new heart and lungs. Mr. Mahoney contacted the local press, and by February 17 the news of a "botched transplant" at Duke became national and then international news.

On February 20, Jesica's precarious status moved her to the top of the transplantation list, and a new set of organs was found and immediately transplanted into her chest. Unfortunately, her cardiopulmonary function deteriorated, and on February 22 she was pronounced dead. Between February 17 and February 25, it was hard to find a newspaper or a television news show that did not feature stories about this terrible, and almost unbelievable, medical error at Duke Hospital.

Inside the medical center and the university, we had committed to doing everything humanly possible to save Jesica's life. We also sought to determine the cause of the error so that it would never happen again, to communicate fully with all regulatory agencies in compliance with a "sentinel event," and, finally, to deal with pressure from the media. Regardless of motives, the press was becoming increasingly fascinated and ferocious with the story of an illegal Mexican immigrant, a teenager, receiving heroic and expensive medical therapy but having the whole process botched by an egregious mistake.

Three lanes of television trucks surrounded Duke Hospital for more than a week, broadcasting the story throughout the world. Whatever we said and did internally, reporters seemed to attribute the worst actions and motivations to the caregivers and the administration. Focusing on what is really important—the life of our patient and the safety of our operations—was of course our main concern, but pursuing our own due diligence in the face of the medically uneducated, frenzied witch hunt outside was overwhelming. Inside the hospital, individuals who had no business being there tried to enter the intensive care units. Members of the press invaded hospital areas and harassed the dispirited clinical staff.

At the height of what the national press called the "botched transplantation at Duke," I made a trip to Washington and visited with Tommy G. Thompson, who was U.S. secretary of Health and Human Services at that time. As he and I talked about new models of patient care and issues related to patient safety, painfully, the television set in the adjacent room was turned to Fox News. The station was featuring stories about Duke, and a reporter was standing in front of Duke Hospital—*my* hospital.

My focus throughout this time was to continue to deliver the best in medical care while also understanding as quickly and completely as possible how this breach in patient safety occurred, keeping up the morale of all those in the medical center, and communicating honestly and effectively with the press so as to minimize negative publicity. The inescapable truth was that a devastating mistake had been made, and the individual most directly involved was the surgeon, Jim Jaggers, who immediately took full responsibility for making it. Jim had assumed that someone else had verified that the organs did indeed match his patient, but this was not the case. What we learned was that in the rush to find a suitable donor for a rare and viable set of heart and lungs, no failsafe mechanisms were in place in this national system to ensure that the tissues matched the recipient. Once again, a tragedy had drawn national attention to patient safety, or lack thereof, in our nation's health system. For our part, we immediately initiated a deep and thorough evaluation at Duke of what went wrong and instituted processes not only to prevent this specific type of medical error but also to enhance safety throughout the institution. We brought in leading experts in developing safer procedures in hospitals and, as in our response to the clinical research shutdown in 1999, did all we could to make Duke a national model for patient safety mechanisms.

During the days before Jesica's death, I received a call from Michael Radutzky, the producer of 60 Minutes. He asked whether I would be willing to appear live on camera to discuss the botched transplant. That program, of course, is known for "sandbagging" individuals on camera and rarely does positive stories because they are essentially not news. Rather, journalists tend to seek audience attention and, at times, adulation through their impact on edgy subjects. That is what led the playwright Tom Stoppard to quip, "The press is a stalking horse masquerading as a sacred cow." Nonetheless, I believed Mr. Radutzky when he said he would do a fair piece and allow Duke to present its side of the story. I discussed this opportunity with university leadership, members of the board, and others and almost uniformly was advised not to do it. Nonetheless, I felt passionate about the fact that we, when presented with our egregious error, did everything possible to do the right thing. I wanted the opportunity to express that truth to a broad audience.

On March 7 and 8, 60 Minutes sent its camera crew, led by journalist Ed Bradley, to interview me, Jim Jaggers, and others on the staff. I found Ed Bradley to be honest and interested in learning the truth without putting a spin on it. The piece, televised on March 16, was seen by more than 13 million people. In June of that year, Allison Faas wrote a piece in Forbes entitled "Duking It Out," reviewing the entire episode and suggesting that Duke's response was similar to Johnson & Johnson's handing of the poisoning of Tylenol capsules: both examples of the benefit of coming clean early.[5]

The tragic transplantation error that led to Jesica Santillan's death had a profound impact on safety at Duke and throughout the United States. A blue-ribbon team worked with the leadership and staff at Duke to develop procedures to prevent errors not only in transplant surgery but also in all potentially dangerous procedures at Duke. We instituted the concept of "time out" and employed checklists similar to those used by pilots before a plane takes off—procedures now broadly used throughout the United States.

One of my most important responsibilities as chancellor was working syn-ergistically with the university. From the time Nan assumed her presidency in 1993 to when we both stepped down in 2004, the process generally went well, but differences in our styles and roles created inevitable conflicts. In 1998, at the time of Nan's review for her second term as president of Duke, Susan B. King, a member of the Duke University board and Nan's review committee, came to visit me. In a lighthearted fashion, Susan indicated that Nan's record was so stellar that the review committee felt they needed to find at least one area in which they could render some advice. They indi-cated that perhaps Nan should devote a greater amount of time to learning more about her medical center and health system. At one university board meeting, James L. Vincent, chairman of the board and CEO of Biogen, Inc., looked Nan in the eye and commented that if one of the health system's network entities went "belly up," she would be held responsible. Indeed, he implied that she needed to be more involved in DUHS affairs.

Given Nan's personality as a high achiever with a spotless record, she took these comments as admonitions. The truth was, however, that she already knew a great deal about the medical center. Thanks in part to our ongoing interactions, she had hardly neglected it. Still, she perceived a need to become more directly responsible for the operations I was leading. She let me know that she would soon become far more involved in the medi-cal center and had tasked her executive vice president, Tallman Trask, and others to embed themselves in the medical center's operations. Nan made it clear, in short, that she wanted to develop her own independent ability to view medical center operations rather than relying on mine.

This new approach created tensions between Nan and me. At times I sensed that she did not trust my leadership and that her representatives undermined my ability to lead. She also seemed uncomfortable with what she perceived as my authoritarian control of that portion of *her* university that dominated all the others economically. As university president, she sought a freer hand in overseeing the medical center, but the nature of her enhanced oversight conflicted with my team's ability to lead. What I could never get Nan to understand was that the corporate nature of the health system required that the CEO really be the CEO and be viewed as such by those within the organization. What I was doing bore little if any similarity to what constitutes the leadership, say, of a political science department.

By the end of her tenure, Nan had developed a strong desire to diminish the authority of the chancellor for health affairs/CEO and president of DUHS. A year before she stepped down in 2004, she commissioned a review of the organizational structure of the Duke University Medical Center and Health System. Lanty L. Smith, a Duke University board member, led the review. The most serious confrontation Nan and I ever had was over a major recommendation of that report, which suggested that, given the creation of DUHS with its own CEO, the role of chancellor for health affairs and the designation DUMC had both lost their raison d'être. Two individuals could and should oversee the entire medical enterprise: the dean of the School of Medicine and the CEO and president of DUHS. The dean of the School of Medicine would report to the provost; the CEO of the health system would report to the university president. This sounded logical in a superficial way, but superficial was exactly what the design of the highly successful DUMC and DUHS was not. A chancellor for health affairs as CEO of the health system was needed to operationalize, strategically bridge, and balance the core missions of education, research, and clinical care. This broad horizon and operational role of the combined chancellor and CEO of the health system allowed Duke to achieve its national leadership position and become a creation of better models of care.

Nan supported the recommendations in the Smith Report, but I opposed the one recommending dissolution of the chancellor's role. I thought it would disassemble a carefully constructed organizational arrangement that gave Duke's medical center and health system a leading position among the nation's most successful and admired academic health systems. Before the report was released, Nan led me to believe that there would be nothing I would find troubling in the report. I felt let down, to say the least.

I received the Smith Report while vacationing in beautiful Mendocino, California. There, on the first page, was an argument for eliminating the medical center. I almost passed out; I couldn't believe what I was reading. This was the only time during our eleven years of working together at Duke when I felt intentionally misled by Nan. I immediately called Ernie Mario, chair of the health system board, to register my dismay. He expressed surprise and concern as well.

When I got back to campus, I spoke with two trusted friends and supporters, Mary Semans and my predecessor, Bill Anlyan, both of whom sat on the Duke Endowment Board. I spoke with them not in their roles as trustees of the Duke Endowment but as knowledgeable and loyal supporters of the medical center. I had no intention to construct a counter–power play. I knew these two people had the experience and understanding to realize how harmful this proposal was. I asked for their advice and told them I needed their help. Both were dismayed by the recommendation and, unbeknownst to me, raised the matter with Russell M. Robinson, II, chair of the Duke Endowment Board. Afterward, Mary and Bill arranged a phone call that included the two of them, Russ, and me. Russ asked, "Ralph, are you wanting the Duke Endowment to intervene in university politics?" I answered, "By no means had I ever envisioned such a thing—absolutely not." I never considered the dismantling of the medical center as an issue for the Duke Endowment, but in retrospect, I can understand how it might have been so construed.

I never found out exactly what happened next, but someone on that phone call or some subset of them, must have spoken to Nan. John Burness, the university senior vice president for public affairs and government relations, later told me: "You smart SOB. You played your trump card and once you did that, what could they do?"

Eventually, whether in private or public I cannot say, many individuals, including Mary Semans, spoke out against the report's recommendations for dissolving DUMC and its chancellor for health affairs. They understood the rationale and the need for a strategic leader whose role is to integrate and leverage the academic and clinical functions. Running them individually would have been a major step backward. This issue was laid to rest, although the primacy of the university president over all of Duke, including its health system, was clarified.

Notwithstanding this painful incident, I consider my eleven-year collaboration with Nan to have been greatly beneficial for the university, including its medical enterprise. In retrospect, I regret that I did not do more to obviate the causes of our disagreements. Our personal differences reflected in part our mutual inability to communicate effectively with one another, but our relationship also involved real differences of personalities, management styles, and views—differences we managed as best we could.

— — —

My initial hope as I began my tenure as chancellor was to see Duke's medical enterprise become a leader in the nation and be recognized as such. I believe this goal was achieved by the time I stepped down. What I learned along the way was how this rise in recognition was associated with totally unexpected events, both positive and negative. I came to view my job as having several major components: overseeing the day-to-day operations of a complex organization, developing strategic plans to improve the operation of the parts of the whole, representing the institution locally and nationally, raising resources needed to succeed, and, finally, responding to crisis. Despite the importance of the first four roles, responding to crisis trumped them all. The sheer unpredictability of the crises we faced and the all-consuming efforts needed to resolve them were among the most difficult challenges I faced as chancellor. I learned that crises can and will occur, and they often provide a useful way to focus on how to prevent them or how to respond more quickly and effectively when they happen. Attention to compliance and to safety for employees, patients, and clinical research subjects became increasingly high priorities and helped us improve as an institution. In a perverse way, these crises also strengthened me as a leader.

16

—

Stepping Down and Lessons Learned

On February 28, 2003, the Duke University Board of Trustees met at the Graylyn International Conference Center in Winston-Salem, North Carolina. From time to time, the Board of Trustees gathered offsite, as it is called, to engage in strategic reviews of the university. This particular meeting focused on the near completion of the "Campaign for Duke," which far exceeded initial expectations of $1.5 billion, ultimately raising $2.36 billion, of which $706 million was for the medical center.

The biggest news at this meeting, however, was Nan Keohane's announcement that she would be stepping down as Duke's thirteenth president at the end of June 2004. Like some members of the board and others, I presume, on the senior leadership team, I was unaware that Nan would make this announcement. Many of us had assumed she would stay on for a third term. Nan decided to leave Duke, however, to become a senior fellow at Princeton, where her husband, Bob, a professor of political science, would be joining the faculty.

Nan's announcement got me thinking that my third term as chancellor for health affairs would also run out at the end of June 2004. Perhaps I should have asked to extend my term for a year or two to allow the new Duke president some time before choosing the next chancellor for health affairs, but I never gave this option serious consideration.

—

As I approached my sixty-fourth year, I came to feel as though I had, since the age of five, almost blindly followed a career path that, although exhilarating, productive, and rewarding in every sense, allowed me little time to experience a life outside of my profession. I had vague dreams of returning to the San Francisco Bay Area but no specific notions of what I wanted to do other than to disengage from the intense lifestyle I had developed as chancellor. Thus, following Nan's announcement and in the face of mounting queries as to whether I wanted to stay on as chancellor beyond 2004, I announced on March 3, 2003, that I would also step down at the end of June 2004. While I was fully committed to effectively serving my third term as chancellor until its very end, I never seriously considered extending my tenure in this role.

There was no winding down, however, during my final year and four months as chancellor. I remained fully engaged not only in facilitating the practical rollout of the health system but also in furthering what I considered to be the second great transformation of medicine, personalized health care. This period also coincided with my services as chair of the AAMC. Moreover, in 2003, I assumed the presidency of the AAP, the leading organization representing physician-scientists and leaders of academic medicine. I thus had a strong national position from which to focus on issues in which I was profoundly invested. These issues included the emergence of clinical research enabling the translation of recent discoveries into practical application, and the concept and implementation of personalized health care, a field that is now dominant in health care but, at that time, was in its infancy.

On September 1, 2003, Nan Keohane announced the creation of a thirteen-member search committee to identify suitable candidates for my replacement. By early spring 2004, three such candidates were identified. On July 1, 2004, Victor J. Dzau, chair of the Department of Medicine at Brigham and Women's Hospital in Boston, became my successor as chancellor for health affairs at Duke University and president and CEO of DUHS.

During my last few months as chancellor for health affairs, I focused on working with the incoming university president, Richard H. Brodhead, to acquaint him with his soon-to-be medical center and health system. Following the selection of Victor, I worked with him as well. My final goals were to complete the memorandum of understanding and commitment to create the Duke-NUS Graduate Medical School, to focus on the performance of the health system, which was rapidly demonstrating that it would be an excellent clinical and financial success, and finally, to roll out Duke Personalized Health Care.

On May 6, 2004, Duke's Board of Trustees hosted a dinner in my honor. At that dinner, I received a gentle but humorous roasting and was given numerous comical gifts by Nan Keohane, one being a cartoon by V. C. Rogers, who had been the editorial cartoonist for the *Durham Herald-Sun*. With Nan at his side, Pete Nicholas, chairman of the board, read a board proclamation acknowledging the accomplishments of my tenure and, in recognition of this, appointed me chancellor emeritus of the university as of July 1, 2004. In addition, the board named the new 120,000-square-foot, $41 million Genome Sciences Research Building in my honor—the Snyderman Genome Science Research Building. I was deeply touched and moved, and I barely recall the remarks I made to the vast group assembled at the dinner. I was overcome with a sense of joy and humility for having been given the privilege to serve Duke University.

On May 8, 2004, I gave my last report on the state of the medical center to the Duke University Board of Trustees. It was humbling yet rewarding to reflect on the experience of being chancellor for health affairs for fifteen and a half years. My final report to the board is included as appendix 3; important statistics related to my fifteen years at the helm of this great medical center are supplied in appendix 4.

Only in the last months of my term did I begin thinking concretely about what I would do after I stepped down. I decided to take a sabbatical that would distance me from the medical center and give Victor a full year to establish his identity without me being anywhere nearby to interfere. I chose to spend the year in San Francisco, doing a sabbatical at the Global Health Institute of the University of California San Francisco. My colleague Haile DeBas, the former dean at UCSF, was on sabbatical himself at that time and kindly offered me the use of his office and staff. Thus, I left the keys to the kingdom with my successor, Victor Dzau, and for the second time during my career at Duke, I packed my belongings, turned off my office lights, and headed west.

Lessons Learned

Twelve years after stepping down, I've had the opportunity to reflect on what I learned during the fifteen and a half exhilarating and often tumultuous years at the helm of Duke's medical enterprise. Most of the lessons are particular to my role as chancellor, others to the careers I had as a physician-scientist and as a senior officer at Genentech.

One lesson may sound counterintuitive to a lot of "alpha" parents out there today, and it is this: attaining important positions of leadership in elite institutions doesn't require the early pedigree of training generally sought after by contemporary parents. I didn't graduate from Choate, Princeton, or Harvard Medical School. Rather, I was the product of largely public education and an excellent, but not elite, college. Nevertheless, by grit, persistence, and some good fortune, I managed to get chances to prove my worth. This may not be the optimal path, but it existed for me, and it worked well.

I am often amused when sitting on boards to find that leaders often are chosen based on the evidence that the individual has done almost the exact job before. Had this been the case for me, I'd never have been a senior vice president at Genentech or chancellor for health affairs at Duke. By the standards of previous success in the same job, I would have been ineligible for both. The candidates who are most qualified for leadership positions may not be experienced at the job at hand but evince proof of prior success in related fields. Those with high energy, drive, a willingness to listen and to learn, and a very high standard for success may be the best bet—at least for institutions or organizations that want innovative leadership.

I have also learned that when one takes on a new job or position, one's prior perceptions of what it will be can never fully do justice to the reality. In choosing to be a physician, a scientist, a biotechnology leader, or a chancellor, I had no clue what the job would really be like. I had a vision of sorts and ultimately was never disappointed that I took the position. Nonetheless, what I actually did and needed to do could only be determined once I took the leap. This, I suspect, is a good thing, as in any career move it is to be expected that the individual will adapt to the needs of the position and grow to meet these needs rather than trying to do the job based on a preconceived vision. Anticipating, learning, being surprised, while growing in a job, is a good thing and a requisite for successful leadership.

In any endeavor, it's valuable to appreciate the golden circle of the what, the how, and the why. An individual or an organization can distinguish itself by what it does, but even more so by how well it does it. What really distinguishes the great from the good, however, is the "why." The why is the core principle that most powerfully drives and sustains the quality and innovation of the what and the how. Commitment to core principles provides a constant guidepost for growth and change. Whenever questions, uncertainties, and sometimes great difficulties arise, having a firm understanding of why one is doing something helps maintain the drive and narrows decisions to the ones that are the most likely to be correct.

In taking on any new position, it is important to learn about the business in depth, to truly understand how it works and whom it serves. It is essential to understand the people, the organizational structure, the constituencies, the products, and the customers, as well as grasping how the parts work and how the funds flow. Doing this early on is important, and although this is seemingly obvious, attending to ongoing issues and immediate needs often diverts leaders from obtaining the necessary knowledge of the core business and the people who drive it. David Packard, co-founder of Hewlett-Packard and a member of the Genentech board, told me of his strong views about the value of management by walking around. I believe in this fully. I enjoyed and learned a great deal by walking around Duke and stopping to talk to employees throughout the medical center. Being in the trenches and understanding the myriad issues facing a complex institution is empowering to the leader and valued by the employees. For most of my tenure as chancellor, I served on clinical rotations as an attending or consulting physician. This allowed me to see firsthand many of the inner workings of the institution. Doing this also allowed me to satisfy my core desire to be a physician while working closely with the people who made the institution run. Some of my great joys came from encounters with staff or patients as I participated as a physician or simply by walking around.

Early on, I tried to benefit from the Carl Furillo story regarding the importance of making an early positive impression. Although starting a new position is initially chaotic, one can look for opportunities to make a positive early impression. Choosing to do something visible and doing it remarkably well creates a feeling of confidence in the leader and makes subsequent decisions a bit more acceptable to others.

As one starts a new role, the initial phase includes a deep learning period during which timely decisions need to be made based on acquired information and advice from trusted associates. After sufficient time on the job, however, patterns emerge and, with experience, personal opinions develop. I've found that it generally takes up to a year before sufficient experience allows the development of personal views of what needs to be done with the sense of "knowing" how things are likely to work out. The capability for accurate pattern recognition is a key to the success of the leader (or any physician, for that matter). While that intuitive feel of "knowing" how to deal with an issue is wonderful and makes the job enjoyable, it is important to appreciate that the opinion may be wrong, no matter how strongly held. Whether it is a physician with a diagnosis or a CEO needing to make a corporate decision, despite the strength of the conviction, it is important to pause and formally consider alternative choices. Over the years, I've found that even my strongly held views have sometimes changed when discussed and tested.

The quality of the people around you is critical to the success of your organization. Never compromise on choosing and retaining only the best people. It is often compelling to retain good, but not outstanding, people just because you like them or because it is so unpleasant to cut loose someone you inherited. This is usually a mistake. With a great team, it is important to listen to and learn from them, and to delegate the independence they need to succeed and hence to help you succeed.

I've found that no matter how much I felt I was listening to others, I often wasn't "listening" enough—or well enough. No matter how much I was communicating, I should always have communicated more. Listening and communicating are critical needs that rarely receive enough attention, even though it is easy to delude ourselves into thinking that they are.

Act decisively when there are sufficient data to do so; postponing a difficult decision is a natural tendency but one that should be avoided. It is often compelling to wait, believing that more time and information can shape a better decision. This may be true, but it is important to be aware that this may be just a way to postpone making a painful choice. Moreover, procrastination feeds the illusion that time is essentially free. But of course it isn't, and making no choice is itself a choice.

Any good leader should understand that he or she is serving an institution, not the other way around. Leadership is service to others and to the missions and goals of the institution served. I've loved Duke since I first joined the faculty in 1972. As chancellor I often felt I was provided with the great privilege of wearing the mantle of the position for a time. During that time, I needed to do my best to honor that role. I clearly understood the need to separate myself from the role I was serving on behalf of the institution. When the need arose to distinguish my own desires from my view of what the chancellor's position ought to be, I tried to choose the latter. I found that embedding the concept of service to a role, with all its responsibilities, helped me make tough choices to weather difficult circumstances. It allowed me to rise above short-term personal wants or needs and to take the strains of the job less personally. It drove me to portray an aspirational role that I believed was good for the institution.

I found it useful to consciously try to maintain a sense of optimism, generosity, humor, and caring for others. In difficult situations, I often engaged in mindfulness to be "in the moment" and sought to identify the good things in my job and my life. Surprisingly to me, this conscious attempt to alter my attitude and sense of well-being often worked. It reminded me of Abraham Lincoln's remark that a person is usually as happy as he or she decides to be. It also set a better example for those around me, who often judged how things were going for the institution by how I seemed to be interpreting them.

I found it to be important, too, to identify several people I respected, liked, and totally trusted. With the individuals in this small group, I could confidentially reveal my thoughts and deepest concerns as well as my joys. Finding colleagues and friends to open up with is difficult when one is an institutional leader. Nevertheless, identifying such a group was essential. In my case, these included Bob Lefkowitz, Bill Donelan, Vicki Saito, and occasionally Joel Fleishman and Bill Anlyan. They helped me get through difficult times and fostered my equanimity and good judgment.

Dear reader, if you have gotten this far and actually read the entire book, you have demonstrated the grit and determination needed to be a successful leader. Hopefully what you have learned from reading this book will help you as you carefully avoid the snares occasionally barring your path to meaningful leadership.

Epilogue

I have often wondered about the source of the intense loyalty that Duke University engenders in so many of the people it touches. Duke breeds intense and compassionate devotion among its faculty, alumni, students and their parents, and many grateful patients of its medical enterprise. It certainly breeds devotion within me, and it began when I first arrived for an internship interview in the Department of Medicine in December 1964. Following my interviews and a grueling experience as a medical student taking "gallop rounds" with the legendary Gene Stead on Osler Ward, the chief resident walked me down through Davison Building and out its front doors. After not more than a dozen steps, as I internalized the beauty and magnificence of the campus and reflected on the bewildering excitement of rounds, I was struck by a deep emotional feeling that Duke was the place for me to come for my medical training. I never lost that sense of wonderment for this institution.

Beyond its awe-inspiring campus and the prowess of its legendary faculty, what makes Duke so special for me is that it allowed a hardworking young man with potential but without pedigree to achieve to the maximum of his ability. As a first-generation American, trained primarily in public schools, who was Jewish and coming from Brooklyn, New York, in 1965, my background made it almost impossible for me to enter most of the country's "top"—and historically privileged—institutions. Duke was different. It opened its arms to hundreds, if not thousands, of people like me from all over the country and allowed us to become all we were capable of being. I sensed this character within the institution and so did my father, an immigrant from the Ukraine who, like so many immigrants during the Depression, struggled to see that his child would have a better life than he had. I recall the pride my father had when he first visited Duke. In truth, one of the reasons I left Genentech to return to Duke as its chancellor was to try to repay the institution for the joy it gave to my parents and my family by allowing me to flourish here—for providing me with a great stage on which to play out my role, whatever it turned out to be.

It's interesting that nearly all discoveries are blatantly obvious to the discoverer. All the advances we made at Duke, everything we did during my time as chancellor, emerged as consequences of what I'd call doing the obvious. What seems obvious, however, is no more obvious to everyone than—to recall Voltaire—common sense is not so common. One has to be both immersed intellectually and engaged emotionally for the obvious to assume its character. So what we found to be obvious emerged from a perspective we had earned, and the result turned out to be transformative innovations that revolutionized not only Duke but health care throughout the world.

Let me leave you with two broad lessons, one logically preceding the other, that emerged from my experience. The first is that the real choice in sound decision management is not between fully articulated plans on the one hand and extemporaneous "winging it" on the other. As President Dwight Eisenhower used to say, paraphrasing the German general Helmuth von Moltke, it's not the *plan* that matters, for it is always the first casualty of war, but rather the *planning*. It is the diligent rehearsing of possibilities, the parsing of options, and learning over time that make the planner-cum-decision maker nimble and confident enough to be bold when the hour to act is at hand.

But to act successfully through boldness and practiced skill presupposes that one knows one's objectives and, as objectives change, that new ones are both worthy and attainable. This is where principle comes in. If objectives and the necessary decisions to attain them are always judged by their adherence to principles, and if these principles are grounded in the ethics of attempting to do good, over time, it is likely that good will be done. Such knowledge and behavior are the sine qua non of real leadership. There are many people who, if told to move an organization from an existing point A to a well-defined point B, can do that with relative ease. It is something else altogether to discern where and what point B is or should be and, once there, to be able to identify and attain even bolder objectives C, D, and beyond.

These lessons about means and ends, after a decade's reflection, are distinctions with meaningful differences. I am grateful to Duke University for allowing me the opportunity to learn them and to act on them in the company of such extraordinarily talented, dedicated, and devoted coworkers. I only hope in return that my service to Duke will be judged with generosity of spirit and a forgiving leniency.

APPENDIX 1

Medical Center Administration Leadership, 1989–2004

School of Medicine

Chancellor for Health Affairs and Dean, School of Medicine
Ralph Snyderman (1989–1998)

Chancellor for Health Affairs, Executive Dean, School of Medicine,
President and CEO, DUHS
Ralph Snyderman (1998–2004)

Vice Chancellor for Medical Center Academic Affairs
Gordon G. Hammes (1991–1999)

Vice Chancellor for Academic Affairs and Dean, School of Medicine
Edward W. Holmes (1999–2000)
R. Sanders Williams (2001–)

Dean for Medical Education
Doyle G. Graham (1987–1992)
Dan G. Blazer (1992–1999)

Associate Vice Chancellor and Vice Dean for Education
Russel E. Kaufman (1999–2002)
Edward C. Halperin (2002–)

Vice Chancellor for Medical Center Administration and CFO
William J. Donelan (1989–1999)

Vice Chancellor for Health Affairs, Executive Vice President,
and COO, DUHS
William J. Donelan (1999–)

Vice Chancellor for Operations, Vice President for Administration, DUHS
Gordon D. Williams (1999–)

Vice President and Chief Financial Officer, DUHS
Kenneth C. Morris (1999–)

Vice President and Chief Medical Officer, DUHS
Gary L. Stiles (1999–2004)

Vice Chancellor for Health Affairs, Science and Technology
Thomas Glenn (1991–1992)
Robert L. Taber (1992–)

Vice President and Chief Information Officer, DUHS and Medical Center
Asif Ahmad (2003–)

Vice Chancellor for Health Affairs
Jean G. Spaulding, MD (1998–2001)

Associate Vice Chancellor for Communications
Vicki Y. Saito (1992–)

Director, Community Relations
MaryAnn E. Black (2002–)

Vice Chancellor for Business Development and Marketing
Alvis R. Swinney (1997–1998)

Associate Vice Chancellor and Chief Operating Officer,
Duke Health Network
Paul M. Rosenberg (1993–1997)

Associate Vice Chancellor for Planning
Steven G. Sloate (1993–1994)

Director, Medical Center Financial Management
Bernard McGinty (1980–1994)

Assistant Vice President for Health Affairs, Planning, and
University Architect
Larry Nelson (1983–1999)

Director of Administration
James L. Bennett, Jr. (1983–1997)

Associate Vice President for Health Affairs
Robert G. Winfree (1980–1997)

DEVELOPMENT

Vice Chancellor for Development
Raymond C. Waters (1973–1992)

Executive Director, Medical Center Development
B. Jefferson Clark (1992–1994)

Vice Chancellor for Development and Alumni Affairs
Joseph S. Beyel (1994–2000)
Steven A. Rum (2000–)

Vice Chancellor for Special Projects
Raymond C. Waters (1994–2004)

DUKE HOSPITAL

Vice Chancellor for Health Affairs and CEO of Duke Hospital
Andrew G. Wallace (1981–1990)

Vice Chancellor for Health Affairs and CEO of Duke Hospital
W. Vickery Stoughton (1990–1991)

Executive Director, Vice Chancellor for Health Affairs and CEO of Duke
Hospital
Mark C. Rogers (1991–1996)

Vice Chancellor for Health Affairs, Vice President and Chief, Hospitals
and Clinical Facilities, DUHS
Michael D. Israel (1996–2002)

CEO of Duke Hospital and Vice President, DUHS
William J. Fulkerson Jr. (2002–)

SCHOOL OF NURSING — DEAN

Dorothy J. Brundage, interim (1987–1991)
Mary T. Champagne (1991–2004)
Catherine L. Gilliss (2004–)

Basic Sciences

BIOCHEMISTRY

Robert L. Hill (1969–1993)
Christian R. H. Raetz (1993–)

BIOLOGICAL ANTHROPOLOGY AND ANATOMY

Richard F. Kay (1988–)

BIOSTATISTICS AND BIOINFORMATICS

(Established in 2000.)
William E. Wilkinson, interim (2000–)

CELL BIOLOGY

Harold P. Erickson, interim (1988–1990)
Michael P. Sheetz (1990–2000)
Harold P. Erickson, interim (2000–2002)
Brigid L. M. Hogan (2002–)

GENETICS

(Established in 1994 when Department of Microbiology and Immunology split; merged with Department of Microbiology to form the Department of Molecular Genetics and Microbiology in 2002.)
Joseph R. Nevins (1994–2002)

IMMUNOLOGY

(Established in 1992 from Department of Microbiology and Immunology.)
Thomas F. Tedder (1993–)

MICROBIOLOGY AND IMMUNOLOGY

(Changed to Department of Microbiology in 1994 when the separate Department of Microbiology and Immunology was established; the Department of Microbiology merged with the Department of Genetics to form Department of Molecular Genetics and Microbiology in 2002.)

Wolfgang K. Joklik (1968–1994)
Jack D. Keene, interim (1994)
Jack D. Keene (1994–2002)

MOLECULAR CANCER BIOLOGY

(Established in 1993; merged with Department of Pharmacology to form Department of Pharmacology and Cancer Biology in 1995.)

Robert M. Bell (1993–1995)
Gordon G. Hammes, interim (1995)

MOLECULAR GENETICS AND MICROBIOLOGY

(Established in 2002 with merger of Department of Genetics and Department of Microbiology and Immunology.)

Joseph R. Nevins (2002–2004)

NEUROBIOLOGY

William C. Hall, interim (1988–1990)
Dale Purves (1990–2002)
James O. McNamara (2002–)

PATHOLOGY

John D. Shelburne, interim (1989–1991)
Salvatore V. Pizzo (1991–)

PHARMACOLOGY

(Merged with Department of Molecular Cancer Biology to form Department of Pharmacology and Cancer Biology in 1995.)

Saul M. Schanberg, acting (1988–1991)
Anthony R. Means (1991–1995)

PHARMACOLOGY AND CANCER BIOLOGY

(Established in 1995.)

Anthony R. Means (1995–)

Clinical Departments

ANESTHESIOLOGY

W. David Watkins (1983–1990)

Joseph G. Reves, interim (1990–1991), chair (1991–2001)

Mark F. Newman (2001–)

DEPARTMENT OF COMMUNITY AND FAMILY MEDICINE

George R. Parkerson, Jr. (1985–1994)

J. Lloyd Michener (1994–)

MEDICINE

Joseph C. Greenfield, Jr. (1983–1995)

Barton F. Haynes (1995–2003)

Harvey J. Cohen, interim (2003)

Pascal J. Goldschmidt (2003–)

OBSTETRICS AND GYNECOLOGY

Charles B. Hammond (1980–2002)

Haywood J. Brown (2002–)

OPHTHALMOLOGY

Robert Machemer (1978–1991)

W. Banks Anderson, Jr., interim (1991–1992)

David L. Epstein (1992–)

PEDIATRICS

Samuel L. Katz (1969–1990)

Michael M. Frank (1990–2004)

PSYCHIATRY

Bernard J. Carroll (1983–1990)

Dan G. Blazer, interim (1990–1992)

Allen J. Frances (1992–1994)

PSYCHIATRY AND BEHAVIORAL SCIENCES

(Established in 1994.)
  Allen J. Frances (1994–1998)
  Ranga R. Krishnan (1998–)

RADIATION ONCOLOGY

(Established in 1991.)
  Leonard R. Prosnitz (1991–1996)
  Edward C. Halperin (1996–2002)
  Leonard R. Prosnitz, interim (2002–2004)
  Christopher G. Willett (2004–)

RADIOLOGY

  Carl E. Ravin (1985–)

SURGERY

  David C. Sabiston, Jr. (1964–1994)
  Robert W. Anderson (1994–2003)
  Danny O. Jacobs (2003–)

APPENDIX 2

Excerpts from the Chancellor's Report to the
Board of Trustees, October 5, 1990

Medicine has undergone a revolution that could not have been envisioned
60 years ago when Duke University Medical Center began. In that relatively
short time, Duke has taken its place within the elite circle of this country's nationally prominent academic health centers. Given the complexity
of the medical center's importance to the university as well as the nation, I
thought it would be useful to describe the medical center in detail and provide an overview of what we are, followed by an assessment of the important challenges we face.

In 60 years we have evolved into an institution that could not have been
imagined back in 1924. The first hospital wards were open wards, with no
partitions between the beds. Baker House was added in 1931. The place
has grown like Topsy, and to those who have seen it grow, it must seem as
though the construction and renovation never stop. But buildings are, of
course, only a small part of the story. Another considerably more important part of the story has been the critical role of people, the importance of
the times, and the need for vision, courage and determination. These have
been necessary ingredients throughout the medical center's history, or we
would not be where we are today. Happily, Duke has definitely been blessed
from the outset in the people who were chosen to begin this grand medical
enterprise.

Today, we have emerged as a major academic health center, impacting
patient care locally, regionally and nationally. We have a very modern

facility that was built through the drive of Bill Anlyan. In Duke North we now have private hospital rooms, no longer the big open ward. The Joseph and Kathleen Bryan Research Building for Neurobiology, a state-of-the-art neurosciences building, opened last February. And in a way, Duke's Life Flight helicopter has itself become a highly visible metaphor for modern medicine. In its coming and going, Life Flight carries with it the implication that therapy at Duke is high-powered and highly technical and necessitates airlifting people as quickly as possible to the hospital to employ this technology to the fullest advantage.

As we look to the future, it is important to understand how the medical center grows, the balance of creativity and how we are to fulfill our responsibilities to the university, to the region, to the nation, and to the world. The medical center has three basic missions: education—to teach; research—to discover new ways of furthering health care; and to heal—to practice medicine. This is a substantial charge, and the size of the medical center reflects that. We have a large budget and a large number of employees; almost 12,000 people work in the medical center.

In terms of our educational mission, it's important to understand how the medical school differs from other professional schools. We do not offer only one degree, although a medical degree is certainly one of the most important, if not the most important degree we grant. However, we also award a doctorate of philosophy in various areas of science, as well as a joint MD/PhD degree to those who are trained as both physicians and researchers, and a master of science in nursing. But our educational mission doesn't stop there. We are heavily involved in post-doctoral training. Scientists with a doctorate degree who want to do research need at least two, and usually four, years of post-doctoral training. Clinical training, as you know, is becoming more and more specialized. We have some of the nation's best internship, residency and fellowship programs, which annually receive thousands of applications for a relatively few available openings. We also stress the increasing importance of continuing education for physicians as they go into practice and Duke has become a major educational resource for them, besides educating a significant portion of the physicians in the Southeast.

The medical school curriculum, which we still call the "new curriculum," actually began in 1966. Dan Tosteson was instrumental in formulating this creative system of teaching medicine. All the basic sciences that are needed to understand human biology, human pathology, and the basis of human diseases are compressed into one, intense year. Most medical schools do this in two years. The Duke approach allows our students to go on the ward and see patients in the second year. The advantage of this is that it pushes students during their first year to be as good as they can be. It also allows them to identify, by taking care of patients early on, science they need to go back to during their third year.

This curriculum affords a significant portion of the class an opportunity to spend a full year doing creative, fundamental research in a laboratory, generally of a well-known investigator. This hallmark of our medical school has distinguished Duke throughout the country and is a unique aspect of the medical curriculum here. The fourth year is devoted to clinical electives, generally reflecting a student's choice of subspecialty.

The primary objectives of our science departments involve teaching and basic research, while our clinical departments, which also conduct research in a more clinically directed environment, teach within the context of various subspecialties. Medical center departments range in size from the five-member Department of Biological Anthropology and Anatomy, which teaches gross anatomy to our medical students yet is a university-wide department, to the Department of Medicine, which has 245 faculty, many of whom are quite junior and turn over rapidly on their way to other academic institutions. The Department of Medicine's annual budget is probably equal to that of some of the smaller countries in the United Nations, which should give you some indication of the medical center's size.

Size does not necessarily connote quality, however. What standards can we use to evaluate how good we are? There are a number of ways to go about it. One is to look at the quality of the research, which is reflected in how competitive we are with similar departments throughout the country in securing grants from the National Institutes of Health. To our credit, in a highly competitive arena, the medical center does very well as a whole and a number of our departments rank among the top 10 in the country when it comes to NIH funding. Our Department of Surgery leads all other U.S. surgery departments in this regard. Biochemistry is eighth nationally, Psychiatry is second, and Pediatrics is very close to the top 10, being ranked 12th. Among the nation's top schools with which we traditionally group ourselves, Duke University Medical Center is ninth in the country in NIH awards. This is a remarkable achievement given our status as a relative newcomer when compared to Harvard, Stanford and other leading schools. I think we will improve our ranking in terms of NIH funds as we more fully develop the science in some of our new departments, providing federal cutbacks don't further erode NIH grant programs.

Another measure of how well we are doing can be found in the number of scientists who are members of major professional societies, perhaps the most prestigious of which is the National Academy of Sciences. We have seven members of the academy in the medical center, and I think the total number in the university is 10. This is not quite as good as some of the schools we like to consider as our equals, and it's an issue I feel I need to spend some time thinking about. At this time we have Bob Lefkowitz, an internationally recognized scientist, probably the most "famous" scientist we have at Duke today; Irwin Fridovich, who is still quite active; and Dale Purves, whom we have just recruited to Duke from Washington University. Many of the others are either emeritus, such as Bernard Amos, are close to retirement, or, as in the case of Jim Wyngaarden, are here in an administrative capacity. Therefore, while we stack up pretty well against other schools, we have room for improvement, and I think this is an area on which we need to focus some attention. The biomedical research field has a plethora of opportunities for major discoveries, and we are laying the groundwork so that Duke will be in a position to contribute its share.

The overall perception of Duke University Medical Center, and we know that perception is really what makes reality, is very positive. We seem to be thought of by the world at large as first-rate in many ways, for very good reasons, and in other ways we may be getting a bit more credit than we deserve. Notwithstanding, I believe we can capitalize on this perception to ensure our strength. Duke University Hospital was rated third nationally by doctors surveyed by *U.S. News and World Report,* which is very good when compared to the other prestigious schools of medicine. It's good for us to know what reality is, and it is advantageous for people outside to think that we are perhaps even better than we are. This ensures a constant effort to live up to the image.

One of the major things we do, and totally within James B. Duke's vision, is to provide health care. This is an important differentiation between a medical center and any other university component. Delivering medical services places us in a competitive, high-dollar environment that is highly entrepreneurial. At the same time, we are delivering services that are also for the welfare of people, for the public good. I think we deliver these services better than any other institution in this region. However, this causes us to be a hybrid organization as it relates to the service of clinical care. We are competing with major enterprises that are trying to dominate the health care industry; therefore, we have to understand our hybrid nature, since clinical care is an integral part of what we do, and health care is a very big industry.

The clinical services at Duke are divided into hospital services, outpatient clinics, and outreach programs, through which we interact with physicians, primarily, throughout the state and region, and the VA Hospital. Duke Hospital is one of the largest private university hospitals in the country, with more than 1,100 beds. It is generally considered to be in the tertiary care sector, which means that we take care of people who have diseases that require high-tech treatment by specialists. Primary care is delivered by a general practitioner, secondary care comes from an internist or a general surgeon, and tertiary care is when you need somebody even more specialized. We have a reputation for providing medical care that is unavailable anywhere else in this region: for example, bone marrow transplantation, heart and liver transplantation, certain types of intensive care and various types of interventional therapy for heart disease, to name a few.

The volume of patient care in the hospital and the clinics is increasing but primarily in outpatient visits. There is a very dramatic tendency towards medicine's becoming more involved in outpatient therapy. However, here at Duke, we are also seeing substantial increases in intensive care, reflecting what appears to be a bifurcation in medicine between those who are very sick and those who can be treated as outpatients. It is necessary to understand that in order to contain medical costs, more and more people are being treated in clinics, which means that those who enter the hospital are very ill indeed.

From a financial point of view, our revenues are definitely increasing, but we are feeling the effects of economic forces that first appeared on the scene back in 1980. I am referring, of course, primarily to the Medicare/ Medicaid DRG reimbursement system though which hospitals are now paid a given amount for a given disease rather than by the old formula of "cost plus." As a consequence, an increasing amount of our costs are unreimbursed. This becomes highly significant when planning for the future. The total amount of net operating income is becoming more difficult to maintain. This year we will bring a little over $6 million to the bottom line, hopefully more; however, as this becomes more difficult, we will need to become more cost-effective.

Our private diagnostic clinics are divided by specialties. An important point that I want to make has to do with the income generation of our ambulatory clinics, our private clinics, which is on the rise. But if you look at the actual expenses, the cost of operation is also on the rise. All revenues above the operating cost flow back into sustaining the system. The building fund is a financial provision that is used to enrich both the basic sciences as well as the clinical sciences. This allows us to develop new programs and build buildings, a vital contribution to the academic function of the medical center, and therefore is a clear cost-shifting of clinical dollars into academic programs. The net income from the Private Diagnostic Clinic is also cost-shifting of clinical dollars into academic programs in the clinical departments. It is crucially important to understand how much we depend on the clinical dollars to support the academic programs of the medical center.

Then, finally, ours is a very relevant institution to the region, as James B. Duke hoped it would be, in terms of the amount of outreach we're doing. We are affiliating and networking with smaller groups of physicians in communities throughout the region. This personal contact is becoming more and more important and is a vital part of medical center strategy. We need to be more accessible to referring physicians and patients alike. Our image is generally good. The perception of Duke has been very positive, as the *U.S. News & World Report* survey shows. We were considered by prominent specialists around the country to have great strength in nine important specialties. It's an image we are striving to improve upon.

In turning to the future, several issues in regard to national health and national health policy are worth mentioning. In order to deliver the best health care, the country not only needs medical personnel, physicians, nurses, all the individuals involved in health care, but the discovery of new diagnostics and therapeutics research discoveries that lead to the next generation of therapies. The clinical facilities that take care of people and new health care policy are currently aimed at increasing the accessibility of health care and decreasing cost. Given that this is the formula for providing the best health care in the world, the academic health center is vitally important to national health policy. We are the creators of medical personnel, almost exclusively, as well as a major source of biomedical discovery of diagnostics and therapeutics. We provide a very important arena for clinical testing. Academic health centers such as Duke deliver 20 percent of the health care in the United States and 40 percent of the indigent care. Academic health centers deliver far more indigent care than any other component of the health care industry, and hopefully in the future we will be considered a more important source for health policy.

The biotechnology revolution is one of the most exciting things that I have witnessed. I admit that I come to this with a certain bias. In the past 10 to 15 years, the development of computers, microelectronics, and molecular biology has totally changed the face of medical practice. Three-dimensional computer graphics have allowed us to determine the structure of molecules, such as a repressor molecule that turns off the action of another molecule. We can understand precisely what the three-dimensional structure of the molecule is due to these graphics and see how it interacts with other molecules. Not only does this give us insight into to how things work, since so often in nature form and function go hand in hand, but it enables professionals in various disciplines to develop new drugs that mimic, for example, repressor molecules and bind to the same site the molecules would. Such drugs have an important, and very specific, pharmacological effect, with few side effects. This is called rational drug design, and many think it's the wave of the future. A number of people at Duke are doing important work in this area.

Thanks to computer technology, we have the ability now to take multiple X-rays and reconstruct on a monitor three-dimensional views of a patient's head, for example. A brain tumor can be viewed three-dimensionally to allow a surgeon to pinpoint it precisely. The power we're developing in medicine is staggering. The ability to miniaturize equipment is manifesting itself in catheters that allow doctors, without the need for major surgery, to guide microsurgical instruments into coronary arteries to remove plaque, the blockage that causes heart attacks. I think within the next five to ten years we will be able to predict who is at risk for having a heart attack and be able as often as not to prevent it.

The molecular biology or the genetic engineering revolution has given medical scientists the laboratory tools to answer almost as many questions as they can think to ask, and this is having a tremendous impact on the practice of medicine. It began about twenty years ago when the structure of DNA was deciphered, which led to the ability to read the blueprint of life. After deciphering the genetic code, scientists then developed enzymes that allowed the language to be cut into specific paragraphs or specific sentences. It could then be removed and replaced in a new sequence that would then create a protein—the building blocks of life.

One of the first impacts that this had in medicine was the creation of a whole new industry, the biotechnology industry, which has the ability to isolate a human gene, remove it and put it into a simple, one-cell organism—a bacterium—that mass-produces the protein according to the implanted genetic blueprint. From this protein biotechnologists can make therapeutic agents based on the human gene. This gave us an industry capable of producing a series of new therapeutics.

Biotechnology is just at the beginning—the opportunities are mind-boggling. Nonetheless, research funding is a great concern to us. Most of the funding to do this research comes ultimately from the government, and as you know, we are facing severe restrictions of governmental dollars. NIH funding for research has grown but in constant dollars remains relatively flat. This is an issue that we have to face. Unless the mood changes substantially in Washington, we must rely more and more on funding from industry. Duke University Medical Center does approximately $100 million a year in discovery research. The academic health center needs to be smarter in dealing with research to make it easier for the pharmaceutical and biotechnology industries to develop those discoveries rapidly into commercially useful products. We need to streamline the transfer of technology between the medical center and industry to make it beneficial, not only for the medical center, but for industry and for the national good as well. After all, the federal government doesn't invest in research for the beauty of science, but for the development of useful products. We are developing a model of how this can be done more effectively.

The health care industry is the single largest industry in the United States, $500 billion and growing. It is expected to be a $1.5 trillion business by the year 2000. The United States spends more money per capita on health care than any other country in the world—far more. Despite that, it's estimated that 3.6 million Americans lack access to the health care system. The system is not adequate. It is not meeting our needs. It is too expensive and in some ways it is too exclusive. I believe it is our responsibility to respond to this need and, given our national platform, to create a policy that eliminates some of these shortcomings.

In the past, up until the 1970s, medicine was a great business to be in because every bill included "cost plus." Whatever you charged a patient for hospital services, the third party payers would pay that cost plus a little more. So you could not lose. Now we are faced with mixed reimbursement. More than 50 percent of our patients no longer pay us based on our charges, but rather on a fixed amount that is determined primarily by the government. If we treat for that amount we break even. If we treat for less, we have the advantage, but if it costs more, we lose money. Last year, the medical center wrote off $120 million in services because of this reimbursement situation. The future promises more of this. Medical care will be paid for based on performance standards, and we will have to understand the competitive nature of this. There are more commercial entities in the market. Kaiser Permanente and others throughout the United States are highly competitive with medical centers similar to Duke. We must be competitive with them. We have to understand our strengths and our weaknesses to do the things that we do well and be even more cost effective than we are today.

Another point that is very important, as I mentioned before, is the bifurcation of medical care—the dichotomy between very high-tech and rather low-tech medicine. Fewer and fewer hospitals will be able to afford to deliver the type of care that we currently provide at Duke. Heart transplantation will not be done at every small hospital throughout the state. There will be two or three centers for heart transplantation. Not every place will be able to do balloon or laser angioplasty. This has important implications for us. We will have even more responsibility as our capabilities continue to make us unique in this region. In addition to that, we will need to develop more extensive low intensity care in the form of ambulatory, outpatient care units.

As far as the current distribution of care at Duke University Medical Center is concerned, about 83 percent is related to acute care and 17 percent to ambulatory care. We are not presently in the home-based or extended care markets. This is somewhat out of sync with predictions for the national scene in the year 2000, with total expenditures expected to average 30 percent for acute care, 45 percent for ambulatory care, and 25 percent for extended care. We need to be aware of this and determine what our role will be in these markets, where our strengths lie, what will allow us to sustain our necessary structure and balance as we expand.

An idea of how important we are in the region is indicated to some degree by the share of total hospital revenues we receive from the region. I doubt many people realize how big our clinical market share is in North Carolina. With 130 hospitals in the state, almost 10 percent of all payments to N.C. hospitals come to Duke. If you combine ambulatory and inpatient revenues, we receive 8.1 percent of payments for health care services in the State of North Carolina.

As we look to the future, our agenda is to have the greatest impact possible, but in a balanced, integrated way with the university, in the region and in the nation. We need to develop a leadership team that appreciates the complexities of our dual identity, as both a health care provider in a highly competitive business and as an academic institution. We must understand how to merge these different purposes successfully. We have redesigned our administrative functions to include a chief of clinical operations, a chief financial officer and head of administration; and an established academician in charge of many of the biomedical research areas. Development and capital formation will also become increasingly important.

In February I'll be talking more specifically about the types of people, programs and facilities Duke will need for the next decade and how we are going about paying for all of this. Duke University Medical Center has emerged nationally as one of the very few academic health centers capable of creating excellence locally within the university and enhancing the functions of the university, but we also recognize our responsibility, as well as our opportunity, to be on a national playing field in terms of U.S. health policy. I think my role as Chancellor for Health Affairs will be, in a balanced, integrated way, to see that we maintain and enhance our position in all of these areas.

APPENDIX 3

The Chancellor's Report to the Board of Trustees, May 8, 2004

As I recall, this is exactly where I stood 15 years ago when I assumed the position of Chancellor for Health Affairs and Keith Brodie asked me to address the Board. It doesn't seem possible that 15 years have passed since that day. As I look around this room, I realize that David Adcock is the only person present today who was in this room 15 years ago. As I leave, you have a new Chancellor for Health Affairs, President and CEO of the Health System coming here from a different institution. There is a lot of new leadership, yet there is quite a bit of stability and I'm glad my partner, colleague and friend, Sandy Williams, is here with me today. Our institution is facing a lot of change, and I thought it would be useful to go through some high points and low points during my 15 years as Chancellor and give you my view of where things were when I assumed the Chancellorship in 1989, where I see things now, and what I see as some of the big challenges for the future.

When I took this job in 1989, I was woefully unprepared. My highest academic administrative experience was as a Division Chief in a Department of Medicine that was roughly 1/12 the size of the Department of Medicine at that time. Fortunately, I spent some time at Genentech, which opened my eyes to other worlds and to how other people think. I came back to Duke primarily for subjective and emotional reasons. Returning here was a very powerful personal draw for me, and my goal was to be an outstanding Dean. It was clear to me when I was a faculty member and as an individual outside of Duke looking in, that this institution—the School of Medicine—was quite frankly viewed as a high second-tier institution. The very top tier at that time included Harvard, Hopkins, Yale, Stanford, Washington University, UCSF, Cornell and Columbia. Some might measure the greatness of a medical school by the number of faculty members who are members of such prestigious organizations as NAS and IOM, as well as NIH funding. We were well below the top tier in those metrics. Some of that is how you play the system, but some of it really is a measure of the quality and the substance of the people in the institution. I think a lot of people felt that Duke was highly regarded, but it didn't have that bulk of outstanding faculty that was required to really be in the very top tier. I saw that as one of my major challenges when I came in.

When I took the position, we had not recruited a basic science chair from outside the institution since 1968. I think Rusty Williams and Sandy Williams will agree that Duke had totally missed out on the recombinant DNA technology revolution. We were not players; we had no part in it, whereas other major institutions like Stanford, UCSF and Harvard were able to lead and capitalize on the revolution. I also recall that at that time, Jack Whitehead, the founder of Technicon, Inc., had created the value of his company at the Durham VA Hospital. That's where the Chem-18 was proven to be effective and in return, he wanted to give a significant gift to Duke (i.e., the Whitehead Institute). This was probably in '85 or '86. He tried to entice an individual to Duke who he hoped would lead the new Whitehead Institute. I remember, in particular, a comment that his choice for Institute Director was made after one of his visits here. He said that he couldn't come to Duke because he couldn't recruit good people here. "Duke isn't quite like going to the desert, but . . . ." So, he would not leave Harvard to come to Duke and Jack Whitehead created the Whitehead Institute in Cambridge. That said something about us at that time.

My goal for the first few years as Chancellor was to build the basic science departments. In my view, the first recruitment would be judged to be symbolic of things to come, and we needed to be successful in that first recruitment. It was neurobiology and the individual we recruited was Dale Purves, who was a member of the National Academy of Sciences. He's still here and I was so pleased last night to take part in the delivery of the Hippocratic oath to our graduating class that included his daughter. After Dale, we recruited two more outstanding basic science chairs; I really thought that was a big part of my job, and at that time it was.

When I started as Dean, my thought was to try to move Duke into that top tier as measured by the usual standards. That is still our goal today and the data that Peter (Lange) showed is very revealing. If we look at the standards by which academic institutions are judged, we are a top tier institution, but I would say we are in the lower portion of a top tier. We are in the top 5, not in the top 3, by the standards that other people use; i.e., members in the National Academy, IOM, NIH grants and various other honorary societies. A point I would make is that the value of standards change. Conventional standards still have a great deal of value, but there are others that are not yet accepted that have the capabilities of defining the quality institutions of the future. We have chosen to take the lead in these new areas that will shape the future of health care. A point I'd make to the Board is that if you think of the companies that comprise the Dow Jones or the top 20 companies today versus 20 years ago, you notice a major difference in the lists. What is most valued today may not have been even thought of 20 years ago. There are certain standards by which we will always judge ourselves, but there are always new kids coming on the block that devise ways of doing things differently, doing them better, and doing them in ways not yet envisioned. This is where I think we have brought Duke from 1989 to today. I'm going to spend a few minutes reviewing some of the achievements that our team has made and new standards we have set.

You don't always end up where you thought you were going to and there is nothing wrong with that. If somebody had said in 1989, "Ralph what is your vision for Duke University Medical Center," I never would have thought of saying a health system, prospective health care, IGSP, DCRI, or a number of other things. The vision in 1989 was much more conventional. It's important to learn along the way. One must learn incrementally and take advantage of opportunities as they present themselves. But the one constant for excellence is to get the very best people.

I don't know how many of you have read the book *From Good to Great* by Jim Collins; I urge anyone interested in management and in leading to put this on their reading list. The book reflects a lot of things that we have focused on and done here. One needs a strong and committed leader and the very best people. Another factor is to determine (and this is something that I advise Deans when they are taking their jobs) whether as a leader, you are going to be a good manager, a good steward of your institution, or an agent of change. If one wants to be an agent of change, it's an entirely different job. A decision was made very early on that we needed and wanted to initiate change. At a minimum we wanted to go from that second tier to being the best at what we do. A word that I find very useful is the word "impact." We wanted to make a difference. We wanted to be a major player. Within our own field of participation, we wanted to make a real difference and when you are talking about health care, that's really substantial.

Dick (Brodhead), I will never forget the comments you made when Victor Dzau was being introduced. You said in your own way, which is so open, honest and revealing, how thrilled you were walking through the Duke Children's Hospital. You were impressed that we really make a difference in people's lives. I just wish everybody would see more directly what we do and how we change people's lives. In addition to all the other academic things, our people improve a lot of lives and do a lot of good. The idea that we needed to be agents of change versus keepers of the status quo came very early in my tenure as Chancellor. Keith Brodie introduced me to the ECAC (Executive Committee of Academic Council) in his office, our first meeting, I hadn't even moved here yet. I described to ECAC that I hoped to see Duke Medical School be the best or amongst the very best in the country. I was very excited about that. Keith spoke to me later and said that ECAC advised me to cool down a little bit—it sounded too much like hype or chest beating. The idea that we want to be "number one," that's just not the way you ought to talk in an academic institution. I was really struck by that, not that I thought it was wrong or mean spirited, but it's a very different cultural feeling than the one I have. In another meeting with ECAC, I remember talking about trying to get all of us to pull together as members of the faculty at Duke and about the importance of our doing things for the institution. One of the members of ECAC responded by saying that "my primary responsibility is to my profession and to my professional societies, not to Duke. I'm a faculty member and I happen to be at Duke, but my obligation is less to the institution than to my profession and to my area of scholarship." Again, that's not wrong, but I think it's important to understand the cultural differences amongst some of the faculty and what they see as their roles within the institution. There is a tremendously different mind-set amongst individuals who are engaged in highly personal scholarship, playing to the outside world, as opposed to individuals who are trying to drive an institution through interactions within that institution. This makes leading a University as you would a company very different indeed. This creates an incredible cultural gap that cannot be trivialized when one tries to lead institutional change in a University. If there is advice that I want to give to the corporate leaders in this room, it is don't trivialize the differences between universities and industry when it comes to leading coherent change. I know that you understand it intellectually, but please don't trivialize it. There are embedded cultural issues that can be changed easily, but others are very hard and take many years. So, the academic mind-set often has individual faculty pursuing their own fields of creativity. Being at Duke, sometimes is just as a matter of convenience. Many are opposed to wanting to develop a structure that thinks and acts like a corporation. We need to understand that these can happen, but it "ain't" easy and we need to understand the mind-set of the cultures within Duke as we implement change.

One of the key features that made a big difference in the nature of my role was the transition from being the Dean of the School of Medicine to the leader of an integrated Health System as well as a Medical Center. This began in the very early 1990s. For the first time, we put together an institutional strategic plan. This had never been done before; it wasn't easy, but we formulated a strategic plan. In that plan, we looked at the three core missions—education, research and clinical delivery—and realized these are all important and necessary in and of themselves, but we felt it would be shallow for us not to apply them to developing better models of health care for society. As an institution, we needed to value our traditional missions, but we also needed to add an overarching mission to serve society. I didn't realize how powerful that overarching mission statement would be. It committed us to say that the derivative of our core activities would create an overarching benefit for society. It also committed us to acting institutionally.

When it became obvious that we needed to have much greater institutional change to meet rapid changes in health care, it became clear that there were certain high-level and empowered people who would need to move aside. I was so politically naive that as I was getting ready for my first review as Chancellor, about three years into a five-year term, I asked two Chairs to step down. The first was the Department of Medicine, our most powerful department. Asking Dr. Greenfield to step down was the right and necessary thing to do but he was determined to fight the decision. This incredibly powerful individual had tremendous loyalty on the part of his faculty. He had been my boss before I was Chancellor. The second was the Chairman of the Department of Surgery, who is an icon in American medicine; I admired this man, Dave Sabiston, and still do. He was about three years beyond his retirement age and due to step down, and it was tough to finally ask him to do so. However, Dr. Sabiston did this gracefully. These decisions created an awful lot of angst amongst some of the faculty and there was a tremendous effort on the part of a group within the Department of Medicine to see I was not reappointed as Dr. Greenfield did not want to step down. The reason I mention this to this Board is to stress how important it is for a leader who is going to engage in change to have the understanding and the support of the Board. Ultimately the Board supported me. It wasn't easy and there were some compromises, but it happened. The mistake that I made was not engaging the Board more early on; so to some degree, in order to back me, they needed to act on faith rather than being involved as much as you are today. I think the enhanced oversight and engagement by the Board that exists today is a big improvement.

We got through that period and were better prepared to meet the challenge of managed care and other forces of change. In aggregate, this was forcing us to act more as a corporate entity. This change to a more corporate academic institution has been a fascinating transition. We have gone into new territories and much of what we have done has never been done before. So much of the success of Duke Medical Center has always depended on the ability of the clinical departments to bring in money from their practice. This was relatively easy before managed care when they did not need to be structured to aggressively grow their practices as clinical businesses. Their approaches were more of an afterthought than a strategy, and in the early '90s, departments began competing with each other for the same patients. There were mini wars breaking out amongst departments attempting to develop similar programs. We needed to get above that, to be able to deliver comprehensive managed care, and to do it as a corporate entity. In the development of the Health System, I am grateful for the support of the leadership of the University, which was very strongly behind us, and I thank Nan for allowing this to happen. The Board was incredibly supportive, including many of you here. Of those not present, I am particularly grateful for the leadership of John Koskinen, Randy Tobias, Ed Sidman, Roy Bostock, Karl von der Heyden, Uwe Reinhardt and Pete Nicholas. Of course, Ernie Mario has played a central role since the beginning. We never could have done it without the strong support of the Board.

During the past 15 years, we developed a number of important institutional entities including the Duke Clinical Research Institute, IGSP, Center for Integrative Medicine, the Clinical Service Unit and, of course, the Health System itself. When we committed to an institutional overarching mission to produce better models of health care, this helped us develop as a corporate entity in addition to the more usual academic component. This led to the development of the institutional building blocks, each of which made sense in themselves (i.e., DCRI) but in the aggregate allowed us to do so much more and these are a thing of beauty. What this allows us to do for the first time in the history of humankind is to deliver a new model of health care, which is derivative of all the core academic missions and makes good business sense. I remember discussing this with this Board, probably going back 3–4 years and hearing the justifiable skepticism of how in the world could this work. In the iterative process of refining it, we have begun to make it workable and are actually beginning to do this at Duke. Despite the fact that people can say it is not yet ready to try to do things that will fundamentally change the practice of medicine, we're actually doing it at Duke; it's very rudimentary, but it is a good working model that could not have been developed unless we had all those other pieces in place. Every one of them was a series of building blocks, including the support of the University Administration. Let me say here again, it isn't easy having a great University like this with a Medical Center and a Health System and somebody like me saying that we are so complicated, you can never understand us and whatever you do, please don't get in our way. I know I can be very difficult—we've had times when the ride has been a little rocky, but we held together, we really did. I think that was based ultimately on sufficient trust and loyalty to the institution, wanting to do good things and having good people. Duke Prospective Health Care and so many of the other things we've done couldn't have been done without Nan's support and we couldn't have done it without the support of Tallman (Trask) and Human Resources. On many of the other things, Peter Lange and I sometimes go head to head, but with me it has always been with a tremendous amount of respect and we ultimately work it out.

I'll end by saying that I have no idea what Victor Dzau's long-term plans for the Health System are. I know he understands the job a lot better than I did when I started, and I think he's very prepared. But, he's going to have to be an agent of change, and I think the main challenge for him will be related to the relationship of the clinical practice plan with the health system. A much more aggressive business-like clinical engine is needed to drive the growth of the health system, but this needs to be done without destroying the academic mission or its culture. I hope that you give Victor the support he needs because if he initiates change, there is going to be resistance, and there will be brush fires. He needs to know that his flanks are covered and people are supportive. I think the Medical Center and the Health System are going to benefit from his leadership. As uncomfortable as I was about a lot of the changes we needed to make, I think we are in a stronger place now than we've ever been. I feel very good in the handoff to Victor. It's not going to be easy for him and at times it will be difficult. Let me say more about Sandy Williams. I think he's one of the strongest academic medical leaders I have ever met. He knows this institution, and he has the highest level of insight, integrity, and sense of quality. I suspect he and Victor will be a great team. This Board is terrific and as I look around I could say something positive about every person here but I just don't have the time. We have world-class leaders here and I will be counseling Victor to take full advantage of the incredible strength of the membership of this Board. These 15 years have been a wonderful voyage for me. I never could have imagined that I would be given the opportunity to lead the Medical Center and I thank you from the bottom of my heart for all the things you have done for me and for Duke. I deeply appreciate your naming a building after me. I find that hard to believe, but I like it, although I haven't totally encompassed it yet. Thank you very much for all you do for Duke.

APPENDIX 4

Fifteen Years of Growth Statistics

EDUCATION	1989	2004
School of Medicine		
Enrollment		
Undergraduate	452	468
Women	30%	51%
Underrepresented minorities	8%	24%
MD/PhD	5%	10%
House staff	871	850
Faculty (total)	1,252	1,495
IOM membership	14	26
Endowment (market value)	$146.2 million	$651.1 million
School of Nursing		
Enrollment	54	374
Faculty	5	36
NIH ranking	Unranked	29
National school ranking	Unranked	29
Endowment (market value)	$1.7 million	$14.0 million

RESEARCH	1989	2004
Tenure-track faculty	709	753
NIH funding	$90.8 million	$245.5 million
Other sponsored research	$19.3 million	$124.3 million
Total sponsored research	$110.1 million	$369.8 million
NIH ranking	8	5
Royalty income	$0.3 million	$3.1 million
U.S. patents issued	7	~50
New research agreements	<100	691
Research space (net assignable)	477,000 sq. ft.	1.02 million sq. ft.

CLINICAL	1989	2004
Inpatients	34,300	59,054
Surgical procedures	22,500	54,543
Outpatients visits	453,900 (includes Emergency Department)	1.4 million (excludes Emergency Department)
Emergency department visits	N/A	60,076
Clinical revenue	$353.3 million	$1.245 billion
Components	Duke Hospital Private Diagnostic Clinic (PDC) Durham Casualty	Duke Hospital Durham Regional Hospital Raleigh Community Hospital PDC Duke University Affiliated Physicians Patient Revenue Management Organization Duke Health Community Care Durham Casualty

FINANCES	1989	2004

School of Medicine

Philanthropy	~$20 million	$75.7 million
SOM endowment (market value)	$146.2 million	$651.1 million
SOM revenue	$202.5 million	$595.8 million
PDC collections	$102.9 million	$288.1 million
Department/central reserves	$107 million	$358.8 million

Duke Hospital

Revenue	$353.3 million	$849.8 million

Annual Operating Budget

Duke University Medical Center (DUMC) including PDC	$312.9 million	$892.8 million
Duke University Health System (DUHS)	$353.3 million (Duke Hospital only)	$1.245 billion

Total	$666.2 million	$2.1 billion

NOTES

CHAPTER 2. HISTORY OF THE ACADEMIC MEDICAL CENTER

1. Abraham Flexner, *Medical Education in the United States and Canada* (New York: Carnegie Foundation, 1910).
2. Vannevar Bush, *Science: The Endless Frontier* (Washington, DC: U.S. Government Printing Office, 1945).
3. *AAMC Data Book: Medical Schools and Teaching Hospitals by the Numbers* (Washington, DC: AAMC, 2014).

CHAPTER 3. EVOLUTION OF THE DUKE UNIVERSITY MEDICAL CENTER

1. James B. Duke, The Duke Endowment Indenture of Trust, 1924, http://dukeendowment.org/sites/default/files/media/images/stories/downloads/tde/Duke-Indenture-MAR-16–2011.pdf.

CHAPTER 10. DUKE CLINICAL RESEARCH INSTITUTE

1. James B. Wyngaarden, "The Clinical Investigator as an Endangered Species," *New England Journal of Medicine* 301 (1979): 1254–59.
2. Ralph Snyderman, "The Clinical Researcher: An 'Emerging' Species," *JAMA* 291 (2004): 882–83.

CHAPTER 11. DUKE UNIVERSITY HEALTH SYSTEM

1. Spencie Love, *One Blood: The Death and Resurrection of Charles R. Drew* (Chapel Hill: University of North Carolina Press, 1996).

CHAPTER 12. INTEGRATIVE MEDICINE

1. Tracy W. Gaudet and Ralph Snyderman, "Integrative Medicine and the Search for the Best Practice of Medicine," *Academic Medicine* 77 (2002): 863.
2. *Integrative Medicine and the Health of the Public: A Summary of the February 2009 Summit* (Washington, DC: National Academies Press, 2009).

CHAPTER 13. PERSONALIZING HEALTH CARE

1. Ralph Snyderman, "Personalized Health Care: From Theory to Practice," *Biotechnology Journal* 7 (2012): 973–79; Ralph Snyderman and Michaela Dinan, "Improving Health by Taking It Personally," *Journal of the American Medical Association* 303 (2010): 363–64.
2. David J. Whellan, et al., "The Benefits of Implementing a Heart Failure Disease Management Program," *Archives of Internal Medicine* 161 (2001): 2223–28; David J. Whellan, et al., "The Metaanalysis and Review of Heart Failure Disease Management Randomized Controlled Clinical Trials," *American Heart Journal* 149 (2005): 722–29.
3. Richard M.J. Bohmer and Laura Feldman, "The Duke Heart Failure Program," Harvard Business School Case 604.038, October 2003. (Revised February 2010).
4. "An Overview of the Human Genome Project," National Human Genome Research Institute. Accessed August 31, 2014. http://www.genome.gov/12011238.
5. Ralph Snyderman and R. Sanders Williams, "Prospective Medicine: The Next Health Care Transformation," *Academic Medicine* 78 (2003): 1079–84; Ralph Snyderman, "The AAP and the Transformation of Medicine," *Journal of Clinical Investigation* 114 (2004): 1169–73.
6. R. Sanders Williams, Huntington Willard, and Ralph Snyderman, "Personalized Health Planning," *Science* 300 (2003): 549.
7. H. Clint Davidson, "Prospective Health: Duke's Approach to Improving Employee Health and Managing Health Care Costs," *CUPA-HR Journal* 55, no. 2 (2004): 11–14; Duke Well History. Accessed August 31, 2014. http://www.dukewell.org/about-dukewell/dukewell-history.
8. Duke Center for Research on Personalized Health Care. Accessed March 14, 2015. http://dukepersonalizedhealth.org.
9. U.S. Department of Veterans Affairs. Blueprint for Excellence. Published September 21, 2014. Accessed March 17, 2016. http://www.va.gov/health/docs/VHA_Blueprint_for_Excellence.pdf.

CHAPTER 14. PHILANTHROPY AND RELATIONSHIPS

1. Email from Sam Katz to Cindy Mitchell dated October 11, 2010.

CHAPTER 15. REPUTATION AND CRISIS

1. Walter E. Campbell, *Foundations for Excellence: 75 Years of Duke Medicine* (Durham, NC: Duke University Medical Center, 2006), 378.

2. John K. Iglehart, "Duke University Conference on the Private Sector," *Health Affairs* 14 (1995): 304–11; John K. Iglehart, "Listening in on the Duke University Private Sector Conference," *New England Journal of Medicine* 336 (1997): 1827–31.

3. E. Marshall, "Shutdown of Research at Duke Sends a Message," *Science* 284 (1999): 1246. Meredith Wadman, "NIH Ethics Office Clamps Down on Duke," *Nature* 399, no. 6733 (1999): 190.

4. Ralph Snyderman and Edward Holmes, "Oversight Mechanisms for Clinical Research," *Science* 287 (2000): 595–97.

5. Allison Fass, "Duking it Out," *Forbes.* June 9, 2003. Accessed March 14, 2016. http://www.forbes.com/forbes/2003/0609/074.html.

ADDITIONAL RESOURCES

CHAPTER 1. FROM BROOKLYN TO DUKE

Chesanow, Neil. "Looking Back on Ralph Snyderman's 15 Years at the Helm." *Duke Med Magazine* 4, no. 1 (Spring/Summer 2004). https://medspace.mc.duke.edu/dukemed -magazine-vol-4-issue-1.

CHAPTER 3. EVOLUTION OF DUKE UNIVERSITY MEDICAL CENTER

Anlyan, William G., MD. *Metamorphosis: Memoirs of a Life in Medicine*. Durham, NC: Duke University Press, 2004.

Campbell, Walter E. *Foundations for Excellence: 75 Years of Duke Medicine*. Durham, NC: Duke University Medical Center, 2006.

Davison, Wilburt Cornell. *Davison of Duke: His Reminiscences*. Durham, NC: Duke University Medical Center, 1980.

Gifford, James, Jr. *The Evolution of a Medical Center: A History of Medicine at Duke University to 1941*. Durham, NC: Duke University Press, 1972.

Williams, Sanders. *The Magic of Medicine at Duke: A History in Our Own Words*. Durham, NC: Duke Medicine Office of Marketing and Creative Services, 2009.

CHAPTER 10. DUKE CLINICAL RESEARCH INSTITUTE

Snyderman, R. "Academic Medicine Can Transform Health Care through Clinical Research." *Academic Medicine* 74, no. 11 (1999): 1224–25.

Snyderman, R., ed. *For the Health of the Public: Ensuring the Future of Clinical Research. Vol. 1, Report of the AAMC Task Force on Clinical Research*. Washington, DC: Association of American Medical Colleges, January 2000.

Snyderman, R., ed. *For the Health of the Public: Ensuring the Future of Clinical Research.* *Vol. 2, Invited Papers.* Washington, DC: Association of American Medical Colleges, November 2000.

CHAPTER 12. INTEGRATIVE MEDICINE

Horrigan, Bonnie. *Voices of Integrative Medicine: Conversations and Encounters.* London: Churchill Livingstone, 2003.

Interview with Christy Mack, Harvey Fineberg, MD, and Ralph Snyderman, MD, on the Institute of Medicine's Summit on Integrative Medicine. *The Charlie Rose Show,* March 28, 2008. http://www.bravewell.org/transforming_healthcare/national _summit/charlie_rose/

Kabat-Zinn, Jon. *Wherever You Go, There You Are: Mindfulness Meditation in Everyday Life.* New York, NY: Hachette Books, 1994.

The New Medicine. http://www.thenewmedicine.org/.

Snyderman, R., and Weil, A. "Integrative Medicine: Bringing Medicine Back to Its Roots." *Archives of Internal Medicine* 106 (2002): 395–97.

CHAPTER 13. PERSONALIZING HEALTH CARE

Burnette, R., L. A. Simmons, and R. Snyderman. "Personalized Health Care as a Pathway for the Adoption of Genomic Medicine." *Personalized Medicine* 2 (2012): 232–40.

Dinan, M., L. Simmons, and R. Snyderman. "Commentary: Personalized Health Planning and the Patient Protection and Affordable Care Act: An Opportunity for Academic Medicine to Lead Health Care Reform." *Academic Medicine* 85 (2010): 1665–68.

Duke Center for Research for Personalized Health Care. http://dukepersonalizedhealth .org/.

Langheier, J. M., and R. Snyderman. "Prospective Medicine: The Role for Genomics in Personalized Health Planning." *Pharmacogenomics* 5 (2004): 1–8.

Simmons, L. A., M. A. Dinan, T. A. Robinson, and R. Snyderman. "Personalized Medicine Is More Than Genomic Medicine: Confusion over Terminology Impedes Progress towards Personalized Health Care." *Personalized Medicine* 9 (2012): 85–91.

Snyderman, R. "Creating Meaningful Health Care Reform." *Journal of Clinical Investigation* 119 (2009): 2855.

Snyderman, R. "Personalized Health Care in 2013: A Status Report on the Impact of Genomics." *North Carolina Medical Journal* 74 (2013): 478–84.

Snyderman, R. "Personalized Medicine 2014: Has Health Care Been Transformed?" *Personalized Medicine* 11 (2014): 365–68.

Snyderman, R. "The Role of Genomics in Enabling Prospective Health Care." In *Genomic and Personalized Medicine,* Vol. 1, edited by Huntington F. Willard, PhD, and Geoffrey S. Ginsburg, MD, PhD, 378–85. San Diego, CA: Elsevier, 2009.

Snyderman, R., and J. Langheier. "Prospective Health Care: The Second Transformation of Medicine." *Genome Biology* 7 (2006): 104.

Snyderman, R., and Z. Yoediono. "Prospective Care: A Personalized, Preventative Approach to Medicine." *Pharmacogenomics* 7 (2006): 5–9.

Snyderman, R., and Z. Yoediono. "Prospective Health and the Role of Academic Medicine: Lead, Follow or Get Out of the Way." *Academic Medicine* 83 (2008): 707–14.

Yoediono, Z., and R. Snyderman. "Proposal for a New Health Record to Support Personalized, Predictive, Preventative, and Participatory Medicine." *Personalized Medicine* 5 (2008): 47–54.

CHAPTER 15. REPUTATION AND CRISIS

"Anatomy of a Mistake: The Tragic Death of Jesica Santillan." http://www.cbsnews.com /news/anatomy-of-a-mistake-16-03-2003/.

"A Week in the Life of a Hospital: On the Front Lines of the War between Money and Medicine?" *Time*, October 12, 1998.

"Discovery Channel Series Features Duke Doctors and Patients." *Chronicle*, September 2000. http://beta.dukechronicle.com/articles/2000/09/20/discovery-channel-series -features-duke-doctors-and-patients.

"Government Halts Duke's Human Research." *Chronicle*, May 19, 1999. http://beta .dukechronicle.com/articles/1999/05/20/government-halts-dukes-human-research.

"Snyderman Defends Hospital." *Chronicle*, February 25, 2003. http://www .dukechronicle.com/articles/2003/02/26/snyderman-defends-hospital#.VYsJt_lViko.

"US Halts Human Research at Duke." *Washington Post*, May 12, 1999, A1. http://www .washingtonpost.com/wp-srv/national/daily/may99/duke12.htm.

"What They Said: Statements on Jesica Santillan." *Duke Today*, February 22, 2003. https://today.duke.edu/2003/02/jesicaquotes0203.html

CHAPTER 16. STEPPING DOWN AND LESSONS LEARNED

Sinek, Simon. *Start with Why.* New York: Penguin, 2009.

PROCEEDINGS FROM THE PRIVATE (HEALTH)
SECTOR CONFERENCE, 1994 TO 2003
(Available at Duke University Medical Center Library)

Snyderman, R., M. Rogers, and V. Saito, eds. *The Academic Health Center and Health Care Reform* New York: Raven Press, 1994.

Snyderman, R., and V. Saito, eds. *The Academic Health Center in the 21st Century.* Durham, NC: Duke University Medical Center and Health System, 1995.

Snyderman, R., and V. Saito, eds. *Academic Health Systems in Transition.* Durham, NC: Duke University Medical Center and Health System, 2000.

Snyderman, R., and V. Saito, eds. *The AHC Responds to Health Care Reform.* Durham, NC: Duke University Medical Center and Health System, 1996.

Snyderman, R., and V. Saito, eds. *Beyond Managed Health Care: The Role of the Academic Health Center*. Durham, NC: Duke University Medical Center and Health System, 1997.

Snyderman, R., and V. Saito, eds. *Enabling Prospective Health Care*. Durham, NC: Duke University Medical Center and Health System, 2002.

Snyderman, R., and V. Saito, eds. *Integrating Health Care Delivery Systems*. Durham, NC: Duke University Medical Center and Health System, 1998.

Snyderman, R., and V. Saito, eds. *Integrated Health Delivery Systems*. Durham, NC: Duke University Medical Center and Health System, 1999.

Snyderman, R., and V. Saito, eds. *Prospective Health Care*. Durham, NC: Duke University Medical Center and Health System, 2003.

Snyderman, R., and V. Saito, eds. *Rational Approaches to Quality: Affordable Health Care*. Durham, NC: Duke University Medical Center and Health System, 2001.

INDEX

Note: Italicized numbers indicate a figure; n indicates an endnote

Academic Consortium on Integrative Medicine, 164, 167–69
academic medical centers: Association of American Medical Colleges (AAMC), 57, 115, 133–34, 165, 182, 205, 222; Association of American Physicians (AAP), 182, 205, 222; center at Duke, 23, 25–31, 34–35, 51–54, 61, 67–69, 132–37; changes in concepts and functions, 1, 3, 17–20, 35, 99–100, 142–43, 153–54; charity and specialty care delivery by, 17, 127; clinical and translational research of, 5, 16, 66, 119, 130–37, 213; decentralized character of early, 19–20, 31–32; depts. and power structures in, 19, 31, 73; as drivers of medical knowledge and innovation, 5, 16, 21, 22–24, 34–35, 66–68, 118, 131–36; as drivers of new industries, 17, 34, 118–19, 136, 179–80, 252; as drivers of specialization, 16, 18–19, 191, 242, 245; economic importance of, 17, 21, 79, 82, 110, 145, 209; financial structures and vulnerabilities of, 20, 53–54, 70, 84, 108, 139–42; health care delivery by, 17, 143, 149–50; health care delivery through Duke University Medical Center (DUMC) and Duke University Health System (DUHS), 141–43, 152–54;

influence of Flexner Report on structures of, 15, 16–17; integrative medicine in, 163–65, 168–69; leading in U.S., 34, 168, 252; national crisis of, 20–21, 32, 43, 67, 138–39, 206; research as basis for reputations of, 34, 46, 134–35, 243–44, 252; U.S. government support of research by, 16, 66–67, 134; vs. medical schools, 18
Activase, 11, 131–32
acute care, 114, 249
African Americans: Dr. Charles Drew case, 146; Maltheus Avery case, 146; community health care programs for, 126; constraints of to Duke's public clinics, 29, 124–25; Danny O. Jacobs, 117, 126, 239; Duke laundry facility (1989), 39–40; "Duke Plantation" (1989), 80, 123, 129, 145; Haywood L. Brown, 117, 126, 238; impact of workforce reduction on at Duke, 110, 125; interactions with local black community, 125–26, 147; lasting socioeconomic impact of discrimination and segregation on local, 124–25, 145–46; legacy of racism at Duke, 123–24, 129, 145–46; in low-paying positions at Duke (1989), 39–40, 80, 145; as medical students at Duke, 123–24, 126–27; minority task force at Duke, 125;

African Americans (*continued*)
recruitment of professionals who were
also, 117, 125–27. *See also* diversity and
inclusion; minorities; race relations
Ahmad, Asaf, 112, 234
Albert Einstein College of Medicine, 164, 168
Albert, Herman (Hy): Herman and Ruth
Albert Lung Cancer Genomics Fund, 200;
relationships to DUMC, 200–201; Ruth and
Herman Albert Eye Research Institute, 200
allied health programs, 17, 27, 31, 37, 60, 62
ambulatory care. *See* outpatient care
Anderson, Robert W. (Bob), 102, 117, 239
Anderson, W. Banks, Jr., 75, 238
Anlyan, William G. (Bill): chancellor and
Dean of School of Medicine (1964–89),
11, 23–24, 37, 38, 44–45, 54–55, 77, 82, 203;
creation of external review of chairs by,
73; establishment of Duke Private Sector
Conference by, 206; fundraising activities of,
194–200, 218–19, 242; role of in employing
Durham's African American residents, 145
anodyne imagery, 157
appointment, promotion, and tenure (APT)
process, 30, 65
Armstrong, Brenda E., 126–27
Association of American Medical Colleges
(AAMC), 57, 115, 133–34, 165, 182, 205,
222
Association of American Physicians (AAP),
182, 205, 222

Barr Committee, 78, 82, 84, 89–90, 92–93,
95, 97–98
basic sciences: changes in tenure criteria
for faculty in, 65; curriculum, 26, 28,
242–43; depts. in, 28, 47, 236–37; faculty
in, 28, 29, 30; funding and space allocation reforms in the, 64, 65, 246; graduate
research and training in depts., 26,
28–29, 62; improvement of as priority
at DUMC, 4, 35–36, 43, 54, 62–65, 252;
inequalities among depts. at Duke, 5, 19,
44–45; interactions of chancellor and
faculty of, 59, 95; participation of faculty
in undergraduate medical education, 27;
recruitment of faculty to improve quality
of depts., 34–36, 45–47, 60, 66, 116, 193
Baugh, Philip J. (Jack), 79, 87, 89–90, 94, 97

Bell, Robert M. (Bob), 47, 89, 237
Bennett, James L., Jr. (Pete), 38, 235
Beth El Congregation (Durham), 88
Beyel, Joseph S., 190, 235
biochemistry, 19, 23, 44, 47, 243
biomedical research: as hallmark of great
academic medical centers, 20, 25, 46, 134,
246; as basis for major industries, 16–17,
34–35, 118–19, 131–36, 248, 252; Bush
report, 16, 263n2; explosion in, 35, 64–65,
118–19, 180, 244, 247; growth at Duke,
34, 48, 62, 65, 114–15, 250; in Singapore,
68, 117–18; transformative influence on
medical knowledge, 16, 131, 166, 179–81;
U.S. government support of, 16, 18. *See also*
research
biostatistics and bioinformatics, 116, 135–36,
180
biotechnology: Activase as first blockbuster
drug produced, 11; Alza Corporation,
154; Duke's participation, 35–36, 59–60,
61; Genentech's leadership in industry,
10, 11, 34–35, 66; genomics as basis for
new approach to health care, 5, 173, 175,
179–82; growth of industry, 16, 17, 34–35,
247–48; leadership of academic medical
centers in utilizing to improve medical
care, 17, 34, 35, 248; radiation technologies,
76, 161, 177; recombinant DNA technology, 34, 35, 66, 252; synthesized proteins,
66, 131, 180, 248; 3D computer graphics
as modeling tool, 247; translational and
clinical research as facilitators of clinical
applications, 5, 119, 136, 222
Black, MaryAnn E., 126, 148, 234
Blazer, Dan G., 74, 107, 162, 233, 238
Board of Trustees: advisory functions, 97, 101,
125–26, 149, 167, 198–99, 208; chancellor's
relationship with Duke, 9, 148–50, 211–12,
223; chancellor's reports to, 57–58, 61, 82,
159, 208, 210, 241–58; decision to close
School of Nursing (1979), 54–55; power
of over APT of faculty and administrators,
30, 77–78, 79, 82, 90, 94; role during
institutional crises, 90, 211–12; as ultimate
governing authority of Duke University,
148, 221
Board of Visitors: membership of Brandt
and Belinda Louie, 200; membership of

Herman and Ruth Albert, 200–201; membership of Milton and Roslyn Lachman, 199–200; membership of Philip and Travis Tracy, 195; membership of Sheppard and Clara Zinovoy, 202; purpose of, 199. *See also* fundraising
bodily humors theory, 14–15
body: form follows function approach to understanding, 107; medical juxtaposition between normal and diseased, 113; mind-body and mind-body-spirit interactions, 157–58, 162–63, 164, 168
Bolognese, Dani P., 78, 97–98
Bravewell Collaborative, 167–68, 169–72
Broad, Shepard and Ruth K., 193
Brodhead, Richard H., 222, 254
Brodie, H. Keith: administrative relationship to chancellor for health affairs, 37, 38; collaboration with Duke's Board of Trustees, 57, 254; Duke University presidency (1985–93), 37; establishment of chancellor's discretionary fund, 41; involvement in faculty appointments, promotions, and renewals, 37, 45, 71, 77–78, 81, 90–91, 94, 97; petitions and letters by faculty members, 45, 87, 89, 90; retirement from Duke's presidency, 79, 92–93
Brown, Haywood L., 117, 126, 238
Brundage, Dorothy J., 55, 236
building construction and facility renovations, 60, 114, 135, 169, 189–91, 194–98, 200, 223, 241–42
Burk, Larry, 156–58

Califf, Robert M., 131–33, 137
"Campaign for Duke", 191, 221
cancer: anticancer drug development at Duke, 68; BRAC-1 and BRAC-2 gene mutations underlying breast, 113; Betty Eldreth case, 41–42; Dana-Farber Cancer Institute (Harvard), 48, 171; Dept. of Molecular Cancer Biology, 47, 237; Duke Cancer Survivorship Program, 177; Duke Comprehensive Cancer Center, 47, 192; Herman and Ruth Albert Lung Cancer Genomics Fund, 200; needs of patients diagnosed with, 161, 171–72, 177; radiation oncology therapy, 76, 161; surgical therapy for, 161, 201

cardiovascular medicine: cardiac rehabilitation programs, 163; cardiomyopathy, 213–14; cardiothoracic surgery and anesthesiology, 73, 116, 153; cardiovascular disease prevention, 160, 163; clinical trials at Duke, 132; congestive heart failure treatments, 178–79, 207; Division of Cardiology, 72, 82, 84, 87, 111–12, 132–33; Duke Cardiovascular Center for Genomic Sciences, 117; Duke Cardiovascular Database, 130; Duke Heart Failure Program, 179; establishment of, 24; heart and lung transplantation, 213–16, 245, 249; heart attack therapies, 131–32; integrative medicine as element of treatment, 163, 169, 207; interdisciplinary clinical program for treatment of cardiovascular disease, 60, 153; pediatric cardiac surgery at Duke, 213; plaque removal and interventional therapies, 245, 247; risk assessment for stroke or heart attack, 180, 247; School of Nursing master's program in cardiovascular care, 114; studies of congestive heart failure, 178; t-PA as drug therapy to unblock coronary arteries, 131–32
caring, compassion, and curing, 113, 116, 173
Carroll, Bernard J. (Barney), 71, 74, 238
cash flows. *See* expenses; margins; referrals; reimbursement; revenues
centralization: as means of making institutional purposes and goals coherent, 4, 20, 60–64, 80, 101–2; absence at DUMC (1989), 19–20, 35, 40–41, 53, 65, 80–81, 101–2, 107–8; advantages and disadvantages of decentralization, 18–20, 25, 140; as efficient means of solving problems, 4–5, 18, 107; as analogous in function to central nervous system, 4, 53–54, 107; coordinative strengths, 80–81, 108–9, 140; hub-and-spokes model, 139, 142, 149, 153; responsiveness of administrative to externally-generated change, 4–5, 13, 25, 53, 80–81, 101–2, 108–9; vs. reflexive, impromptu growth and organization, 18, 141
certificate programs, 26–27
Champagne, Mary T., 55, 108, 114, 236
chancellor for health affairs: advisory groups and committees of, 59, 153; appointment powers over administrative staff, 30;

chancellor for health affairs (*continued*)
APT powers over faculty, 30–31; direct report administrators, 26, 27, 29, 107–8; discrepancy between powers and responsibilities of (in 1989), 30; and external reviews of depts., 73–76, 81, 95; financial powers of, 31, 40–41; reporting responsibilities of, 59, 105, 148–49, 159; responsibilities as CEO of DUHS, 150–53; responsibilities of, 23, 25–32, 37, 78, 148. *See also* Snyderman, Ralph

change: academic curriculum, research, and training as targets of, 59–60, 62, 134–36; anticipation as tool for managing, 84, 101–2, 119; communication as tool for implementing, 79–80, 84–88, 91, 100–101, 149, 255–56; cost-effectiveness as driver of, 54; discovery as basis for technological, 24, 179–80, 182–83, 247; diversity and inclusion as drivers of change in recruitment, 63, 123, 125–29; flexibility and adaptability as institutional tools for surviving, 12, 20, 25, 43–44, 96–97, 101–2, 106–7, 254–56; in American health care as influence on academic medical centers, 4, 18, 20, 32, 36, 43–44, 84, 87; individuals as agents of, 54, 70–75, 78, 88–92, 100, 162–63, 253–54, 257–58; innovation, improvement, and problem-solving as bases for, 134–36, 161, 173–74, 175–82, 185, 253, 257; magnitude of as influence on its implementation, 96–97; managed care as impetus for institutional, 84, 99–100, 138–42; resistance and anxiety as inevitable responses to, 4, 78–79, 81–83, 85–90, 141, 182; thinking and attitudes as factors in achieving, 181–85, 225, 230, 254–55; unpredictable elements of, 100, 158–61, 226

chemistry, 15, 22

children. *See* Dept. of Pediatrics; pediatrics

chronic diseases: annual national costs of treatments, 175–76, 178; asthma, 128; diabetes, 128, 169; hypertension, 128; rheumatoid arthritis, 159–60

Clark, B. Jefferson (Jeff), 190, 235

clinical care margins. *See* margins; reimbursement

clinical depts.: changes in tenure criteria for faculty, 65, 135; clinical opportunities as influences on expansion of, 19; collaboration with basic sciences depts., 26; committees, 59, 108; competition for revenues among, 52–53; cross-subsidization among, 52, 246; decentralized, uncoordinated nature of, 53–54; dependence of on patient referrals, 53, 139–40; external reviews of, 72–76; faculty responsibilities in, 27–29, 31, 108, 135, 143; financial restructuring of in response to managed care reforms, 84–85, 139–43, 256; graduate research and training in, 27, 29, 243; growth and creation of at Duke, 19, 76; inequalities among at Duke, 19, 45, 51, 54; political tensions in, 70–72, 78–79, 81–82, 89–91; power of chairs of, 41, 45, 50–51, 54, 76, 109, 140; recruitment of faculty to improve quality of, 60, 72, 75–76, 116–17; reforms and modernization in, 50–51, 59, 70, 72–76, 78, 106–9; relationship of with DCRI, 132–35; relationship of with DUAP, 143; relationship of with PDC, 29–30, 31, 51, 53, 108, 140; revenue sources of, 31, 51–53, 64, 70, 138, 256; subspecialties of the, 238–39

clinical research, 130–36, 209–13

Clinical Research Forum, 135

Clinical Research Training Program, 113–14, 136

clinical trials: commercial contract research organizations (CROs), 131; crisis at Duke (1998–99), 208–13; drawbacks of corporate-sponsored, 131, 136; Duke congestive heart failure study, 178–79; Duke Institutional Review Board (IRB), 208–13; at Duke University (as of 1998), 209; importance of procedural documentation in, 212; national and international, 134, 135; objective data, 131, 132, 136; protection of human subjects in, 209–13; purpose of, 131–32, 134; tests of Activase and streptokinase, 131–32. *See also* investigators and investigation

closed versus open systems, 100–101

Cohen, Harvey J., 117, 238

collaboration: DUHS model for, 139, 141–42, 152; enhancing as goal of Long Range Plan, 62, 74; institution-wide, 58–59, 62; interdepartmental within DUMC, 70, 76, 84, 102, 128; interdisciplinary programs,

59, 107, 113, 114, 194; of DUMC with other entities at Duke University, 28–29, 62, 75; of DUMC with outside entities, 66–69, 118, 134, 194

collegiality, 45, 49, 71, 72, 76

Columbia University, 168, 173, 252

commercial hospital chains, 139, 147, 249

communications: as means of facilitating media access to Duke, 205, 215; African American community as special target for, 125, 126, 147; committees, 95, 108; expansion of as element of reform, 95, 107, 203–4; functions of dept., 203–4; importance of communicating vision of change, 4, 84; importance of honesty, 215; importance of listening, 98, 100–101, 226; need for clear and frequent, 100–101; open hospital forums as means of improving, 79–80, 95; publications, 95, 207–8; regular meetings with chairs, faculty, and staff as means of sustaining, 69–70, 84, 87–88, 95; reputation as concern of, 203, 204, 214–15; walk-arounds as tool for meeting employees in their environments, 39–40, 95

community: communication and interactions of DUMC with local, 5, 84, 101, 125, 147–49; community hospitals, 132, 142, 144–49, 152, 260; community outreach, 60, 84, 126–28, 148, 234, 245, 246; community physicians, 143; PrimaHealth, 143

complementary and alternative medicine (CAM) therapies, 156, 161–68, 177

computers, 62, 112, 130, 134, 247

Consortium of Academic Health Centers for Integrative Medicine, 164, 166–68

continuing medical education, 60, 62, 114, 242

core mission: faculty participation in, 20, 28–29, 31, 33–34, 36; financial support for educational and research elements of, 20; influence of on Long Range Plan, 61, 101–2, 119, 203, 255; of Duke University Medical School, 13, 22, 25, 218; relevance to societal needs, 13, 35, 61

costs: cost-cutting initiatives at Duke, 109, 183–84, 206–7, 245–46, 249; cost-effectiveness, 54, 60, 62–65, 101–2, 109, 113, 139; cost management for chronic disease patients, 175–76, 178–79; cost-plus

billing model for clinical services, 51, 245, 249; cost recovery per square foot of research space, 64; cost shifting of clinical revenues, 20, 27, 35, 51, 65, 138, 245–46; health care, 106–7, 180–84, 206, 245–46; high of specialized and intensive medical care, 149, 245; personalized health care as means of reducing medical, 180, 182–83; reimbursement of medical by insurance carriers, 20, 128, 138–40, 149, 176, 179, 184, 207; research, 20, 49–51, 60; savings through Promising Practices program, 127–28; technological developments as means of reducing medical, 180–82

crisis: caused by job layoffs to cut costs, 110, 125; Greenfield's civil war, 83–86, 90–94; importance of communication in, 203–4; in academic medicine provoked by managed care, 21, 32, 43; management of, 210, 220; of organ transplant error, 213–16; Office for Protection from Research Risks (OPRR), 208–12

cross-subsidization, 20, 27, 31, 35, 51–2, 65, 138

curriculum: basic science of medical students, 28, 113, 242–43; updating of Duke's medical school, 26, 38, 59–60, 62, 113, 169

Davison, Wilburt C., 22–23, 197–98

deans: AAMC advisory program for, 57; AAMC Council of Deans, 115, 133–34, 165, 205; for admissions, financial aid, and student affairs, 26; dean of medical education, 38, 74; dean of Duke-NUS Graduate Medical School (Singapore), 116; dean of Graduate School of Nursing, 27, 30, 55, 114; dean of School of Medicine, 20, 26, 30, 38, 45, 77, 114–17; dean of School of Nursing, 20, 27, 55, 59, 108, 114, 236; dean of undergraduate medical education, 26, 27, 30, 59, 62; role of academic in coordinating curriculum development, 26, 27, 28

dept. chairs: autonomy at Duke, 31–32, 44, 50–51, 63, 139–41; centralization and new restraints on powers of, 62–66, 98, 101, 108–9, 139–41; chancellor's role in recruitment of, 45–46, 60, 71–76, 81, 92, 101–2, 252; collegiality among, 45, 72, 76; and development of Long Range Plan,

dept. chairs (*continued*)
57–61, 63–65; "dwarfs" and "giants", 45,
63; external review process, 73–76, 81, 95;
inequalities in power of, 19, 40, 44–45;
influence of over revenues, 20, 31, 41, 51,
70; longevity of, 50–51, 73, 83; and medical
center funding and space allocations for
research, 64–65; personal politics of, 71,
81–90; powers of over recruitment, 63;
relationship to CEO of Duke Hospital, 54,
108–11; relationship to chancellor, 30–32,
40–41, 59, 69–70, 73–76, 89–92, 157;
replacement of, 60, 71–75, 81, 115–16, 255;
role in building medical depts., 19–20, 36,
45–46, 66, 73–74, 116–17; role in PDC, 30,
31, 70, 139–41; tensions between, 44–45,
52, 70–72, 76
Dept. of Anesthesiology, 52, 70, 73, 157
Dept. of Biochemistry: chair of, 19, 23, 44,
47–48, 60, 78, 236; national ranking of,
243; new faculty appointments, 63
Dept. of Biological Anthropology and
Anatomy, 117, 236, 243
Dept. of Biostatistics and Bioinformatics, 116,
135–36, 236
Dept. of Cell Biology, 45, 46–47, 81, 116, 129,
193–94, 236
Dept. of Community and Family Medicine,
60, 76, 128
Dept. of Genetics, 236, 237
Dept. of Immunology, 48, 236–37
Dept. of Medicine: chairmanship of Joe
Greenfield, 52, 69, 72, 75–76, 79, 81–86,
255–56; chairs of the, 24, 50, 115, 117, 130;
coordination of with other depts., 70;
financial vulnerability of under managed
care system, 84; leadership of in developing
field of clinical investigation, 131–33, 178;
politics in (1989–93), 75–76, 79, 81–82,
87, 90; relationship of to Duke Clinical
Research Institute (DCRI), 132–33; relationship of to DUHS; revenue-generating capacity of the, 52, 84, 243; strengths of (1989),
33–34, 44
Dept. of Microbiology and Immunology, 48,
60, 65, 236–37
Dept. of Molecular Cancer Biology, 47, 237
Dept. of Molecular Genetics and Microbiology, 236, 237

Dept. of Neurobiology: chair of the, 45–46,
81, 116–17, 237, 252; interdisciplinary
research program in neurosciences, 60;
Kathleen Bryan Research Building for
Neurobiology, 242; research in Alzheimer's
disease at, 193
Dept. of Obstetrics and Gynecology: chair of
the, 71–75, 81, 117, 126, 151, 238; external
review of the, 73–75; financial losses by
the, 51, 70, 71, 74, 75
Dept. of Ophthalmology, 60, 75–76, 81, 200,
238
Dept. of Pathology, 41, 47, 52, 70
Dept. of Pediatrics: chair of the, 73, 75, 81,
238; external review of the, 73; financial
losses by the, 51, 70, 196; national ranking
of the, 243; philanthropic support for the,
196–98
Dept. of Pharmacology, 47, 237
Dept. of Pharmacology and Cancer Biology,
45, 47, 81, 237
Dept. of Psychiatry: chair of the, 51, 60,
71–74, 81, 103, 157, 162, 238–39; external
review of the, 73; financial losses by the, 51,
70; national ranking of the, 243
Dept. of Radiation Oncology, 76, 117, 239
Dept. of Radiology: chair of, 44, 52, 70–71,
75, 81, 89, 239; external review of the, 73,
75; radiology versus radiation oncology
services, 76
Dept. of Surgery, 52, 70–71, 83, 102, 117,
126, 239
departments: as basis for establishing institutional reputation, 45–47, 60–61, 102,
106, 243–44; as focal point of loyalty for
some faculty, 31; as agents of stagnation or
progress, 34–36, 45–47, 50–51, 60; basic
science at Duke, 26–29, 47, 54, 62, 64–65,
236–37, 243; broadening of institutional
oversight of, 60–64, 98, 101–2, 139–43,
252; chairs as major influence on character
and development of their, 19, 31, 44–48,
50–52, 63, 71; clinical at Duke, 26–29,
50–54, 65, 128, 139–41, 238, 243; collaboration between as goal of reform, 59,
76, 84, 102, 133, 139–43, 243; departmental
components of Long Range Plan, 58–61;
early model of autonomous, nonintegrated
academic medical, 5, 19–20, 31, 51–53,

63, 69–72, 140, 256; external reviews of, 73, 75; finances of individual, 51–53, 64, 69–70, 84, 138, 143, 246, 256; inequalities among as function of their disciplinary nature, 19, 31, 41, 51–52, 70–71, 196, 243; new at Duke, 47, 76; opportunistic nature of development of, 6, 18–19, 51; as organizational basis for academic medical faculty, 19; as point of origin for appointments, promotion, and tenure granted to faculty, 30–31; research space allocations for, 64

development: contributions from Ruth and Shepard Broad Foundation, 193; Lucille P. Markey Charitable Trust., 193–94; mission of dept. for institutional, 190–91; role of Vice Chancellor Raymond C. "Bucky" Waters, 38, 48, 107, 190, 196, 199, 235; Joseph S. Beyel, 190, 235; B. Jefferson Clark, 190, 23; Steven A. Rum, 191, 235. *See also* fundraising

diagnosis: cancer, 161, 177; development of new technologies for, 16, 246; diagnostic clinics, 124, 246; diagnostic procedures, 15, 52, 70; predictive diagnostics, 175, 180–85; psychiatric, 74

discoveries: basic discovery research, 66, 134; as basis for advances in medicine, 22, 34–35, 118–19, 247–48; contribution of medical to improvements in health care, 5, 159, 242, 246–47; financial value of medical research, 18, 21, 66–67; funding for promising research, 51, 134, 248; investigator-led biomedical research as major source of, 134, 136; patents, licenses, and intellectual properties, 67–68; reputational value of medical research, 18, 23–24, 34, 134; research fields ripe for production of, 46, 66, 118, 244; translation and commercialization of medical, 5, 66–67, 119, 131, 136, 222

disease: burdens of, 2, 177; cancer, 118, 177; cardiovascular, 24, 60, 114, 130, 153, 160; caring as element of treatment for, 159–60, 177; chronic, 128, 159–60, 169, 175–76, 178; complex, multifaceted, 162, 176; environment as factor in manifestation of, 180; evolution of, 118, 181; financial costs of, 177–79, 183, 245; genetic factors

underlying risk, 118, 173, 180–83; "germ theory" of, 14; inflection curve of development, 181; integrative medicine approach to treatment of, 5, 169, 173; interdisciplinary approaches to study and treatment of, 60, 153; medical specialization and, 16, 18, 27, 28, 139–40, 243; microorganisms as causative agents of, 14; pathophysiological approach to study of, 16, 113, 242–43; personalized health care approach to, 175–78, 180–84; prevention of, 173, 175–76, 180–82; reactive, "find-it, fix-it" approach to treatment of, 1–2, 161–62, 175–76, 180; rheumatoid arthritis, 159; scientific discovery as influence on knowledge and treatment of, 16, 18, 64–65, 66, 159, 180; specialized and tertiary treatment of, 35, 114, 138, 140–42, 144, 149, 245–46; synthetic molecules as tools for treatment of, 15, 131, 247–48; theory of bodily humors and cause of, 14

diversity and inclusion, 5, 116–17, 126–29. *See also* African Americans; diversity and inclusion; race relations

Division of Cardiology, 72, 73, 117, 132–3

Division of Rheumatology and Immunology, 10, 38, 44, 48, 56, 102

DNA: deciphering of human genome, 247–48; Duke data bank, 118; recombinant technology, 34, 35, 66, 252

Donelan, William J. (Bill), 38, 40, 58, 107, 132, 142–44, 227, 234

drugs: blockbuster, 11; development and design of, 68, 131, 136–37, 247; FDA licensing of, 11, 47–48, 131

Duke Center for Genetic and Cell Therapeutics, 68

Duke Center for Human Genetics, 118

Duke Center for Integrative Medicine (DCIM), 162–63, 165–66, 168–69

Duke Children's Health Center (McGovern-Davison Children's Health Center), 190–92, 197–98

Duke Clinical Research Institute (DCRI): computerization and big data manipulation at, 134, 135; early reactions to in academia, 133–34, 135; genomics as field of study by the, 134, 137; graduate research at the, 113, 136; origins and expansion of the,

Duke Clinical Research Institute (*continued*)
130–35; patents and licensing revenues
generated by the, 68–69, 135, 136; role of
in establishing national clinical research
standards, 135–37; role of Robert L. Taber
in establishing the, 67–69
Duke Eye Center (Ruth and Herman Albert
Eye Research Institute), 192, 200, 201
Duke Health Sector Conference, 179, 206–7
Duke Hospital: as research and training site,
26, 27, 29, 178; CEO of, 29, 30–31, 38, 54,
86, 108–12, 152, 235; clinical service units
(CSUs) at, 153; DUMC faculty at, 29, 31,
139–40; governance of, 23, 29–32, 37, 38,
54, 86, 109–12; health care facilities and
services of, 29, 191, 213–16, 245; influence
of clinical dept. chairs on functions of, 31,
89, 90; legacy of racism at, 123–24, 146;
Long Range Plan reforms at, 54, 58–59,
80, 107–11, 139–42; nonreimbursed and
underreimbursed medical care by, 127;
nursing care at, 142, 245; operational elements of, 29–30, 39–40, 99–100, 108–9,
124, 140–42; origins of, 22; oversight of by
chancellor as Dean of School of Medicine,
30, 37, 148; Promising Practices Program
at, 127–28; relationship of PDC to, 29–31,
139–41; relationship to DUHS, 148–53, 260;
revenues of, 30, 31, 70, 138–42, 261
Duke Hospital Raleigh. *See* Raleigh Community Hospital
Duke–National University of Singapore
(Duke-NUS) Graduate Medical School, 68,
103, 117–18, 134
Duke Personalized Health Care, 183–84,
222–23
Duke Private Sector Conference, 179, 206–7
Duke University Academic Council, 77, 94,
254
Duke University Affiliated Physicians (DUAP),
143, 152, 260
Duke University Health System (DUHS):
ad hoc advisory group for, 153; Board
of Directors of (1998), 151–53, 181–82;
financial and reputational contributions
of to DUMC, 154–55, 207, 261; governance
of, 111–12, 150–53, 217–19; incorporation
of, 105, 149–52; influence of on concepts
of health care delivery, 176–85; relation-

ship of to Duke University, 105–6, 149–50,
153; research relationship of with other
university components, 154; scale of health
care services provided by, 176–77
Duke University Medical Center (DUMC):
1990 assessment of the, 57–58, 241–50;
aspirations of Chancellor Snyderman for
the, 33, 36–37, 66–67, 87, 113–14, 118–19;
Building Fund of the, 30, 40, 246;
changes, initiatives, and recruitment for
the, 61–69, 79–81, 84, 107; core missions
of the, 13, 20, 25, 35, 61, 101–2, 119, 218;
diversity and inclusion initiatives in the,
123–29; Duke Endowment Indenture of
Trust, 22, 263n1; economic significance
of in North Carolina, 17, 79, 82, 110,
145; external review of depts. in the,
72–76, 81; functions of (1989), 25–30;
governance of the, 30, 31–32, 37, 69–70,
73, 107–12, 114–18; health care delivery
initiatives by the, 139–46, 148–52, 207;
Long Range Plan for the, 59–66, 72,
88, 107, 139; operations of the, 38–41,
50–55, 261; origins of the, 22; overarching mission of the, 61; political tensions
in (1993), 81–84, 86–90; relationship of
PDC to, 29–30, 53, 139–41; relationship
of to Duke University, 25, 30, 38, 66–67,
148–50; reputation of the, 22–23, 25, 50,
204, 206, 208; responsibilities of chancellor to the, 30–37
Duke University president. *See* Brodie, Keith;
Keohane, Nannerl O.
Duke University Preventive Approach to
Cardiology (DUPAC), 163
Durham: Beth El Congregation, 88; community relations between DUMC and, 125–26,
127–28, 146–8; diversity and inclusion initiatives by DUMC, 124–7; Durham County
Commissioners, 126, 145, 147–48, 152;
economic importance of DUMC to, 17, 79,
110, 145, 169; employee relations initiatives
by DUMC, 38, 39–40, 79–80, 95; *Herald-
Sun* newspaper, 82, 85–66, 87, 223; legacy
of racism in, 123–24, 145–7; PrimaHealth
physicians in, 143; Promising Practices program for residents of, 127–8; relationship
of DUHS to, 144, 148, 152; Rotary Club, 85;
Union Baptist Church, 147

Durham Regional Hospital: African American professionals at, 126; financial difficulties of (1995), 127, 144–45; operational oversight of by Duke University, 126, 144–48, 152, 260; segregation at, 123, 146–47

Durham Veterans Affairs Hospital, 10, 27, 48, 252

Dzau, Victor J., 222, 223, 254, 257–8

emergency medical care, 17, 127, 184, 260

employees: advisory task force of African American, 125; dignity and respect as primary concerns of Duke, 80; Duke Plantation, 80, 123, 129, 145; morale, 79–80, 82–83, 86; open forums with, 79–80; personalized health care plan for Duke, 5, 183–84; plight of African Americans at bottom of Duke hierarchy of, 40, 80, 123, 145; population of at DCRI, 134; population of at DUMC, 37, 242; training programs for, 40; walk-arounds by chancellor to meet, 39–40, 225; workforce diversification and inclusion initiatives at Duke, 95, 125, 129; workforce reduction crisis at, 40, 79, 82–83, 109–10, 125, 208

enrollments, 26, 27, 114, 259

Epstein, David L., 76, 238

Erickson, Harold P., 116, 236

excellence: as institutional goal, 61, 109, 113, 136, 190, 253; communications as means of facilitating sense of, 203, 205–6, 208

expenses, 27, 29, 109–10, 180, 246. *See also* revenues

faculty: academic rights of, 31, 67, 136–37; as influence on development of clinical specialization, 18, 19, 139–40; APT of, 30, 65; autonomy of, 53, 139–40; clinical at Duke, 15, 19, 28–29, 31, 124, 139–40; committees, 59, 67, 77–78, 95, 108; dept. chairs as influence on fellow, 63, 69, 70, 72, 80–82, 102, 140; diversity and inclusion initiatives, 126, 128–29; influence of Flexner Report on, 17–18; institutional loyalty of Duke's, 35, 229; joint appointments of, 29; Long-Range Plan as influence on development, 59–66, 72, 88, 107, 139; medical at Duke, 15–16, 19, 22, 28; mindsets of medical, 44, 53, 58, 69, 254–55; nursing at

Duke, 27, 55, 114; DCRI, 134–36; Institute for Genome Sciences and Policy (IGSP), 119; Private Diagnostic Clinic (PDC), 29–30, 31, 108, 139–40; Office of Science and Technology support functions for, 67; organization of by depts., 19, 31, 58, 99; political environment created by, 39, 42, 45, 70–72, 78–80, 84–87, 90–91; productivity, 19, 64, 134; professional societies for medical, 17; recruitment as driver of institutional change, 36, 49–50, 59–60, 63–64, 66, 193–94; reputation as influence on recruitment of, 18, 22–23, 33–34, 36, 46, 229, 251–52; retirement, 51, 71, 73, 81, 83, 89, 255–56; School of Medicine at Duke, 22, 28, 269; School of Nursing (1989), 27, 269; sources of income for medical school, 20, 51, 60, 64–65, 69–70, 135, 139–40; space allocations and cost recovery per square foot, 64, 80; status of DUAP, 143; tenure, 28, 64, 65, 128–29, 135–36, 260; Whitehead Scholars Program, 49–50, 64

fellowship programs, 27, 28, 59, 113–14, 123–24, 242

Fetzer Institute (Kalamazoo), 163–64

financial sustainability: adequate revenues as fundamental to institutional, 5, 25, 80–81, 142, 144, 178–79, 206, 246; external funding as source of, 19, 189; lack of inherent to decentralized academic medicine, 3–4, 20–21, 43, 51–54, 80–81

"find-it, fix-it" model, 162, 176, 177

Fleishman, Joel L., 88, 192–93, 227

Flexner, Abraham, 15–16, 22

Flexner Report and Flexner model, 15–16, 17, 19, 22, 25, 99–100

Food and Drug Administration (FDA), 11, 48, 131, 137

Francis, Allen J., 74, 103

Frank, Michael M., 75, 238

Fulkerson, William J., Jr., 112, 236

funding: as metric in calculating space allocations, 64; allocations to basic science depts., 64–65; as influence on faculty recruitment and quality, 18, 34; for clinical translation, 136; corporate and philanthropic for medical and biotechnological research, 18, 68, 248, 260; federal for

integrative medicine (*continued*)
growth of in United States, 156–57; in medical curriculum, 169; role of Jon Kabat-Zinn as national advocate of, 163–64; role of Bravewell Collaborative in national advocacy of, 167–68, 169–72; role of C. J. Mack Foundation in national advocacy of, 165, 167–70, 172; role of George Foundation in national advocacy of, 166–67; role of Tracy W. Gaudet in developing Duke's program for, 165, 168–69; roles of Martin J. Sullivan, Larry Bark, and Jeff Brantley in bringing to Duke, 156–57

intensive care, 17, 214, 215, 245
internship program, 27, 29, 126, 242
intervention. *See* medical intervention
investigators and investigation: academic clinical, 130–36; practical contributions of clinical, 131, 137; productivity of as basis for lab space allocations, 64, 65; recruitment of junior, 49–50, 51, 65; training requirements for academic clinical, 135–36. *See also* clinical trials; research
Israel, Michael D. (Mike), 109, 111–12, 152, 236

Jacobs, Danny O., 117, 126, 239
Jaggers, James, 213–16
Johns Hopkins University, 16, 19, 22, 23, 34
Johnson, Charles (Charlie), 126
Joklik, Wolfgang K. (Bill), 44, 48, 237

Kabat-Zinn, Jon, 158–60, 163, 164, 166, 171
Katz, Samuel L. (Sam), 75, 196–97, 238
Kaufman, Russel E., 210, 233
Kay, Richard F., 117, 236
Keene, Jack D., 48, 237
Keohane, Nannerl O. (Nan): administrative and financial interests of in DUMC, 104–6, 105–6, 118, 150–52, 157, 217–18, 256; Duke University presidency of (1993–2004), 66, 79, 96, 217, 221; familial and educational background of, 103, 105; leadership style of, 104, 105, 217–19; relationship of chancellor with, 103–6, 109–10, 115, 173–74, 217, 219, 222–23; role of in initiatives to promote diversity and inclusion at Duke, 105, 128–29; role of in five-year review of chancellor, 79, 92–96; role of in political

tensions in DUMC, 87, 89–90, 92–93; Smith Report, 218–19; support of creation of DUHS by, 105–6, 150, 256; support of creation of IGSP by, 119

Krishnan, Ranga R., 103, 239
Krzyzewski, Mike, 191, 197

Lachman, Milton and Roslyn, 199–200
leadership: academic versus corporate, 217–18, 254–5; as embodiment of institutional commitment, 61, 213; anticipation and responsiveness as crucial traits for managing change, 81, 112–13, 150, 226, 230–31; centralized as basis for creating institutional focus, 61, 219; centralized as basis for setting institutional priorities, 61, 125–26, 128; chairs as influence on development of their depts., 19, 46, 70–72, 74–75, 92; characteristics and attitudes that facilitate effective, 224; committees as tools for integrating institutional elements, 108; communication, interaction, and public relations as crucial to, 61, 85–86, 101, 203–5, 212–13, 216, 225–26; comprehension of institutional structures and functions as vital to, 25, 37–41; crises and unexpected events as challenges inherent to, 98, 208, 213, 219–20; definition of one's role as leader, 253–54; Duke chancellor for health affairs, 23, 31, 78, 220; Duke's quest for as innovator, 113–14, 130, 135, 150, 153, 162–63; Duke's quest for as outlined in its 1991–1996 Long Range Plan, 60; Duke's quest for in emerging areas of medical research, 24–25, 34–35, 36, 45–46, 119, 132, 194; Duke's quest for status as national leader in medicine, 53, 54, 87, 113, 168, 218, 219; external positions as institutional asset of, 115, 204–5; five-year review as tool for assessing need for change, 77; fundraising and institutional development duties of, 119, 192, 199–200; importance of transparent, objective budgeting process, 64; importance of assessing of institutional components, 38–39, 43, 99, 225; importance of finding opportunities to build quality and reputation, 45; importance of frankness in interactions, 111–12, 147; importance of having honest advisors

Medicare and Medicaid, 138, 169, 179, 245
meditation. *See* mindfulness
mentoring: of medical students and faculty, 26, 28, 126, 129, 197, 200; of patients, 168, 177
Michener, J. Lloyd, 76, 238
microbiology, 14, 19, 44, 47–48, 60, 65, 81, 236–7
mind-body, 157–58, 162–63, 164, 168
mindfulness and meditation: as therapy at DCIM, 162–63, 165–66; as approach to disease, 160–61; as element in treatment of cancer patients, 161, 177; inclusion of in Duke medical curriculum, 113, 169; mental conditioning and, 158; programs for at University of Massachusetts, 158, 160; role of in integrative medicine, 161–63, 165–66; therapeutic effects of caring and compassion, 160–63, 177; work in and advocacy of by Jon Kabat-Zinn, 158–59, 163–64
minorities: affirmative action, 129, 203–4; discrimination against, 105; initiatives to address concerns of at DUMC, 91, 95, 125; promotion and tenure tracking of, 125–27; recruitment of, 63, 129; statistics concerning, 127, 259. *See also* African Americans; diversity and inclusion; race relations
Miraval retreats, 164, 166–7
molecules: as fundamental topic in medical school curriculum, 113; computer modeling of, 247; impact of molecular biology on medical research and practice, 247; molecular detection in development of disease, 181; protein, 66, 131, 180, 248; synthesized as tools of medical treatment, 15
Morris, Kenneth C., 111, 234

National Academy of Sciences, 23, 34, 46, 62, 244, 252, 253
National Institutes of Health (NIH): Clinical Translational Science Awards (CTSA), 136; degree program in clinical research with Duke, 113–14, 136; funding of clinical research projects by the, 134–35; grants for biomedical research from the, 16, 28, 46, 65, 67, 243–44, 248; grants from as indicator of educational quality, 24, 46, 243–44, 252, 253; Human Genome Project, 179–80;

sharing of pharmacological research data by, 136–37; statistics, 259–60
Nelson, Larry, 38, 58, 108, 235
networks: clinical trial, 132, 134; constraints of medical on referrals, 139–40; DUAP, 143; DUHS, 4, 105–12, 139–43, 149–55, 176–77, 181–84, 217; physician, 110, 139–43, 176–77, 245–46; PrimaHealth physicians, 143; role of primary physicians in managed care, 32, 138–39; United Network for Organ Sharing (UNOS), 214
neurosciences, neurobiology, and neurosurgery, 23, 45–46, 60, 81, 193, 242, 252
Nevins, Joseph R. (Joe), 47, 89, 236, 237
Newman, Mark F., 116, 238
nursing education, 1, 27, 54–55, 60, 62, 114

Obamacare, 185
Office for Protection from Research Risks (OPRR), 208–12
Office of Science and Technology, 67–69, 132, 234
open versus closed systems, 100–101
opportunity: challenge as, 54, 84–85, 206, 216; change as, 36, 45–46, 74, 107; emergence of through scientific discoveries, 34–36, 46, 64, 66, 118–19, 244, 248; entrepreneurial, 52, 68; perception of, 39–41, 55, 57–61, 68, 136, 205, 225; planning, reaction, and, 13, 18–20, 25, 36, 45; principles as guidelines for seizing, 13, 160, 250, 253. *See also* risk
outcomes: clinical trial, 130–1; health care, 127–28, 161, 183, 185
outpatient clinics, 27, 29, 124, 178–79, 245, 249

Parkerson, George R., Jr., 76, 238
participatory medicine, 1–2, 113, 175–81, 184, 185
patents and licensing, 67–69, 260
patients: as source of revenues, 20, 51–52, 149, 246, 249, 250, 256; ability of to benefit from new discoveries, 159–60, 247; anodyne imagery as benefit for, 157; broader, nonmedical needs of, 5, 119, 127, 176–77, 181; cancer, 161, 177; care of as one element of mission of academic medical centers, 20, 140; caring and compassion as influences on wellbeing of, 159–61, 177;

physicians (*continued*)
of toward CAM, 162, 164–65, 168, 171–72;
clinical services functions of physicians-
in-training, 29; clinical specialization
among, 16, 18, 139–40, 242, 245; clinical
trials as sources of evidence for, 131;
continuing education for, 242; DUAP,
143, 260; Flexner model for training, 15,
17–18; integrative medicine as treatment
option for, 168; Long Range Plan goals
for training, 113; managed care regulations, 138–39; personalized health care
by, 181, 183–84; physician networks, 110,
139–43, 176–77, 245–46; physician-patient
relationships, 91, 159–60, 161–62, 172,
176, 181; physician-scientists, 10–11, 24,
36, 87, 159, 174, 224, 242; PrimaHealth
network, 143; primary care, 18, 32, 53, 108,
138–44, 165, 183; referrals system at Duke,
53, 80, 108–9, 139–42; as researchers, 20;
revenue-generating role of at DUMC, 51, 53,
80, 140–42; technological discoveries as
influence on, 14; women, 125–29
physics, 15, 22
Pizzo, Salvatore V., 47, 89, 237
planning: action stage of, 45–48, 61–5; communications and marketing as tools for
facilitating plans, 80, 107; departmental
plans and broader institutional, 58–61;
flexibility and adaptability as essential to
good, 230; learning as basis for, 38–39, 45;
listening as crucial to, 100–101, 226; long-
range, 35–36, 43–44; personalized health,
179–85; principle-based decision-making
as element of, 12–13; revenue sources, 41,
245–46; risks, unexpected crises, and, 72,
87, 89, 110, 125, 213, 245–46; strategic,
centralized, 4, 35–36, 53–54, 109, 139, 142.
See also goals and priorities
postdoctoral training, 28, 29, 128
predictive medicine, 175–76, 180–81, 182–85,
247. *See also* personalized health care
preventive medicine: as alternative to reactive
approach to disease, 175, 176, 180; as element of Duke's pilot program for personalized health care, 183–85; cardiovascular
prevention, 160, 163, 247; chronic disease
as focal point of, 175–76, 178; fee-for-
service insurance reimbursement as dis-

couragement to, 183, 184; goals of, 127, 154,
172–73, 181; Promising Practices, 127–28.
See also personalized health care
primary care physicians: DUAP, 143; Duke's inability to respond to referrals from (1989),
53, 108, 139, 149, 245; empowerment of
through managed care, 32, 53, 138–39;
PrimaHealth network, 143; primary care
as money-losing area of medical practice,
53; primary care as most accessible medical practice option for women, 128; role
of in Duke's model of personalized care,
183; role of in Duke's new hub-and-spokes
health system, 139, 141–43; training of, 18
Private Diagnostic Clinic (PDC), leadership of
the, 30–32, 75, 98, 106
Promising Practices, 127–28
Prosnitz, Leonard R. (Len), 76, 117, 239
prospective health care, 5, 112, 175, *181*, 183,
253, 257
protection. *See* safety
protein: genetically engineered, 131; tissue
plasminogen activator (t-PA), 131
proteomics, 180
public relations, 203–4
publication: of annual Duke health conference proceedings, 206, 207–8; corporate
restrictions on findings from contracted
clinical research, 131, 136; of faculty
research results, 67; journal articles regarding innovations at Duke, 135, 212–13; of
clinical research findings, 131, 134, 136.
See also media
Purves, Dale, 46, 89, 116, 237, 244, 252

race relations, 79, 124, 125, 126–27, 147.
See also African Americans; diversity and
inclusion; minorities
radiation oncology, 76, 161, 177
radiology, 76
Raetz, Christian R. H., 47, 236
Raleigh Community Hospital, 144, 260,
148152
Ravin, Carl. E., 44–45, 70–71, 75, 89, 117,
151, 239
recombinant DNA technology, 34, 35, 66, 252
recruitment: as basis for institutional reputation, 22–23, 49–51, 59–60, 62–66, 74, 102,
193–94; chancellor's role in, 30, 35–36,

45–46, 49, 61–63, 76, 102, 252, 253; diversity and inclusion as influences on, 63, 117, 126–29; Whitehead Scholars Program, 63–64, 149–50, 193
referrals: departmental collaboration in responding to, 70, 76, 140–41; difficulty of getting appointments at Duke (1989), 80, 108; enhancement of Duke's system through DUAP, 143; enhancement of Duke's system through PrimaHealth, 143; financial importance of receiving, 53, 149; influence of changes in reimbursement policies on, 84, 139; managed care empowerment of primary physicians over, 138–39; medical network restrictions on, 139–40; patient as major source of income, 53, 84, 139–40; reform of Duke's system for, 109, 142–43, 149, 246; unaffiliated primary care physicians as major source of Duke's, 53, 80–81, 108, 139
reimbursement: as entrepreneurial incentive in academic medicine, 52; changing patterns of, 84, 179, 183, 185, 249; cost-plus model, 245, 249; cross-subsidization, 51–52; discrepancies in between inpatient and outpatient care, 179; discrepancies in between invasive and non-invasive procedures, 52; fee-for-service model, 20, 183, 249; insurance company biases regarding, 141, 177–78, 179, 183–85, 207, 245–46; low for non-invasive procedures, 52; low-margin and low-reimbursement as endemic to certain kinds of health care, 51, 53, 75, 127, 196; Medicare and Medicaid, 138, 169, 179, 245; nonreimbursed care for indigent patients, 127; Obamacare, 185; shrinkage of under managed care, 84, 138, 141; underreimbursement for emergency care, 127. See also margins
Reinhardt, Uwe E., 152, 207, 256
reputation: as responsibility of chancellor of health affairs, 6, 33, 36; best academic medical centers (1989), 20, 34, 252; influence of on institution's ability to attract faculty, students, and funding, 18, 45–46, 50–51; of Duke as medical research center, 22–24, 33–36, 45–46, 130; of DUMC, 108, 175, 204, 206, 208, 245; and risks of visibility, 208, 210, 211, 214–16, 219–20;

self-reinforcing nature of, 18, 50–51; value of, 41
research: in cardiovascular physiology, 24; clinical, 134; Clinical Research Forum, 135; DCRI, 67–69, 113, 132–36; investigator-initiated laboratory, 67, 133–34, 136, 243; Office of Science and Technology, 67, 132; patents and licensing derived from, 67–69, 260; pharmacological, 137; translational, 5, 119, 136, 222. See also biomedical research; investigators and investigation; medical research
residency program, 10, 29, 59, 242
revenues: as source of power for clinical dept. chairs, 31, 41, 44, 133; budget cuts and workforce reduction as responses to reduced, 79, 109–10; commercialization of academic research discoveries as source of, 21, 66–67; competition between clinical depts. for, 52; compounding of staff and services as means of increasing, 20–21; coordinated functions of clinical depts. as source of tensions and of, 70; cross-subsidization as source of, 64, 133, 138, 246; external research grants as source of for basic science depts., 64, 260; generated by DCRI, 133, 135, 209; generated by DUHS, 5, 154–55; generated by DUMC, 29, 66, 250, 260; generated by royalties, 69, 260; income from PDC via 5(b) transfers as source of, 30, 31, 140, 261; insurance reimbursement policies as impediment to generation of, 20–21, 32, 179, 207, 245–46; managed care as curb on medical, 32, 85, 139–42; patents and licensing as source of, 69, 260; philanthropy as source of, 21, 48–50, 190–91, 261; practices and events that impede generation of, 20, 76, 84, 108, 139–40, 176; referrals as source of, 53, 70, 84, 139–40, 241–42; self-enforcing effect of for lucrative clinical practices, 18–19, 37, 70; specialization as source of increased, 18, 108, 245, 246; tuition as source of, 20, 26–27, 189. See also expenses; margins
Reves, Joseph G. (Jerry), 73, 95, 116, 238
Rex Hospital, 144, 148
risk: assessment and mitigation of for individual patients, 175, 180–81, 183–84, 247; innovation as, 164–65; institutional at

Santillan, 213–16; on planning, 57–61, 230; on principles, 13, 230–31; recruitment goals of for dept. chairs and faculty, 46, 74, 193; renewal crisis of (1993), 77–79, 81–84, 92–95; research associateship at NIH, 10; residency at Duke, 10, 24, 89, 130; role of in establishing DCIM, 162–69, 174; running as element of personal maintenance for, 158; senior management team for DUHS (1996), 111–12; senior management team for Duke Hospital (1993), 107–8; senior management team functions, 58–64; senior managers: direct reports (1989), 38; Smith Report crisis, 218–19; on taking responsibility, 210–12; work of at Durham Veterans Affairs Hospital, 10. *See also* chancellor for health affairs; leadership

Spaulding, Jean G., 125–27, 151, 234

Spaulding, Kenneth, 125

specialists: faculty specialization, 16, 18, 112, 117; growth of clinical specialization, 16, 18–20, 191, 242; medical referrals to, 20, 108, 139–42, 245, 246

Stead, Eugene A., Jr. (Gene), 24, 89, 130, 229

Stiles, Gary L., 111–12, 183, 234

Stoughton, W. Vickery (Vick), 54, 86, 109, 110, 235

strategic planning. *See* planning

students: clinical practice exposure for medical, 15–16, 229, 243; curriculum and areas of study available to medical, 62, 113, 169, 243; degree options available for pursuit, 26, 113; Duke-NUS, 117–18; faculty training and mentoring of, 15–16, 22, 28, 29, 197; Flexner model for training medical, 15, 16–17; initiatives to promote diversity and inclusion among medical, 124, 126–27, 129; nursing, 27, 114; participation of in medical research, 17–18, 24, 113; populace at Duke University Medical School, 26–27, 126–27; reputation as tool for recruitment of, 18

Sullivan, Martin J. (Marty), 156–58, 160, 162

SUNY Downstate Medical Center, 10, 117

Swinney, Alvis R. (Al), 111, 142, 234

synthesized molecules, 15, 66, 131

Taber, Robert L., 67–68, 132, 234

teaching: advances in teaching of medicine and of nursing, 62, 114, 242–43; emer-

gence of research and clinical care as priorities over, 17–18, 139; influence of Flexner Report on medical, 17; of personal health practices, 128; as one of several responsibilities of medical faculty, 15–16, 28, 47, 126, 140, 243; teaching hospitals, 16–17, 22, 27, 29

technology: as benefit to patient information and knowledge, 179–81; embrace of by DUMC, 60, 62, 112; information, 112, 134; leadership of academic medical centers in introducing new forms of, 5, 16–18, 35, 60, 68–69, 131; three-dimensional computer graphics, 247

Tedder, Thomas F., 48, 236

tenure. *See* faculty

therapeutics: academic medical centers as innovators behind new, 16–17, 131, 137, 246; biotherapeutics, 135; diagnostics as guide to new, 15, 246; discoveries as essential to improvement of, 16, 66, 246; genetic and cell, 68, 248; role of clinical trials in development of, 134–35, 137; role of integrative medicine in development of, 160, 163, 166; synthesized molecules as basis for new, 15, 66

therapy: acupuncture as, 171–72; aromatherapy, 171–72; chemotherapy as cancer, 161, 171–72, 177; CAM, 156, 161, 168, 177; gene, 59; for human body based on concept of bodily humors, 14; influence of psychological wellbeing on, 161, 172; interventional, 245; massage, 161, 162; mindfulness meditation as complement to, 160, 177; occupational, 27; personalization of, 175, 177, 181, 182–83, 185; physical, 27, 113; radiation oncology as cancer, 76, 161, 177; reiki, 168; role of in "find-it, fix-it" medicine, 161–62; selection of least risky as medical concern, 91; surgery as for cancer, 161, 177; targeted, 185; tissue plasminogen activator (t-PA) as myocardial infarction, 131

Thomas Jefferson University, 164, 168

Thomas, R. David (Dave), 197–99

Tracy, Philip R. and Travis, 195

transparency, 64, 95, 131, 136–7

transplantation: blood type compatibility for organ, 213–14; bone marrow, 245;

transplantation (*continued*)
Jesica Santillan case, 213–16; concept of procedural "time out", 216; interdisciplinary program in, 60; organ, 23–24, 245, 249; United Network for Organ Sharing (UNOS), 214
Truman, President Harry S, 210, 211–12
tuition: as source of revenue, 20, 26–27, 189; for School of Nursing (1989), 27

undergraduates: medical program for, 19, 26–27, 28, 59, 62; nursing program for, 27, 114; statistics concerning Duke, 259
University of California, San Francisco, 34, 76, 164, 168, 173, 252
U.S. Dept. of Health and Human Services. *See* Office for Protection from Research Risks (OPRR)

veterans: Durham Veterans Affairs Hospital, 10, 27; Veterans Health Administration, 185

Wallace, Andrew G. (Andy), 38, 41, 54, 235
Washington College, 10
Waters, Raymond C. (Bucky), 38, 48, 107, 190, 196, 199, 235
Watkins, W. David, 71, 73, 238

wellness, 127, 154, 168
Whitehead, Edwin C. (Jack), 34, 48–50, 64, 193, 252
Whitehead Institute (MIT), 34, 48–49, 50, 252
Whitehead Scholars Program, 49–50, 64, 193
Wilkinson, William E., 116, 236
Willett, Christopher G., 239
Williams, Gordon D., 111, 234
Williams, R. Sanders (Sandy), 116–17, 182, 233, 251, 252, 258
Winfree, Robert G. (Bob), 38, 58, 235
women: discrimination against, 105; initiatives to address concerns of at DUMC, 91, 95, 126, 128–29; promotion and tenure tracking of, 128–29; recruitment of, 63, 129; statistics concerning, 128, 259
workforce. *See* employees
Wyngaarden, James B. (Jim): as advocate of high-quality clinical investigation, 130, 135, 137; as chair of Dept. of Medicine, 24; creation of Duke's Research Training Program by, 24; role in recruiting outstanding researchers to Duke, 24, 50, 51, 102

X-ray technology, 15, 22, 247

Zinovoy, Sheppard and Clara, 202